Surgical Infections

Editors

TRACI L. HEDRICK
ROBERT G. SAWYER

SURGICAL CLINICS
OF NORTH AMERICA

www.surgical.theclinics.com

Consulting Editor
RONALD F. MARTIN

December 2014 • Volume 94 • Number 6

ELSEVIER

1600 John F. Kennedy Boulevard • Suite 1800 • Philadelphia, Pennsylvania, 19103-2899

http://www.surgical.theclinics.com

SURGICAL CLINICS OF NORTH AMERICA Volume 94, Number 6
December 2014 ISSN 0039–6109, ISBN-13: 978-0-323-32632-2

Editor: John Vassallo, j.vassallo@elsevier.com
Developmental Editor: Colleen Viola

Surgical Clinics of North America (ISSN 0039–6109) is published bimonthly by Elsevier Inc., 360 Park Avenue South, New York, NY 10010-1710. Months of publication are February, April, June, August, October, and December. Business and Editorial Offices: 1600 John F. Kennedy Blvd., Suite 1800, Philadelphia, PA 19103-2899. Periodicals postage paid at New York, NY and additional mailing offices. Subscription prices are $370.00 per year for US individuals, $627.00 per year for US institutions, $180.00 per year for US students and residents, $455.00 per year for Canadian individuals, $793.00 per year for Canadian institutions, $510.00 for international individuals, $793.00 per year for international institutions and $250.00 per year for Canadian and foreign students/residents. To receive student/resident rate, orders must be accompanied by name of affiliated institution, date of term, and the *signature* of program/residency coordinator on institution letterhead. Orders will be billed at individual rate until proof of status is received. Foreign air speed delivery is included in all *Clinics* subscription prices. All prices are subject to change without notice. POSTMASTER: Send address changes to *Surgical Clinics*, Elsevier Health Sciences Division, Subscription Customer Service, 3251 Riverport Lane, Maryland Heights, MO 63043. **Customer Service (orders, claims, online, change of address): Telephone: 1-800-654-2452 (U.S. and Canada); 314-447-8871 (outside U.S. and Canada). Fax: 314-447-8029. E-mail: journalscustomerservice-usa@elsevier.com (for print support); journalsonline support-usa@elsevier.com (for online support).**

Reprints. For copies of 100 or more, of articles in this publication, please contact the Commercial Reprints Department, Elsevier Inc., 360 Park Avenue South, New York, New York 10010-1710. Tel. 212-633-3874, Fax: 212-633-3820, E-mail: reprints@elsevier.com.

The Surgical Clinics of North America is also published in Spanish by McGraw-Hill Interamericana Editores S.A., P.O. Box 5-237 06500 Mexico D.F. Mexico; and in Portuguese by Interlivros Edicoes Ltda., Rua Comandante Coelho 1085, CEP 21250, Rio de Janeiro, Brazil; and in Greek by Paschalidis Medical Publications, Athens Greece.

The Surgical Clinics of North America is covered in *MEDLINE/PubMed (Index Medicus), EMBASE/Excerpta Medica, Current Contents/Clinical Medicine, Current Contents/Life Sciences, Science Citation Index*, and *ISI/BIOMED.*

Contributors

CONSULTING EDITOR

RONALD F. MARTIN, MD
Staff Surgeon, Department of Surgery, Marshfield Clinic, Marshfield, Wisconsin; Clinical Associate Professor, University of Wisconsin School of Medicine and Public Health, Madison, Wisconsin; Colonel, Medical Corps, United States Army Reserve

EDITORS

TRACI L. HEDRICK, MD
Section Colon and Rectal Surgery, Department of Surgery, University of Virginia, Charlottesville, Virginia

ROBERT G. SAWYER, MD, FACS, FIDSA, FCCM
Professor of Surgery and Public Health Sciences, Division of Acute Care Surgery and Outcomes Research, Department of Surgery, University of Virginia, Charlottesville, Virginia

AUTHORS

MAJDI N. AL-HASAN, MD
Director of Antimicrobial Stewardship and Support Program, Division of Infectious Diseases; Associate Professor, Department of Medicine, Palmetto Health Richland, University of South Carolina School of Medicine, Columbia, South Carolina

JOHN C. ALVERDY, MD, FACS
Center for Surgical Infection Research and Therapeutics, University of Chicago Medicine, Chicago, Illinois

REZA ASKARI, MD, FACS
Associate Trauma Director, Brigham and Women's Hospital, Harvard Medical School, Boston, Massachusetts

ANTONIA F. CHEN, MD, MBA
Rothman Institute, Philadelphia, Pennsylvania

PETER CHEN, PhD
Sunnybrook Research Institute, Sunnybrook Health Sciences Centre, Toronto, Ontario, Canada

JEFFREY A. CLARIDGE, MD, MS
Director, Division of Trauma, Critical Care, Burns, and Acute Care Surgery; Associate Professor, Department of Surgery, MetroHealth Medical Center, Medical Director, Northern Ohio Trauma System, Case Western Reserve University School of Medicine, Cleveland, Ohio

JOHN J. COMO, MD, MPH
Associate Professor, Department of Surgery, MetroHealth Medical Center, Case Western Reserve University School of Medicine, Cleveland, Ohio

CHARLES H. COOK, MD, FACS, FCCM
Division of Acute Care Surgery, Trauma and Surgical Critical Care, Department of Surgery, Beth Israel Deaconess Medical Center, Harvard Medical School, Boston, Massachusetts

JENNIFER DEFAZIO, MD
Center for Surgical Infection Research and Therapeutics, University of Chicago Medicine, Chicago, Illinois

THERESE M. DUANE, MD, FACS, FCCM
Department of Surgery, JPS Health Network, Ft. Worth, Texas

HEATHER EVANS, MD, MS
Associate Professor, Harborview Medical Center, Seattle, Washington

IRMA D. FLEMING, MD
Center for Surgical Infection Research and Therapeutics, University of Chicago Medicine, Chicago, Illinois

ELIZABETH D. FOX, MD
Resident, General Surgery, Department of Surgery, Brown University, Rhode Island Hospital, Providence, Rhode Island

CHRISTOPHER A. GUIDRY, MD
Division of Acute Care Surgery and Outcomes Research, Department of Surgery, University of Virginia, Charlottesville, Virginia

DAITHI S. HEFFERNAN, MD, AFRCSI
Assistant Professor of Surgery, Division of Trauma and Surgical Critical Care, Department of Surgery, Brown University, Rhode Island Hospital, Providence, Rhode Island

SNIR HELLER, MD
Rothman Institute, Philadelphia, Pennsylvania

MARC G. JESCHKE, MD, PhD
Department of Immunology, University of Toronto; Division of Plastic Surgery, Department of Surgery, University of Toronto; Director, Ross Tilley Burn Centre, Sunnybrook Research Institute, Sunnybrook Health Sciences Centre, Toronto, Ontario, Canada

RACHEL G. KHADAROO, MD, PhD, FRCSC
Assistant Professor, Division of General Surgery, Department of Surgery; Division of Critical Care Medicine, University of Alberta, Edmonton, Alberta, Canada

JASON A. LUCIANO, MD, MBA
General Surgery Resident, Department of Surgery, University of Pittsburgh, Pittsburgh, Pennsylvania

SARA A. MANSFIELD, MD
Division of Trauma, Critical Care, and Burn, Department of Surgery, The Ohio State University College of Medicine, Columbus, Ohio

PATRICK J. O'NEILL, PhD, MD, FACS
Associate Trauma Medical Director, West Valley Hospital, Goodyear, Arizona; Clinical Associate Professor of Surgery, University of Arizona School of Medicine – Phoenix, Phoenix, Arizona; Assistant Professor of Surgery, Mayo Clinic College of Medicine, Rochester, Minnesota

MOHAMED F. OSMAN, MD
Brigham and Women's Hospital, Harvard Medical School, The University of Toledo College of Medicine

JULIE OTTOSEN, MD
Surgical Critical Care Fellow, Harborview Medical Center, Seattle, Washington

JAVAD PARVIZI, MD, FRCS
Rothman Institute, Philadelphia, Pennsylvania

RAJESH RAMANATHAN, MD
Virginia Commonwealth University Medical Center, Richmond, Virginia

DANIEL RAYMOND, MD, FACS
Cleveland Clinic Foundation, Cleveland, Ohio

NITIN SAJANKILA, BS
Medical Student, Department of Surgery, MetroHealth Medical Center, Case Western Reserve University School of Medicine, Cleveland, Ohio

ROBERT G. SAWYER, MD, FACS, FIDSA, FCCM
Professor of Surgery and Public Health Sciences, Division of Acute Care Surgery and Outcomes Research, Department of Surgery, University of Virginia, Charlottesville, Virginia

BADDR SHAKHSHEER, MD
Center for Surgical Infection Research and Therapeutics, University of Chicago Medicine, Chicago, Illinois

GINA R. SHIRAH, MD
Surgical Critical Care Fellow, Division of Trauma & Critical Care Surgery, Department of Surgery, Maricopa Medical Center, Phoenix, Arizona

MILE STANOJCIC, MSc
Sunnybrook Research Institute, Sunnybrook Health Sciences Centre, Toronto, Ontario, Canada

CHRISTOPHER M. WATSON, MD, FACS
Chief of Surgery and Director of Surgical Trauma ICU, Division of Acute Care Surgery; Clinical Assistant Professor, Department of Surgery, Palmetto Health Richland, University of South Carolina School of Medicine, Columbia, South Carolina

PANG Y. YOUNG, MD
Resident, Department of Surgery, University of Alberta, Edmonton, Alberta, Canada

OLGA ZABORINA, PhD
Center for Surgical Infection Research and Therapeutics, University of Chicago Medicine, Chicago, Illinois

BRIAN S. ZUCKERBRAUN, MD
Associate Professor, Department of Surgery, University of Pittsburgh; Department of Surgery, VA Pittsburgh Healthcare System, Pittsburgh, Pennsylvania

Contents

> Sepsis can be defined as a systemic inflammatory response syndrome occurring in the presence of an infectious source. Over the past 25 years, numerous guidelines have been established to clarify definitions and improve the overall management of clinical sepsis. In light of these multiple paradigm shifts, this review attempts to summarize the innate immunologic alterations that manifest during sepsis, establish and compare mouse models of sepsis with the clinical course, and discuss the authors' views on additional elements that should be considered in modeling and predicting clinical sepsis from the standpoint of a basic research setting.

> This article summarizes emerging concepts on the role of the intestinal microbiome in surgical patients. Revolutionary research over the past decade has shown that human beings live in close and constant contact with boundless communities of microbes. Recent innovations in the study of the human microbiome are reviewed. To demonstrate the applicability of these studies to surgical disease, the authors discuss what is known about the role of microbes in the pathogenesis of perioperative complications. Enhanced awareness of the human microbiome will empower clinicians to adopt novel practices in the prevention and treatment of a variety of surgical conditions.

> Infections remain a significant problem among surgical patients. Technological advances, especially in the arena of nano-technology, have markedly improved the ability to detect, prevent and treat surgical infections. No longer limited to culture-based methods of pathogen detection or standard antimicrobial therapies, options for management of surgical infections are rapidly expanding. Such advances are critical in this era of rapidly developing resistant and virulent strains of organisms. Further, our understanding of the host pathogen interaction grows exponentially with the development of computer-based modeling, aiding in expediting research endeavors.

It is critical for health care personnel to recognize and appreciate the detrimental impact of intensive care unit (ICU)-acquired infections. The economic, clinical, and social expenses to patients and hospitals are overwhelming. In order to limit the incidence of ICU-acquired infections, aggressive infection control measures must be implemented and enforced. Researchers and national committees have developed and continue to develop evidence-based guidelines to control ICU infections. A multifaceted approach, including infection prevention committees, antimicrobial stewardship programs, daily reassessments-intervention bundles, identification and minimization of risk factors, and continuing staff education programs, is essential. Infection control in the ICU is an evolving area of critical care research.

Although originally described in *Staphylococcus aureus*, resistance among bacteria has now become a race to determine which classes of bacteria will become more resistant. Availability of antibacterial agents has allowed the development of entirely new diseases caused by nonbacterial pathogens, related largely to fungi that are inherently resistant to antibacterials. This article presents the growing body of knowledge of the herpes family of viruses and their occurrence and consequences in patients with concomitant surgical disease or critical illness. The focus is on previously immunocompetent patients, as the impact of herpes viruses in immunosuppressed patients has received thorough coverage elsewhere.

There has been a good deal of dialogue about pay for performance and linking outcomes with reimbursement, especially given the recent national health care legislation. Many such concerns are caused by upcoming changes that have been outlined in the Affordable Care Act. This article discusses these upcoming changes and reviews some of the literature that supports them, specifically those related to surgical infections. Likewise, the lack of support for some of these changes in the academic literature is discussed. Finally, some of the proposed key benchmarks and the methodologies behind the design of those benchmarks are discussed.

It is estimated that more than 575,000 individuals develop bloodstream infections (BSI) annually in North America, accounting for nearly 80,000 deaths. Central line–associated BSI (CLABSI) is a major contributor to the cost of health care. Although primary BSI may be seen by the surgeon, a secondary BSI is more likely to be encountered, especially CLABSI. Prompt identification of the source of infection in patients with secondary

BSI is paramount. This practice allows early source control and initiation of appropriate antimicrobial therapy, with subsequent improvement in outcomes. An understanding of evidence-based preventative measures and bundles is important.

problematic and controversial. Aspiration pneumonia is often included as a subtype of HAP but may be related to community-acquired aspiration events. Scoring systems exist and new surveillance guidelines have been implemented to make early recognition of pneumonia more precise and objective. Management and prevention should follow recommendations, including early empirical therapy, targeted therapy, and limited duration of treatment. Patients with trauma present a challenge to the diagnosis and management of pneumonia, because of increased risk for aspiration and underlying chest and pulmonary injury.

SURGICAL CLINICS
OF NORTH AMERICA

DOWNLOAD Free App!

Review Articles
THE CLINICS

NOW AVAILABLE FOR YOUR iPhone and iPad

Foreword

Surgical Infections

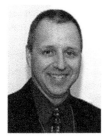

Ronald F. Martin, MD
Consulting Editor

In another moment I had scrambled up the earthen rampart and stood upon its crest, and the interior of the redoubt was below me. A mighty space it was, with gigantic machines here and there within it, huge mounds of material and strange shelter places. And scattered about it, some in their overturned war-machines, some in the now rigid handling-machines, and a dozen of them stark and silent and laid in a row, were the Martians—dead!—slain by the putrefactive and disease bacteria against which their systems were unprepared; slain as the red weed was being slain; slain, after all man's devices had failed, by the humblest things that God, in his wisdom, has put upon this earth.

—H.G. Wells (War of the Worlds)

You have to learn the rules of the game. And then you have to play better than anyone else.

—Albert Einstein

The timing of this issue of the *Surgical Clinics of North America* on infection was not by any means planned to coincide with the rapid expansion of the Ebola virus outbreak in Western Africa. Yet, at the time I am typing this, there are now reports of over 2000 fatalities from this viral disease. In addition, four American health care workers have reportedly been transferred home for treatment after contracting the virus in Western Africa. Two of the health care workers were treated at Emory and have already been released. Another, quite coincidentally a former medical school classmate of mine, is being treated in Nebraska and appears to be improving. The fourth patient has not been named, and I have no information about her or him.

Remarkably, it appears that this "uniformly lethal" disease may not be so lethal if you have access to the right types of treatment. How much of this is due to good basic, and perhaps beyond basic, supportive care, and how much may be due to some "super serum" as has been speculated about in the press, I have no idea. Still, what appears to be clear is this: if one lives in Africa, in places that cannot provide excellent support-ive care, one is likely to fare far worse if infected with Ebola than someone who lives in

Surg Clin N Am 94 (2014) xiii–xv
http://dx.doi.org/10.1016/j.suc.2014.09.016
0039-6109/14/$ – see front matter © 2014 Published by Elsevier Inc.

surgical.theclinics.com

a region with reliable care. Furthermore, if one lives in a place where cultural practices and sanitation standards, such as the handling of medical waste, enhance the likelihood of disease transmission, one is more likely to see a local outbreak of disease that is harder to control. This latter concept isn't exactly new. It has been well-understood in theory since John Snow wrote his essay, "On Cholera," that describes the relationship of the disease prevalence to the proximity of contaminated water supplies. So, in brief, both infrastructure *and* human behavior matter when it comes to disease transmission.

Why should that matter to those of us in the developed world, particularly in the United States? After all, we in the United States claim to have the most advanced medical facilities and practices in the world—right? Well, maybe or maybe not; it depends on where you are. In many ways, it wouldn't matter if we did, because there is much room for improvement. There are still too many barriers to infection prevention and infection control. Many hospitals still have "semi-private" rooms (which is a little like being semi-pregnant—not really a state that exists; it's either private or not). Hand-washing facilities are highly variable; wall-mounted dispensers are not the same as hand-washing, and a whole range of other issues and practices fosters cross-contamination. Of course, the barriers to improving these issues are largely financial and inertial, with emphasis on the former. Perhaps more troubling is the question of why a financial barrier exists. In short, it is most likely because the investors (eg, the hospitals or facilities) are expected to fund the improvements, but society at large is likely to reap the bulk of the financial rewards. Should that be a barrier to "doing the right thing"? No, probably not, but it is. In an era of declining reimbursement and increasing expectations, the system buckles and fails somewhere.

Even if we could magically improve the treatment facility issues, we still have our own practices and the behavior of the patients as well—everything from the clothes we wear (or don't), to the use of stethoscopes, to chart and computer handling. In response to this recognized problem, we have a multitude of mandated practices that are "sure" to prevent infection and so forth. Many of them make sense, and some are just plain silly. Perhaps more troubling, though, is the rigidity that we sometimes apply to these rules in the absence of data due to the difficulty of assessing their impact while simultaneously imposing financial penalties that may or may not be fostering the best care. Combine this with the host (spelled patient) factors that go along with making infections more likely or challenging—such as obesity, poor diabetes mellitus control, tobacco use, intravenous drug abuse, hesitancy or resistance to use well-established vaccines, and other generally risky behaviors that foment infectious disease—and it doesn't take long to realize that infection prevention and control is not something that begins and ends in the inpatient health care environment. It is a collective process.

While attribution of causation may be a problem, it is no cause for nihilism. As Einstein said (and as is quoted above), you have to know the rules of the game and then play a better game. Drs Sawyer and Hedrick have amassed a group of people to spell out the rules of the game as well as we can. Some of this may seem like stuff you have seen before, but I suspect that for many people, there will be much here that is eye-opening. For the astute reader, this material should well-position you to play the game wherever you may live and work. It will remain up to you, however, to be the advocate for change where necessary. You must play better and convince your colleagues and associates to play better as well.

We are not likely to eradicate infection. The micro-organisms have been around a lot longer than we have and most likely will be around at least as long if not longer than we will be. It is our job to work on the relationship. I hope by the time this issue is delivered to your door, we have better news on the outbreak in Africa and that my former class-mate is well and reunited with his family.

Ronald F. Martin, MD
Department of Surgery
Marshfield Clinic
1000 North Oak Avenue
Marshfield, WI 54449, USA

E-mail address:
Martin.ronald@marshfieldclinics.org

Preface

Surgical Infections

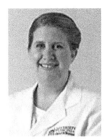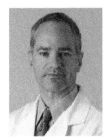

Traci L. Hedrick, MD   Robert G. Sawyer, MD
Editors

Prior to the germ theory, surgery was commonly used in a last ditch attempt to cure various advanced infectious maladies. Infected limbed were amputated after traumatic injury; boils were drained, and malodorous tumors removed. Elective surgery was out of the question before the advent of antibiotics, given that a surgical site infection was fatal. In the past century, however, the relationship between surgery and infectious disease has evolved, resulting in the ability to perform ever more complicated procedures.

A series of early advances proved invaluable in paving the road for the modern infectious disease revolution, including Semmelweis' discovery that hand washing could prevent postpartum infections. This was followed by Lister's description of "hospital disease," which he successfully prevented with carbolic acid for asepsis. With Flemings' discovery of the antibacterial properties of penicillin in 1928, the ability to treat severe infections further opened the possibility to modern surgical advancement. Only 20 years after the introduction of penicillin however, penicillin-resistant *Staphylococcus aureus* was reported, leading to significant surgical morbidity. With the advent of mechanical ventilation and other advances in critical care, we saw the emergence of ventilator-associated pneumonia, catheter-related sepsis, and bloodstream infection. Superimposed was the evolution of the immunocompromised host as the result of advances in chemotherapy and organ transplantation and the emergence of the human immunodeficiency virus. This has invariably led to the development of unexpected and new infections created entirely by modern medicine, such as *Clostridium difficile* and multiresistant pathogens.

The methods of discovery in the field of surgical infections and theories related to their development are expanding in exponential fashion. The delicate balance between medical progress and the emergence of unexpected infections will continue. As such, a good working knowledge of surgical infections is paramount to strive to prevent any unnecessary biologic cost of our interventions. Perhaps the most effective and efficient way to improve surgical infectious disease outcomes is to strive for the appropriate, judicious, and evidence-based use of antibiotics for the prophylaxis and treatment

Surg Clin N Am 94 (2014) xvii–xviii
http://dx.doi.org/10.1016/j.suc.2014.09.015
0039-6109/14/$ – see front matter © 2014 Published by Elsevier Inc.

surgical.theclinics.com

of infection. A concise review of the most commonly encountered surgical infections and the latest in modern infectious disease discovery are the focus of the current issue.

Traci L. Hedrick, MD
Section Colon and Rectal Surgery
University of Virginia
P.O. Box 800709
Charlottesville, VA 22908-0709, USA

Robert G. Sawyer, MD
Department of Surgery
Division of Acute Care Surgery and Outcomes Research
University of Virginia
P.O. Box 800709
Charlottesville, VA 22908-0709, USA

E-mail addresses:
th8q@hscmail.mcc.virginia.edu (T.L. Hedrick)
rws2k@hscmail.mcc.virginia.edu (R.G. Sawyer)

Differences Between Murine and Human Sepsis

Peter Chen, PhD[a,1], Mile Stanojcic, MSc[a,1], Marc G. Jeschke, MD, PhD[b,c,d,*]

KEYWORDS

- Sepsis • Systemic inflammatory response syndrome • Proinflammatory
- Anti-inflammatory • Cytokines • Leukocytes

KEY POINTS

- Murine models do not accurately reflect human sepsis.
- Detection of clinical sepsis usually occurs during the late phases of the disease progression, and is often associated with irreversible damage to patients.
- Most of the existing mouse models of sepsis reflect only the immunologic aspect of the disease, and this xenogeneic comparison is suitable only when comparing the early phases of this clinical disorder.
- Instead of the conventional biphasic approach to modeling sepsis, sepsis should be perceived as a triphasic phenomenon by incorporating a preinfected state as a part of the pathologic simulation.
- Progression of sepsis may be foreshadowed by the immunologic state of the patient before infection, which is determined by the net effect of proinflammatory and anti-inflammatory modulators.

INTRODUCTION

Sepsis and severe sepsis continue to burden the health care system and are among the greatest medical concerns, with a mortality rate ranging from 30% to 50% in North America.[1] Sepsis is the most common cause of death in intensive care units and has

This work is supported by grants from the National Institutes of Health (R01 GM087285-01); Canadian Institutes of Health Research Funds (123336), CFI Leader's Opportunity Fund (Project #25407); Physician's Services Incorporated Foundation: Health Research Grant Program.

[a] Sunnybrook Research Institute, 2075 Bayview Avenue, Toronto, Ontario M4N 3M5, Canada; [b] Department of Immunology, University of Toronto, Toronto, Ontario, Canada; [c] Division of Plastic Surgery, Department of Surgery, University of Toronto, Toronto, Ontario, Canada; [d] Ross Tilley Burn Centre, Sunnybrook Research Institute, Sunnybrook Health Sciences Centre, 2075 Bayview Avenue, Toronto, Ontario M4N 3M5, Canada

[1] These authors contributed equally.

* Corresponding author. Ross Tilley Burn Centre, Sunnybrook Research Institute, Sunnybrook Health Sciences Centre, 2075 Bayview Avenue, Room D704, Toronto, Ontario M4N 3M5, Canada.

E-mail address: marc.jeschke@sunnybrook.ca

Surg Clin N Am 94 (2014) 1135–1149
http://dx.doi.org/10.1016/j.suc.2014.08.001
0039-6109/14/$ – see front matter Crown Copyright © 2014 Published by Elsevier Inc. All rights reserved.

surgical.theclinics.com

been shown to result in an annual health care cost of $14 to $16 billion.[1,2] Between 1979 and 2000, sepsis accounted for an incidence rate of 500,000 cases in the United States. More recently, that figure has increased to onward of 750,000 cases annually.[3] Sepsis can be defined as a systemic inflammatory response syndrome (SIRS) occurring in the presence of an infectious source.[4] The most frequently observed gram-positive and gram-negative bacteria in septic patients include *Staphylococcus aureus*, *Streptococcus pyogenes*, *Escherichia coli*, *Klebsiella* species, and *Pseudomonas aeruginosa*.[5–7] It has long been understood that gram-negative bacteria are the most common sources of bacteremia in sepsis; however, Martin and colleagues[8] showed that the last 25 years has witnessed a shift in gram-positive dominance, with an average annual increase of 26% in cases within the study period.

In 1992, as part of an international effort to standardize the classification process, the American College of Chest Physicians and Critical Care Consensus Conference proposed diagnostic guidelines for SIRS, sepsis, severe sepsis, and septic shock.[9] Generally speaking, the SIRS response is triggered by nontraumatic causes; sepsis can be considered the activation of SIRS inflicted by microbial infections (eg, bacterial, fungal, viral); severe sepsis has the inclusion of multiple organ dysfunction; and the manifestation of hypotension with a lack of responsiveness to fluid resuscitation is septic shock. The specific criteria for each condition are listed later in this article. In 2003, another consensus panel revisited these in an attempt to clarify categorical ambiguity. It was determined that some of the symptoms of SIRS, such as tachycardia, manifest in other septic and nonseptic conditions, and are poor at differentiating it from other conditions. Thus, the terms sepsis and severe sepsis can be used interchangeably when there are organ complications present as a result of infection.[10] More recently, the Surviving Sepsis Campaign produced updated guidelines in an effort to improve the management of sepsis.[11] Suggestions were noted for all categories of sepsis, with an emphasis placed on early quantitative resuscitation of the septic patient within the first 6 hours of positive blood cultures. In light of these multiple paradigm shifts in defining clinical sepsis, this review attempts to provide a summation of the innate immunologic alterations that manifest during sepsis, establish and compare mouse models of sepsis with the clinical course, and discuss the authors' views on additional elements that should be considered in modeling and predicting clinical sepsis from a basic research setting.

Systemic Inflammatory Response Syndrome

A patient must demonstrate at least 2 of the following criteria:

- Temperature less than 36°C or greater than 38.3°C
- Heart rate greater than 90 beats/min
- Respiratory rate greater than 20 breaths/min or $Paco_2$ (partial pressure of arterial carbon dioxide) less than 32 mm Hg
- White blood cell counts less than 4000 cells/µL, greater than 12,000 cells/µL, or more than 10% bands

Sepsis

SIRS with the inclusion of an infection.

Severe Sepsis

Sepsis with the association of hypotension, hypoperfusion, or multiple organ dysfunction.

Septic Shock

Sepsis with hypotension (blood pressure <90 mm Hg) or a deviation from baseline of 40 mm Hg or greater despite fluid resuscitation.

IMMUNE PATHOPHYSIOLOGY

The traditional and most widely accepted perspective regarding the immunologic alterations during the septic response includes the hyperinflammatory response initiated from multiple factors. More recently, this paradigm has shifted with a competing theory regarding a compensatory response. Both of these theories along with the pathophysiology of sepsis are discussed in this section.

The host immune response initiates a surge of proinflammatory cytokines that collectively encompass the "cytokine storm." Endotoxins found on the bacterial cell wall serve as danger-associated molecular patterns (DAMP) and pathogen-associated molecular patterns (PAMP) that are detected by pattern recognition receptors of the innate immune system.[12] For example, the lipopolysaccharide (LPS) component of gram-negative *Pseudomonas aeruginosa* is recognized by toll-like receptor (TLR)4 on the cell surface of antigen-presenting cells (monocytes/macrophages), which in turn stimulates the production of proinflammatory mediators such as tumor necrosis factor (TNF), interleukin (IL)-1β, and IL-6. The severity of this response has been attributed to numerous factors including comorbidities, pathogen load, and virulence.[13] This response elicits a cascade of systemic and tissue-specific events including homing of chemokines to the injury site, phagocytosis, and vascular damage.[14–16] The response is not limited to the site of infection; elevated levels of IL-6 stimulate the liver's production of C-reactive protein, which functions as an acute-phase reactant and is a biomarker of interest for predicting sepsis.[10,17,18] This sequence of events contains numerous alterations on immune cell behavior and function, outlined in **Table 1**.

Another paradigm that has gained increasing acceptance is a delayed and potentially prolonged anti-inflammatory response that succeeds the initial hyperinflammation. The inability of SIRS to explain all of the pathologic alterations, and the lack of sepsis prevention after reducing hyperinflammation occurring in conjunction with anti-inflammatory mediator release,[19] raised the possibility of a fundamental disconnect for a unilateral understanding of sepsis. This process was later described as

Table 1
Overview of systemic inflammatory response syndrome and sepsis effects on innate and adaptive immune cells

	Apoptosis	Cytokine Production	Reference
Macrophage		↑↓ Pro- (early/late) ↑ Anti-	Cavaillon and Annane,[21] 2006 King et al,[53] 2014 Hotchkiss et al,[54] 2002
Dendritic cell	↓	↓	Hotchkiss et al,[54] 2002
Neutrophil	↓ (delayed apoptosis)	↑↓ Pro- (early/late) ↑ Anti-	Drifte et al,[55] 2013 Taneja et al,[56] 2004
Natural killer cell	↑	↓	Reviewed in Stearns-Kurosawa et al,[57] 2011
T cell	↑	↑	Hotchkiss et al,[58] 2001 Venet et al,[59] 2004
B cell	↑	↑ Antibody production	Hotchkiss et al,[58] 2001

the compensatory anti-inflammatory response syndrome (CARS).[20] This biphasic view of the septic response has shed light on the increased susceptibility to secondary complications and immune dysfunction at variable times during the course of infection.[14,21] Specifically, CARS has been described to include the following components[20,22]:

- Reduced cytokine response in monocyte activation
- Lymphocyte apoptosis and dysfunction
- Reduction in monocyte human leukocyte antigen (HLA)-presenting receptors
- Increased expression of anti-inflammatory IL-10

The cytokine components of the compensatory response include release of IL-10, IL-1 receptor antagonist (IL-1RA), and transforming growth factor-β (TGF-β),[23–25] collectively representing a normal homeostatic response to limit inflammation.[26] Other studies have used the CARS model to show that septic patients with low proportions of HLA-DR (a measure of immune challenge and hallmark of sepsis) produced low amounts of proinflammatory cytokines in response to bacterial challenge.[27] IL-10 levels have been shown to correlate with multiple organ dysfunction and mortality.[28] Lastly, when considering both models of the septic response, a high IL-10 to TNF ratio was a predictor of mortality in patients admitted with fever.[29] Contrasting evidence for the capacity of anti-inflammatory soluble mediators to have therapeutic value has generally been limited to animal models (see later discussion). A prospective single-center clinical study conducted by Gomez and colleagues[30] did not show any support for a 2-phase model underlying the pathophysiology of sepsis and, as expected, was only able to conclusively show that immune variables behaved in a "mixed and time-dependent manner."[30] Thus, neglecting all of the aforementioned studies supporting both sides of the spectrum, the compensatory response can be simplified to an adaptive reaction of the immune system to dampen inflammation (**Table 2** summarizes the immune mediators). However, the distinguishable elevation in anti-inflammatory cytokines at early stages of trauma raises questions regarding the adaptive nature of this response, discussed further in subsequent sections.

WHAT ARE ANIMAL MODELS ACTUALLY MODELING?

Clinically, sepsis is physiologically defined by 2 hemodynamic phases: an early hyperdynamic phase and a subsequent late hypodynamic phase.[31] Although the underlying mechanisms of these phases are beyond the scope of this review, it is pertinent that

Table 2
Overview of compensatory anti-inflammatory response syndrome (CARS) effect on innate and adaptive immune cells

	Apoptosis	Cytokine Production	Reference
Macrophage		↑ Anti-	Opal and DePalo,[60] 2000
Dendritic cell	↑	↑ Anti-	Ward et al,[22] 2008
Neutrophil	↓	↓ Pro- ↑ Anti-	Reviewed in Hotchkiss and Karl,[13] 2003
Natural killer cell	↑	↓	Reviewed in Hotchkiss and Karl,[13] 2003
T cell	↑	↓	Reviewed in Adib-Conquy and Cavaillon,[19] 2009
B cell	↑	↓	Reviewed in Adib-Conquy and Cavaillon,[19] 2009

the hyperdynamic phase is characterized by low systemic vascular resistance (SVR) and increased cardiac output (CO), whereas the hypodynamic phase causes a decline in CO and SVR remains constantly low.[32] As the hallmark of clinical sepsis, this parallel phenomenon is often used as the gold standard in animal models of sepsis to evaluate its clinical relevancy.[33,34] However, in addition to the hemodynamic phases, extensive reports from the past 2 decades have suggested a complex and rivaling role of the immune-inflammatory responses of sepsis in defining the accuracy of these animal models in recapitulating human sepsis. Therefore, subsequent sections of this review are dedicated mainly to discussing the immunologic similarities and differences between mouse models and clinical sepsis.

IMMUNOLOGIC MOUSE MODELS OF SEPSIS

Fervent attempts to study and develop novel clinical therapeutics for sepsis have led to the implementation of mouse models. At present, there are 3 different approaches to induce sepsis in mice that are commonly practiced: exogenous administration of a toxin (such as LPS, other endotoxins, or zymosan); exogenous administration of live bacteria; and disturbance of the animals' endogenous protective barrier (introducing colonic leakage to allow migration of bacteria). However, despite the definitive progression of our understanding about the physiologic and immune responses to sepsis with these models, the practicality of translating this knowledge to clinical applications is controversial. The source of this controversy lies within the inherent discrepancy of these models to recapitulate the course of human disease in the clinic. Specific types of models (eg, exogenous toxin administration) may depict only a particular type of sepsis or partial pathophysiology of septic patients. Thus, the main challenge faced by researchers is to select the appropriate model that most accurately reflects the human disease. Applying the knowledge generated from these models to dictate the mechanistic course for therapeutic development continues to be the overall goal. This section presents a comprehensive overview of the different mouse models of sepsis and their relevance to human sepsis.

Toxemia

The toxemia model is established by the injection of TLR agonists such as LPS (TLR4 agonist[35]) or CpG DNA (TLR9 agonist[36]) into mice via intravenous or intraperitoneal routes. The efficacy of this model in recapitulating clinical sepsis is summarized in **Table 3**. One of the major deviations from clinical sepsis of this model is the differences in the immune response, whereby a single bolus of endotoxin administration in mice results in a transient and rapid "spike" of systemic cytokine production, whereas clinical sepsis exhibits a prolonged elevation of systemic cytokine production

Table 3 Comparison of the toxemia model with clinical sepsis	
Similarities with Human Disease	**Differences with Human Disease**
Endotoxin induces shock state in both mice and humans	Humans more sensitive than mice to endotoxin
	The dose of lipopolysaccharide (LPS) resulting in 50% death (LD_{50}) in mice is approximately 1–25 mg/kg body weight,[61–63] whereas an LPS dose of 2–4 ng/kg body weight in humans can inflict severe sickness[64,65]
	Model does not recapitulate the clinical hemodynamic phases
	Different cytokine responses

and is typically lower in serum concentration by multiple orders of magnitude. Further-more, neutralization of proinflammatory mediators ameliorated septic pathophysi-ology in endotoxicosis mouse models, whereas no success was observed in clinical trials.

In general, the culprit of the numerous discrepancies observed between the toxemia models of sepsis in comparison with clinical pathology is inherently attributed to the differential physiology between humans and mice. For example, hemopexin, an iron-binding acute-phase protein that is present in mouse serum but absent from hu-man serum, may account for the difference in LPS sensitivity between mice and humans.[37] These soluble factors have been suggested to suppress the production of proinflammatory cytokines by peripheral blood mononuclear cells when challenged by endotoxins such as LPS, or other exogenous danger signals recognized by pattern recognition receptors.[38]

Live Bacteria Infection

Another method to induce sepsis in mice is by inoculating viable bacteria into animals. Depending on the experimental design, single or mixed bacterial flora can be intro-duced into mice through either the intravenous or intraperitoneal route. In addition, topical administration of live bacteria at the injury site (eg. burns, trauma models) is also an option to mimic post-injury infections observed in clinical settings. However, when compared with clinical pathology, this method of sepsis induction still pos-sesses several major pitfalls. In mice, low bacterial inoculant leads to clearance, whereas high bacterial load results in complement fixation, resulting in rapid bacteria lysis.[39] Therefore, it is very difficult for this model to recapitulate the physiologic con-sequences of bacterial growth in the host and organ infiltration reported in the clinic, as the septic-like response observed in the mouse model is mainly inflicted by endotoxemia.

In addition to the aforementioned caveat, there have been reports describing differ-ential routes of bacterial inoculation leading to unique cytokine responses. For example, bacterial inoculation into the blood compartment of animal models results in the strong generation of proinflammatory cytokines (eg, TNF-α, IL-6, IL-1), whereas peritoneal administration does not lead to such a robust cytokine response.[40,41] Inter-estingly the anti-inflammatory cytokine IL-10 has a protective role in sepsis induced by peritoneal administration of bacteria, in contrast to its worsening effects in the lung infection models.[42–44] Collectively, these differences suggest that there may be an organ-specific or site-specific immunity mounted against microbial infections, and these unique responses may account for the reported differences between mouse models of sepsis and clinical incidents, as outlined in **Table 4**.

Host Barrier Disruption

The most credible animal model of sepsis involves the perturbation of endogenous physical barriers, consequently granting bacterial access to sterile compartments originally inaccessible (eg, peritoneal cavity). Two major host barrier-disruption mouse models are currently implemented in laboratory settings: cecal ligation and puncture (CLP)[45] and colon ascendens stent peritonitis (CASP).[41] Owing to the extensive amount of information and complexity of these models, a point-by-point depiction of the relevant details is listed here.

Cecal ligation and puncture: similarities with human disease

- Considered the gold standard for sepsis research
- Mimics human appendicitis or perforated diverticulitis

Table 4
Comparison of the live bacterial infection model with clinical sepsis

Similarities with Human Disease	Differences with Human Disease
Induces a similar shock state that is observed in human bacterial infections	High inoculating bacterial dose in mice often results in rapid lysis of bacteria by complement[39]
This model is more accurate in recapitulating a clinical infectious scenario in contrast to the artificial LPS administration approach	Pathologic phenotypes observed in model is likely due to endotoxemia and not infection
Dosage and the viable phases of bacteria inoculant can be manipulated to mimic clinical infection, sepsis, or SIRS in mice	Route of bacterial administration (peritoneal cavity, blood, lungs) may have confounding roles in cytokine functions and the mediation/alleviation of sepsis pathology

- Model established by midline laparotomy followed by the exteriorization of cecum, ligation of the cecum distal to the ileocecal valve, and finally the puncturing of the ligated cecum[45,46]
- Creates a "hole" in the cecum whereby the animal is infected by mouse stool gradually leaking into, and accumulating, in the intra-abdominal space of the animal, serving as an inflammatory source, and subsequently generates necrotic tissue (further propagates the inflammation)
- Severity of the disease (assessed by mortality) can be manipulated by the size of the "hole", which is determined by the needle gauge used for puncture, or the amount of punctures given to the animal[46]
- This model can mimic both the early and late (irreversible) phases of sepsis, as surgical excision of necrotic tissue beyond certain time points is unable to improve survival
- The CLP model recreates the hemodynamic, metabolic, and immunologic phases of human sepsis[45]

Cecal ligation and puncture: differences with human disease

- Variable outcomes reported between laboratories, whereby some CLP models using 20-gauge needles for the puncture show higher survival rates than those using 22-gauge needles (would hypothesize the opposite)[47]
- The strains of bacteria that cause the infection in CLP may not represent the flora that are commonly depicted as the culprits of infection, which leads to clinical sepsis (eg, *P. aeruginosa*)
- Most reports of clinical sepsis and patients that exhibit septic shock are pediatric or elderly patients,[1] whereas adult mice are the usual candidates when using mouse models; the age discrepancy of model versus clinic should not be overlooked

Cecal ligation and puncture: possible explanations for the observed differences

- Despite the model being able to recapitulate the hemodynamic, metabolic, and immunologic phases of human sepsis, it is still very difficult to stage human sepsis with this model alone (especially the end stage of sepsis, such as severe sepsis and septic shock), because of the lack of the common and regular physiologic monitoring of these models that is available to humans in the clinic

- The infectious bacterial flora in CLP may be different from those in natural infections, so the immunologic responses observed in these models in comparison with the clinic can obviously be different
- The age discrepancy between mouse models of sepsis and clinical sepsis may suggest a differential composition and efficacy of their immune system in response to bacterial insult; therefore, results from adult mouse models may not match clinical reports, and should be interpreted with caution when extrapolating to pediatric/elderly patients

Colon ascendens stent peritonitis: similarities with human disease

- A stent is inserted into the colon ascendens of the animal, which causes a continuous leakage of fecal matter into the peritoneal cavity[41,46]
- The diameter of the inserted stent determines the pathologic severity of the sepsis: the bigger the diameter the greater the stool leakage, incidence of infection, and sepsis progression[41]
- Lethality observed in CASP is usually a consequence of sepsis-induced multiorgan failure (lung, liver, and kidney), which is highly reminiscent of clinical reports of sepsis-induced death
- CASP mimics the proinflammatory profile of clinical sepsis, as demonstrated by the rapid elevation of proinflammatory cytokines (eg, TNF-α, IL-1) 3 hours after stent insertion[41,48]

Colon ascendens stent peritonitis: differences with human disease

- Does not recapitulate the hemodynamic phases of clinical sepsis[46]
- The anti-inflammatory cytokine response occurs simultaneously with the proinflammatory (3 hours after stent insertion), which deviates from the 2-phase immune profile (proinflammatory [SIRS] followed by anti-inflammatory [CARS]) of clinical sepsis[41,48,49]
- Like CLP, multiple bacterial flora originating from fecal matter of the animal will act in concert to induce sepsis, which may confound when comparing with the culprit bacterial species of clinical sepsis

Colon ascendens stent peritonitis: possible explanations for the observed differences

- In comparison with other models, the CASP model is not as well characterized in its representation of the hemodynamic, metabolic, and immunologic phases of human sepsis

Cecal ligation and puncture versus colon ascendens stent peritonitis

- In CLP the disruption of the host barrier cannot be easily reversed (or reversed at all); in CASP the stent can be removed, thus reducing or eliminating the source of bacterial accumulation in the peritoneal cavity
  - The option of reversing the disrupted host barrier in mouse models is to mimic surgical interventions in clinical sepsis
- In CLP the site of infection is the intra-abdominal space, as shown by the abscess formation postsurgical maneuver; in CASP, the peritoneal cavity is the susceptible niche where bacterial accumulation and infection takes place
  - Therefore, CLP and CASP actually model 2 different kinds of disease that will both eventually lead to sepsis

- As the pathogenesis between the models differs (peritoneal vs intra-abdominal), it is evident that the immunologic responses observed in both models can be different, and will be difficult to compare
- CASP is more surgically challenging than CLP

DISCUSSION

As described earlier, the primary concern of using mouse models to simulate clinical sepsis is that a single model usually depicts only a particular type of sepsis, or delineates partially the clinical pathophysiology of septic patients. After surveying the common sepsis mouse models used in research laboratories, it is apparent that at least immunologically, most of these models can only mimic the acute septic response. This information may be trivially interesting, but lacks clinical applicability, considering that most clinical sepsis indicators are reported during the late or irreversible phases of sepsis. Nonetheless, this realization provides a rationale for explaining the poor efficacy thus far of pharmacologic interventions attempting to treat clinical sepsis, which mostly involve the neutralization of the acute proinflammatory response.[50] It is inherently flawed to attempt to translate acute-phase sepsis regimens used in mouse models at the bench in the hopes of rescuing late-phase sepsis in the clinic.

The outstanding, yet fundamental question that still remains is: how do we accurately model clinical sepsis in animals to design appropriate and effective therapeutics? This question can potentially be approached in 2 ways: the development of additional mouse models to more accurately reflect the late phases of clinical sepsis; or finding a set of biomarkers that can detect clinical sepsis in the acute phase, which can be implemented to make comparisons with the abundance of acute-phase–centered sepsis data generated over the last 2 decades. In terms of developing or improving mouse models, progress by the scientific community has abated since the development of CLP and CASP, which were introduced and published in 1980[45] and 1998,[41] respectively. Although these barrier-disruption models are acknowledged as the gold standard of laboratory sepsis models, they each possess multiple flaws in the simulation of clinical sepsis, particularly with the late phases. Lastly, a recent extensive study comparing the genomic regulation in response to trauma, burns, and infections between humans and mice showed very little correlation between the 2 species,[51] suggesting, at least in the context of these insults, that a xenogeneic comparison of mouse with human may not be suitable.

Therefore, perhaps the best method to treat clinical sepsis should derive from a clinical research–based approach: the identification of a collection of biomarkers in preseptic patients that can predict their vulnerability to septic onset. Take, for example, a hypothetical course of hospitalization and complication of a thermally injured patient. Here, thermal injury serves as a clinical model whereby burned patients are now susceptible to opportunistic infections because of a damaged skin barrier. Subsequently, the immunologic profiles of these burned patients who eventually develop sepsis can be compared with their thermally injured, nonseptic counterparts (either infected or noninfected). The course of this patient study should be divided into at least 3 sections: preinfected (immediate post-thermal injury), infected, and septic, with blood work collected at all 3 stages. Preinfected, infected, and septic cytokine profiles of these patients can be generated via high-throughput enzyme-linked immunosorbent–based assays.

This approach offers several advantages over mouse modeling of sepsis: First, it circumvents the flaws of the mouse-human xenogeneic comparison (eg, genetic differences due to speciation, the confounding effects of clinical resuscitation maneuvers not given to mice). Second, the comparison of patient data can be stratified so that only patients of identical age range, gender, severity of burns, and sepsis diagnosis will be compared. Lastly, once a large enough sample size is achieved, statistical models can be tailored and implemented (eg, multiparameter analysis of variance) to evaluate the validity of this scientific design, while addressing the effects of the confounding factors such as comorbidities, ethnicities, and

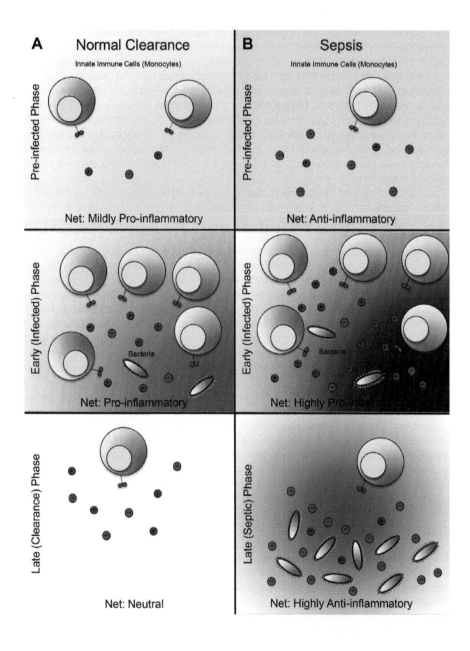

the different genetic background of this patient pool. Unpublished data (Chen et al. 2014) from the authors' laboratory shows that there is a 5- to 7-fold increase of several anti-inflammatory cytokines in the plasma of preinfected burned patients who eventually develop sepsis (blood collected 96 hours after burn injury with no reported infection) in comparison with thermally injured patients who never develop sepsis. A robust plasma proinflammatory cytokine profile was detected in both groups, with no statistical difference.

Albeit preliminary, what do these data mean? The authors hypothesize that perhaps the pivotal determinant of sepsis progression may not be the proinflammatory response, but the degree of foreshadowing anti-inflammatory response before or during bacterial infection, which will ultimately affect the extent of bacterial clearance in these hosts. As shown in **Fig. 1**A, clinical patients who do not develop sepsis have a blood microenvironment that is characterized by a slightly proinflammatory state in the preinfected phase (the net result of medium-grade

◀——————————————————————————————————————

Fig. 1. Systemic immunologic profile as a predictor of sepsis: a working model. (*A*) Microbial clearance of a patient who experiences opportunistic infection. In the preinfected phase, the patient blood microenvironment is in a mild proinflammatory state resulting from the mounted immune response against danger-associated molecular patterns (DAMP) molecules (generated in the process of the trauma or burn). This low-grade proinflammatory state primes the patient's immune system to sense external insults, thus facilitating efficient detection of microbial infiltration. During the early, or infected phase, the invading bacteria are detected by the circulating leukocytes that were recruited to combat the original insult (trauma, burn). This detection results in a heightened proinflammatory response, which leads to additional proinflammatory cytokine production and recruitment of leukocytes, ultimately leading to bacterial eradication. In the late or clearance phase the invading microbes are eliminated, and the immune system is restored to a neutral state by a balance of proinflammatory and anti-inflammatory signals. (*B*) Sepsis development in an infected patient. In the preinfected phase, the net anti-inflammatory state of the blood microenvironment is defined by low-grade proinflammatory response mounted against the DAMP molecules, and an abundance of anti-inflammatory cytokines, produced possibly by the liver (the trigger for this response remains elusive). During the early/infected phase, a proinflammatory response is mounted against the invading microbes by the recruited leukocytes. However, because the blood microenvironment before the infected phase was anti-inflammatory, these recruited leukocytes must produce aberrantly higher levels of proinflammatory cytokines to achieve a net proinflammatory state to offset the effects of the preexisting anti-inflammatory soluble factors. As a result, these leukocytes will likely overexert their effector function and rapidly deplete their effector function potential, leading to immune exhaustion. This state is reminiscent of the systemic immune response syndrome (SIRS), or the classic cytokine storm that is observed in the acute phases of sepsis. Importantly this strong, yet relatively brief proinflammatory state does not lead to sterile immunity, which would lead to bacterial evasion from the host's immune surveillance. In the late/sepsis phase, the immune system is exhausted and is therefore unable to produce additional proinflammatory mediators, despite having the residual bacteria from the infected phase. Furthermore, to counter the spike of proinflammatory signals in the infected phase, a massive surge in anti-inflammatory response is produced, resulting in a net anti-inflammatory microenvironment, similar to the compensatory anti-inflammatory response syndrome, which is conducive to bacterial growth, dissemination, and, ultimately, sepsis. Spheres with plus symbols denote proinflammatory mediators; spheres with minus symbols denote anti-inflammatory mediators. The immunologic state of each phase is determined by the ratio of proinflammatory mediators relative to anti-inflammatory mediators (mildly proinflammatory, 2:1; proinflammatory, 3:1; neutral, 1:1; anti-inflammatory, 1:3; highly proinflammatory, 5:1; highly anti-inflammatory, 1:5).

proinflammatory and low-grade anti-inflammatory response). This concept is intuitive because most burned patients (or trauma patients) have suffered some form of insult, which will lead to the production of proinflammatory cytokines in response to endogenous DAMP molecules as a result of inflammasome activation.[52] These patients, usually with wound openings, are now more susceptible to microbial infections in comparison with healthy individuals. On bacterial invasion of the wound site, the microbes will elevate and perpetuate the proinflammatory response of the host, thus facilitating bacterial clearance. After bacterial clearance an anti-inflammatory response follows, resulting in the neutralization of the proinflammatory response, ultimately restoring the neutral immunologic state of the host. By contrast, an abundance of anti-inflammatory cytokines is already present in the plasma of patients who eventually develop sepsis (see **Fig. 1**B). In this scenario, the blood microenvironment is in an anti-inflammatory state. If bacteria invade the wound of this host, the host's immunologic status is not conducive to bacterial clearance; thus the bacterial may be able to escape the immune surveillance of the host, and quickly establish logarithmic growth phase in the host, consequently leading to organ infiltration and, ultimately, sepsis.

Although there are several unanswered questions about this model (eg, what is the factor or factors that are triggering the initial production and accumulation of anti-inflammatory cytokines in the septic patient?), the primary goal of this schematic is to highlight the potential importance of the preinfected, or prelude, phase of sepsis pathology, which seems to have been be underappreciated in the past. Here the authors propose to adjust the conventional biphasic definition of sepsis (defined by early and late) into a multiphasic trilogy (preinfected, infected/early, sepsis onset/ late) via the incorporation of this prelude phase. In conjunction with the immunologic cytokine profiles associated with each phase, it may help shed light on the development of novel animal models that can more accurately reflect clinical sepsis, which one day might serve as the foundation for the development of effective regimens for septic patients.

REFERENCES

1. Angus DC, Linde-Zwirble WT, Lidicker J, et al. Epidemiology of severe sepsis in the United States: analysis of incidence, outcome, and associated costs of care. Crit Care Med 2001;29(7):1303–10.
2. HCUP Facts and Figures, 2006. Statistics on hospital-based care in the United States. Rockville (MD): Agency for Healthcare Research and Quality (US), 2008.
3. Funk DJ, Parrillo JE, Kumar A. Sepsis and septic shock: a history. Crit Care Clin 2009;25(1):83–101, viii.
4. LaRosa SP, Opal SM. Sepsis strategies in development. Clin Chest Med 2008; 29(4):735–47, x–xi.
5. Opal SM, Garber GE, LaRosa SP, et al. Systemic host responses in severe sepsis analyzed by causative microorganism and treatment effects of drotrecogin alfa (activated). Clin Infect Dis 2003;37(1):50–8.
6. Ramachandran G. Gram-positive and gram-negative bacterial toxins in sepsis: a brief review. Virulence 2013;5(1):213–8.
7. Ranieri VM, Thompson BT, Barie PS, et al. Drotrecogin alfa (activated) in adults with septic shock. N Engl J Med 2012;366(22):2055–64.
8. Martin GS, Mannino DM, Eaton S, et al. The epidemiology of sepsis in the United States from 1979 through 2000. N Engl J Med 2003;348(16): 1546–54.

9. American College of Chest Physicians/Society of Critical Care Medicine Consensus Conference: definitions for sepsis and organ failure and guidelines for the use of innovative therapies in sepsis. Crit Care Med 1992;20(6):864–74.

10. Levy MM, Fink MP, Marshall JC, et al. 2001 SCCM/ESICM/ACCP/ATS/SIS International Sepsis Definitions Conference. Crit Care Med 2003;31(4):1250–6.

11. Dellinger RP, Carlet JM, Masur H, et al. Surviving Sepsis Campaign guidelines for management of severe sepsis and septic shock. Crit Care Med 2004;32(3):858–73.

12. Calfee CS, Matthay MA. Clinical immunology: culprits with evolutionary ties. Nature 2010;464(7285):41–2.

13. Hotchkiss RS, Karl IE. The pathophysiology and treatment of sepsis. N Engl J Med 2003;348(2):138–50.

14. Boomer JS, Green JM, Hotchkiss RS. The changing immune system in sepsis: is individualized immuno-modulatory therapy the answer? Virulence 2013;5(1):45–56.

15. Casey LC. Immunologic response to infection and its role in septic shock. Crit Care Clin 2000;16(2):193–213.

16. Giamarellos-Bourboulis EJ, Raftogiannis M. The immune response to severe bacterial infections: consequences for therapy. Expert Rev Anti Infect Ther 2012;10(3):369–80.

17. Christ-Crain M, Morgenthaler NG, Struck J, et al. Mid-regional pro-adrenomedullin as a prognostic marker in sepsis: an observational study. Crit Care 2005;9(6):R816–24.

18. Gabay C, Kushner I. Acute-phase proteins and other systemic responses to inflammation. N Engl J Med 1999;340(6):448–54.

19. Adib-Conquy M, Cavaillon JM. Compensatory anti-inflammatory response syndrome. Thromb Haemost 2009;101(1):36–47.

20. Bone RC, Grodzin CJ, Balk RA. Sepsis: a new hypothesis for pathogenesis of the disease process. Chest 1997;112(1):235–43.

21. Cavaillon JM, Annane D. Compartmentalization of the inflammatory response in sepsis and SIRS. J Endotoxin Res 2006;12(3):151–70.

22. Ward NS, Casserly B, Ayala A. The compensatory anti-inflammatory response syndrome (CARS) in critically ill patients. Clin Chest Med 2008;29(4):617–25, viii.

23. Fischer E, Van Zee KJ, Marano MA, et al. Interleukin-1 receptor antagonist circulates in experimental inflammation and in human disease. Blood 1992;79(9):2196–200.

24. Marchant A, Deviere J, Byl B, et al. Interleukin-10 production during septicaemia. Lancet 1994;343(8899):707–8.

25. Marie C, Cavaillon JM, Losser MR. Elevated levels of circulating transforming growth factor-beta 1 in patients with the sepsis syndrome. Ann Intern Med 1996;125(6):520–1.

26. Munford RS, Pugin J. Normal responses to injury prevent systemic inflammation and can be immunosuppressive. Am J Respir Crit Care Med 2001;163(2):316–21.

27. Astiz M, Saha D, Lustbader D, et al. Monocyte response to bacterial toxins, expression of cell surface receptors, and release of anti-inflammatory cytokines during sepsis. J Lab Clin Med 1996;128(6):594–600.

28. Doughty L, Carcillo JA, Kaplan S, et al. The compensatory anti-inflammatory cytokine interleukin 10 response in pediatric sepsis-induced multiple organ failure. Chest 1998;113(6):1625–31.

29. van Dissel JT, van Langevelde P, Westendorp RG, et al. Anti-inflammatory cytokine profile and mortality in febrile patients. Lancet 1998;351(9107):950–3.

30. Gomez HG, Gonzalez SM, Londono JM, et al. Immunological characterization of compensatory anti-inflammatory response syndrome in patients with severe sepsis: a longitudinal study. Crit Care Med 2014;42(4):771–80.

31. Parker M, Parrillo J. Septic shock. Hemodynamics and pathogenesis. JAMA 1983;250(24):3324–7.

32. Abraham E, Shoemaker W, Bland R, et al. Sequential cardiorespiratory patterns in septic shock. Crit Care Med 1983;11(10):799–803.

33. Fink M, Heard S. Laboratory models of sepsis and septic shock. J Surg Res 1990;49(2):186–96.

34. Deitch EA. Animal models of sepsis and shock: a review and lessons learned. Shock 1998;9(1):1–11.

35. Poltorak A, He X, Smirnova I, et al. Defective LPS signaling in C3H/HeJ and C57BL/10ScCr mice: mutations in Tlr4 gene. Science 1998;282(5396):2085–8.

36. Hemmi H, Takeuchi O, Kawai T, et al. A Toll-like receptor recognizes bacterial DNA. Nature 2000;408(6813):740–5.

37. Liang X, Lin T, Sun G, et al. Hemopexin down-regulates LPS-induced proinflammatory cytokines from macrophages. J Leukoc Biol 2009;86(2):229–35.

38. Warren H, Fitting C, Hoff E, et al. Resilience to bacterial infection: difference between species could be due to proteins in serum. J Infect Dis 2010;201(2):223–32.

39. Cross AS, Opal SM, Sadoff JC, et al. Choice of bacteria in animal models of sepsis. Infect Immun 1993;61(7):2741–7.

40. Evans GF, Snyder YM, Butler LD, et al. Differential expression of interleukin-1 and tumor necrosis factor in murine septic shock models. Circ Shock 1989; 29(4):279–90.

41. Zantl N, Uebe A, Neumann B, et al. Essential role of gamma interferon in survival of colon ascendens stent peritonitis, a novel murine model of abdominal sepsis. Infect Immun 1998;66(5):2300–9.

42. Greenberger MJ, Strieter RM, Kunkel SL, et al. Neutralization of IL-10 increases survival in a murine model of Klebsiella pneumonia. J Immunol 1995;155(2):722–9.

43. van der Poll T, Marchant A, Buurman WA, et al. Endogenous IL-10 protects mice from death during septic peritonitis. J Immunol 1995;155(11):5397–401.

44. van der Poll T, Marchant A, Keogh CV, et al. Interleukin-10 impairs host defense in murine pneumococcal pneumonia. J Infect Dis 1996;174(5):994–1000.

45. Wichterman KA, Baue AE, Chaudry IH. Sepsis and septic shock—a review of laboratory models and a proposal. J Surg Res 1980;29(2):189–201.

46. Buras JA, Holzmann B, Sitkovsky M. Animal models of sepsis: setting the stage. Nat Rev Drug Discov 2005;4(10):854–65.

47. Baker CC, Chaudry IH, Gaines HO, et al. Evaluation of factors affecting mortality rate after sepsis in a murine cecal ligation and puncture model. Surgery 1983; 94(2):331–5.

48. Maier S, Traeger T, Entleutner M, et al. Cecal ligation and puncture versus colon ascendens stent peritonitis: two distinct animal models for polymicrobial sepsis. Shock 2004;21(6):505–11.

49. Emmanuilidis K, Weighardt H, Maier S, et al. Critical role of Kupffer cell-derived IL-10 for host defense in septic peritonitis. J Immunol 2001;167(7):3919–27.

50. Fink MP. Animal models of sepsis. Virulence 2013;5(1):143–53.

51. Seok J, Warren HS, Cuenca AG, et al. Genomic responses in mouse models poorly mimic human inflammatory diseases. Proc Natl Acad Sci U S A 2013; 110(9):3507–12.

52. Stanojcic M, Chen P, Harrison R, et al. Leukocyte infiltration and activation of the nlrp3 inflammasome in white adipose tissue following thermal injury. Crit Care Med 2014;42(6):1357–64.
53. King EG, Bauza GJ, Mella JR, et al. Pathophysiologic mechanisms in septic shock. Lab Invest 2014;94(1):4–12.
54. Hotchkiss RS, Tinsley KW, Swanson PE, et al. Depletion of dendritic cells, but not macrophages, in patients with sepsis. J Immunol 2002;168(5):2493–500.
55. Drifte G, Dunn-Siegrist I, Tissieres P, et al. Innate immune functions of immature neutrophils in patients with sepsis and severe systemic inflammatory response syndrome. Crit Care Med 2013;41(3):820–32.
56. Taneja R, Parodo J, Jia SH, et al. Delayed neutrophil apoptosis in sepsis is associated with maintenance of mitochondrial transmembrane potential and reduced caspase-9 activity. Crit Care Med 2004;32(7):1460–9.
57. Stearns-Kurosawa DJ, Osuchowski MF, Valentine C, et al. The pathogenesis of sepsis. Annu Rev Pathol 2011;6:19–48.
58. Hotchkiss RS, Tinsley KW, Swanson PE, et al. Sepsis-induced apoptosis causes progressive profound depletion of B and CD4+ T lymphocytes in humans. J Immunol 2001;166(11):6952–63.
59. Venet F, Pachot A, Debard AL, et al. Increased percentage of CD4+CD25+ regulatory T cells during septic shock is due to the decrease of CD4+CD25- lymphocytes. Crit Care Med 2004;32(11):2329–31.
60. Opal SM, DePalo VA. Anti-inflammatory cytokines. Chest 2000;117(4):1162–72.
61. Glode LM, Mergenhagen SE, Rosenstreich DL. Significant contribution of spleen cells in mediating the lethal effects of endotoxin in vivo. Infect Immun 1976;14(3):626–30.
62. McCuskey RS, McCuskey PA, Urbaschek R, et al. Species differences in Kupffer cells and endotoxin sensitivity. Infect Immun 1984;45(1):278–80.
63. Reynolds K, Novosad B, Hoffhines A, et al. Pretreatment with troglitazone decreases lethality during endotoxemia in mice. J Endotoxin Res 2002;8(4):307–14.
64. Barber AE, Coyle SM, Fischer E, et al. Influence of hypercortisolemia on soluble tumor necrosis factor receptor II and interleukin-1 receptor antagonist responses to endotoxin in human beings. Surgery 1995;118(2):406–10 [discussion: 410–1].
65. Suffredini AF, Reda D, Banks SM, et al. Effects of recombinant dimeric TNF receptor on human inflammatory responses following intravenous endotoxin administration. J Immunol 1995;155(10):5038–45.

The Opposing Forces of the Intestinal Microbiome and the Emerging Pathobiome

Jennifer Defazio, MD[1], Irma D. Fleming, MD[1],
Baddr Shakhsheer, MD[1], Olga Zaborina, PhD,
John C. Alverdy, MD*[,1]

KEYWORDS

- Microbiome • Bacteria • Anastomotic leak • Sepsis • Infection • Metabolomics
- Proteomics

KEY POINTS

- Colorectal surgery has evolved overtime, and yet the incidence of surgical site infections and anastomotic leaks persists.
- The microbiome has an emerging role in human health and various diseases, such as anastomotic leak, gut-derived sepsis, and wound infection.
- Current investigations using high-throughput functional metagenomics approaches have significantly advanced our knowledge of the host-microbiome interaction.

INTRODUCTION

For centuries, humans have dismissed the importance of microbial organisms whose mere existence is essential to our ability to survive and remain healthy. Microbes and the complex community structures in which they assemble and function have remained invisible for decades, only occasionally garnering recognition during times of plague and strife. Over time, however, research has shown that human beings live in close and constant contact with boundless communities of microbial organisms. These organisms are not only our cohabitants but they are also most of the live forms around and within us, outnumbering all other living beings on earth. The human body is

This work was supported by National Institutes of Health grant 5R01 GM062344-11 and DDRCC grant P30 DK42086.
There are no financial disclosures.
Center for Surgical Infection Research and Therapeutics, Department of Surgery, Pritzker School of Medicine, University of Chicago, 5841 S Maryland Ave, MC 6040, Chicago, IL, USA
[1] Individuals contributed equally to this work.
* Corresponding author. University of Chicago Medical Center, 5841 South Maryland Avenue, MC 6090, Chicago, IL 60637.
E-mail address: jalverdy@surgery.bsd.uchicago.edu

a vessel to trillions of microbes, and it has been estimated that the number of microbes in or on the human body outnumber the total number of human cells by a factor of 10. The human body consists of around 10 trillion cells, whereas 100 trillion bacteria[1] colonize its surfaces and intestinal tract directly participating in health maintenance. For every gene in the human genome, there are 100 bacterial genes. The human-associated bacterial communities and their genomes are collectively referred to as the *microbiome* and are present in the gut, mouth, skin, and all surfaces exposed to the external environment, including the lungs. The role of the microbiome in health maintenance is emerging as having a profound influence on overall homeostasis. Human behavior, in turn, can have a significant impact on the structure and function of the microbiome. Thus, humans and their microbiota are engaged in a mutualistic relationship that is crucial for the well-being of both living bodies. Everything from the food or medications ingested to the way an individual is born influences the species, community structure, and function of microbiota that take up residence in our bodies. The recent recognition that the pharmacodynamics and efficacy of cancer chemotherapy depend on the structure and function of our microbiota[2,3] is forcing a reconsideration of the way we approach disease and its treatment. Therefore, it is becoming increasing untenable to dismiss the health of the microbiota when considering both the pathogenesis of disease and its treatment. For this reason, we are forced to adopt new life practices as well as reevaluate the many established methods of medical and surgical management of disease. The purpose of this article is to summarize what is currently known about the role of the microbiome in health and disease and to provide instances in which consideration of the host-microbiota interaction might affect future research and care of surgical patients.

RISING INCIDENCE OF SURGICAL INFECTIONS, ANTIBIOTIC RESISTANCE, BOWEL PREPARATIONS, AND BEYOND

Before the past 70 years, surgical infection radically limited surgeons' ability to perform advanced operations. Before the 1850s, postoperative "irritative fever" developed in most patients, leading to overwhelming sepsis and death.[4] Surgeons seldom washed their hands, and students were encouraged to place bare hands in the operative field for educational purposes.[5] The famed surgeon William Halsted went so far as to operate in tents placed outdoors at Bellevue Hospital for better infection control.[6] In the midnineteenth century, Joseph Lister introduced antisepsis, providing the foundation for modern aseptic technique. By the end of the century, Louis Pasteur's germ theory was gaining acceptance. The combined work of these two pioneers led to significantly decreased perioperative morbidity and mortality.

In the 1950s, prophylactic antibiotics came into use for surgery. Despite inconsistent results from early clinical trials, Burke[7] demonstrated that the timing of antibiotic administration relative to the beginning of the procedure was crucial with respect to decontaminating the skin. In the 1960s, Bernard and Cole[8] furthered the earlier work by performing a randomized controlled trial demonstrating the benefit of preoperative intravenous antibiotic prophylaxis in gastrointestinal tract operations. Work in the 1970s to the 1990s helped to define the role of the intestinal microflora on postoperative sepsis in general and on wound infection specifically. However, these studies were limited by results generated by culture alone and have not been repeated using newer genome-based identification methods.[9,10] There is concern that we are using antibiotics with broader coverage than is necessary, which has the unwanted consequence of selecting out for more resistant organisms while at the same time destroying the health-promoting microbiota. During critical illness such as occurs following trauma and burn injury, a countermeasure to the unavoidable use and consequences of broad antibiotic coverage has been to administer selective digestive decontamination (SDD) with oral nonabsorbable antibiotics to eliminate potential pathogens that remain in the gut. This approach has not been widely accepted because of the fear of resistance. Another approach has been to repopulate the gut microbiota with probiotic organisms administered orally during critically illness. The use of such probiotic organisms has been controversial and the results disappointing. Both SDD and probiotic feeding to critically ill patients suffer because they are based on empirical evidence and there still exists major gaps in knowledge to explain how the microbiome maintains health during physiologic stress. Clinical trials of SDD suffer from a lack of detailed understanding of the precise effect it has on the community structure, taxa, and function of the intestinal microbiota. Numerous human and animal studies using 16S rRNA-based genomic analysis of the microbiota demonstrate that loss of the core microbiome during physiologic stress and critical illness directly affects immune function and is associated with poor outcomes. To date there are no studies that have examined the effect of SDD on the function, structure, and detailed taxa of the gut microbiome at multiple time points during critical illness. Whether microbial genes, such as virulence genes and antibiotic resistance genes, are activated within the transcriptome of the microbiota during SDD develops remains unaddressed. Similarly, the effect of a single strain of probiotic bacteria, or even several strains, can recapitulate the core functionality of the microbiota on the immune system during critical illness remains unstudied. Use of genomic, metagenomic, transcriptomic, and metatranscriptomic approaches to define how to best eliminate threatening microbes and preserve those that are health promoting is now available. These approaches represent an immense opportunity to shift from the empiricism of correlating a broadly kill or selectively repopulate approach to clinical outcomes to one in which the robustness and resilience of the core microbiome can be defined and maintained.

A similar line and approach of investigation could be applied to bowel preparation before elective gastrointestinal surgery. It has taken decades for surgeons to accept that mechanical cleansing of the bowel with purgative agents may be unnecessary, even harmful in elective gastrointestinal tract surgery.[11–14] Historically, cleansing mechanical bowel preparations (MBP) were used to decontaminate the gastrointestinal tract as well as make the bowel easier to work with intraoperatively. However, MBP does little to decrease the concentration of bacteria in the bowel mucosa and lumen; it does, however, serve to upset the local microbiome allowing opportunistic pathogens the opportunity to thrive.[15–17]

The use of oral antibiotics in elective colon surgery has varied tremendously as a result of the work performed on MBP. Use of oral antibiotics to modify the intestinal microflora before surgery started in the 1930s and continued over the ensuing 40 years as more antibiotics came into use. In the 1970s, Clarke and colleagues[18] perform a randomized control trial at the Veterans Administration hospitals in which patients received either oral erythromycin-neomycin or placebo after MBP. No intravenous antibiotics were used on the control group. The results showed a decrease from a 35% surgical site infection rate in the placebo group to a 9% rate in the oral antibiotic group ($P<.05$). Further studies confirmed this early finding, and oral antibiotics became the standard of care. Although fecal cultures were examined initially, they proved to be of little use in directing subsequent practices and antibiotic choices. As mortality rates and surgical site infections decreased from 1970 to 2000, oral antibiotics were eliminated, intravenous antibiotics were empirically chosen, guidelines were developed, and the science to verify all these changes and choices was left abandoned. As clinical outcomes slowly improved, the need to understand the causality between antibiotic choice and outcome faded in interest. The downside of this disinterest is the emergence of antibiotic resistance, persistent surgical site infections, anastomotic leaks, sepsis, and a lack of understanding of why they continue to occur.

The past 100 years has seen colorectal surgery transformed from a uniformly deadly endeavor to an intervention that can be performed with minimally invasive techniques. Yet, despite these advances, the incidence of surgical site infections and anastomotic leaks persists and plague clinical practice. Although surgical site infections following gastrointestinal surgery are most certainly attributed to exposure to the intestinal microbiota, this mechanism for anastomotic leak is less well accepted despite compelling data supporting it (vide infra). The complications of surgical site infection and anastomotic leak carry a substantial mortality risk.[19–21] The relative risk of death is increased by a factor of 2.2, and the average length of stay is increased by 5 days.[22] The role of MBP in conjunction with oral antibiotics remains to be fully elucidated. Further characterization of the microbiome and its interactions with the host can potentially lead to novel targets to further decrease the surgical site infection rate. Yet this approach will require a more genomic understanding of the community structure, taxa, and function of the microbes we need to preserve and those that we need to eliminate. More importantly is realizing when, in terms relative to surgery, and where, meaning orally or locoregionally, to do this.

EMERGING IMPORTANCE OF HUMAN MICROBIOME IN HEALTH AND DISEASE

The emerging role and importance of the microbiome in human health and disease is being discovered across various medical and surgical problems. Subtle perturbations in the microbiome are now being found to influence diseases and their progression and resolution. Technological advances in genomics, proteomics, and metabolomics have begun to reveal the immense impact that our microbiome has on our health and development of disease and its complex relationship with the host.

Our coexistence with the gut microbiota is a dynamic and mutually beneficial relationship. Commensal bacteria are critical in the regulation of digestion. The bacteria of the gut regulate host energy metabolism and body mass index. In this way, they have been linked to obesity. For example, gut flora aid in digestion and degradation of nondigestible plant polysaccharides and fiber in our diet.[1] Enzymes capable of digestion of nutrients otherwise inaccessible have been found in the genomes of gut bacterial species (eg, *Bacteroides thetaiotaomicron*). Gut bacteria have also been found to impact the storage of fat. Normal flora has been shown to stimulate triglyceride storage by inhibiting fasting-induced adipocyte factor, a protein inhibitor of lipoprotein lipase.[1,23] It has been hypothesized that altered gut flora may limit the ability of lipoprotein lipase to adequately process triglycerides and thereby lead to obesity. Recent studies have shown that when the cecal microflora of obese mice and transferred to lean mice, there is a significant weight gain in the previously lean mice.[24,25] Similarly, germ-free mice are leaner than conventionally raised mice despite increased food intake.[26,27] They must consume 30% greater calories in order to maintain the same weight as their counterparts.[28] If these germ-free mice then receive a microbiota transplant from obese mice, they develop a 60% increase in body fat.[27] Studies have then looked at human subjects and found that when following a fat-restricted or carbohydrate-restricted diet, *Bacteroides* species increase overtime relative to the Firmicutes.[29] Importantly for surgeons, patients who had a Roux-en-Y gastric bypass were found to have a decreased abundance of Firmicutes in their gut as compared with their obese counterparts.[25,30]

Recent studies have shown that the commensal bacteria and their products are vital in regulating the development, homeostasis, and function of the host immune system.

It has been shown that in mice who have their microbiome removed via antibiotics, the reduction in MyD88-mediated innate immune signals leaves the mucosa more permeable to commensal bacteria and less capable of postinjury repair.[31] The intestinal commensals have also been found to stimulate the expression of antimicrobial factors, such as RegIIIγ, which protect the epithelium from invasion by bacteria and control the balance of members of the microbial community.[32] The microbiota also stimulate the production of cytokines that strengthen the immune system (interleukin [IL]-10, IL-22) and facilitate the clearance of pathogens.[32] The normal microbiota play a clear and definite role in shaping and directing both the local and systemic immune system in order to maintain homeostasis and defend itself against invading pathogens.

GENOMICS, METAGENOMICS, PROTEOMICS, AND METABOLOMICS: THE FUTURE OF SURGICAL RESEARCH

Our microbial companions perform several metabolic reactions that are not encoded in the human genome but are necessary for human health. Consequently, when considering the human genome, there should be an inclusion of human genes and those of our microbes. As a result of innovations in high-throughput sequencing technologies, it is now possible to study the microbiome on a massive scale that was not possible years ago. Most microbial species present in and on the human body have never been isolated, cultured, or sequenced, largely because of the inability to reproduce necessary growth conditions in the laboratory.[33] Fortunately, advances in technology and the understanding of bacteria growth have allowed for the recreation of such conditions. There are numerous microbial processes waiting to be discovered.

After identifying the components of the human microbiome, it is then necessary to study their activities and functionalities in their environment by high-throughput functional metagenomic approaches.[34] Metagenomics, or the study of microbial communities, takes advantage of the advances in sequencing technology and analysis methods to comprehensively examine microbial communities directly from their natural habitats, potentially revealing the previously unseen.[33] Accordingly, the National Institutes of Health (NIH) has established the Human Microbiome Project (HMP) as a road map initiative.[33] The HMP uses 16S rRNA and metagenomic sequencing to characterize the complexity of the human microbiome at various body sites. This project has generated extraordinary amounts of data about the complexity of the human microbiome and provides a foundation for further research into the influence of the microbiome on human health and disease. With the support of the HMP, an enormous amount of consideration has been put toward defining which microbes are normal and which may be associated with disease pathogenesis.[1] The translational significance of microbes is relevant not only to research within every NIH institute but certainly to every surgical discipline.

Although phylogenetic and metagenomic approaches may reveal candidate species and genes that may be important in certain conditions or diseases, they do not provide evidence for the actual involvement of these species or genes. In other words, metagenomics allows for the identification of microbial genes but fails to provide information about downstream molecules that are actually produced in their environment. Hence, functional approaches are needed that aim to identify the active molecules and species. These functional studies also provide the basis for studying the environmental interactions between the microbe and their host, which is of significant importance as functional studies could reveal molecular mechanisms and, therefore, lead to developing treatment strategies for diseases associated with the human microbiota. With this concept in mind, researchers have introduced transcriptomics, proteomics, and metabolomics.[35,36] Transcriptomic, proteomic, and metabolomic approaches at the community level, also termed *meta-omics*, have all been applied to observe molecular activities of the human microbiota.[37] Unfortunately, metatranscriptomic studies, analyzing bacterial mRNA, are difficult as the prokaryotic mRNA is highly unstable. Similarly, metabolomics, metabolite analysis, is also considerably difficult because all body fluids are in contact with cells, and, thus, metabolites are rapidly absorbed. Moreover, metabolite analysis is rather challenging requiring a series of high-throughput instruments and large databases for which many metabolites are unknown and, hence, would require initial identification.[37] In contrast, metaproteomics analyzes proteins, which are generally quite stable and can correlate directly to the genetic code, with the advantage that prokaryotes are known to have limited post-translational processing. Therefore, metaproteomics is likely to illustrate a highly reliable picture of microbial function with relation to the host environment.

APPLICATION OF NEXT-GENERATION SEQUENCING TECHNOLOGY TO SURGICAL PROBLEMS
Anastomotic Leak

Although anastomotic leak is most commonly framed as a problem of surgical technique, there is compelling evidence that its etiopathogenesis is microbial. Although clinical studies as early as 1939 implicated the intestinal microbiota as causative agents in anastomotic leak by virtue of a reduction in leak rates with oral antibiotics, it was not until 1955 that Cohn and Rives[38] demonstrated in dogs that the microbial content of the intestine causes leak.[38] This notion was confirmed later by a rat study in which oral versus intravenous antibiotics were tested to prevent anastomotic leak with results that clearly showed that oral antibiotics eliminated leaks, whereas intravenous antibiotics with a similar spectrum of activity did not.[39] These studies were largely ignored, as leak rates, surgical site infection rates, and mortality following colon surgery decreased from 1970 through to 2000. Therefore, oral antibiotics have been largely eliminated and anastomotic leaks persist in high-risk regions. Recently several randomized prospective studies have proven that oral antibiotics decrease anastomotic leak rates; however, the microbiologic detail around these empirical observations remains undefined. The authors' group has recently demonstrated that intestinal microbes can cause anastomotic leak in rats via mechanisms that involve their phenotypic transformation to high-collagenase producers. Despite decades of work in this area, the application of oral antibiotics in gastrointestinal surgery remains controversial and largely abandoned. There are no groups worldwide studying a microbial mechanism of anastomotic leak using new-generation technology. Again, an immense opportunity to define the role of microbes in anastomotic leak is being overlooked. Furthermore, the choice and route of the currently recommended antibiotics for gastrointestinal surgery is based on incomplete data that are culture based and more than 40 years old.

Gut-Derived Sepsis

Normal homeostasis of the gut is maintained through complex interactions between the microbiome and its environment. Humans and their microbiome generally maintain a well-tolerated symbiotic relationship.[40] However, during prolonged critical illness, the gut is exposed to numerous stressors, including antibiotics, vasopressors, hypoxia, and so forth, which contribute to the development of a community of virulent pathogens in the gut, which the authors refer to as the *pathobiome*.[41–43] The authors of this review hypothesize that this pathobiome then interacts with the gut epithelium and immune system to drive the immunopathology of sepsis.

The normal microbiome is composed of a wide variety of bacterial species. The authors' laboratory has found that the bacterial composition of the gut as measured through the feces of normal subjects is diverse with protective anaerobes predominating and very low amounts of proteobacteria. However, when the stool of intensive care unit (ICU) patients with severe sepsis is examined, there is an almost complete loss of those protective anaerobes and diversity. These patients undergo prolonged exposure to multiple antibiotics throughout their ICU admission. Despite the treatment they received, the authors were still able to culture virulent and drug-resistant pathogens from the stool throughout their hospital course.

This pathobiome that can develop in the gut of critically ill patients can cause dysfunction within the immune system. Given the limitation of antibiotics to eliminate all potential pathogens and to suppress the mutability of microbes, other strategies to contain rather than eliminate pathogens is needed. It is not the mere presence of the pathogen itself that leads to lethal inflammation but rather whether pathogens are cued to express virulence. The authors' laboratory has made the novel observation that during extreme physiologic stress, such as occurs during critical illness, host compensatory cues are released into the local gut microenvironment that are gathered, processed, and transduced by certain pathogenic species leading to triggering of their virulence circuits. Therefore, a dynamic in vivo virulence activation mechanism among intestinal pathogens exists whereby pathogens are cued by host factors to express enhanced virulence. In animal models of lethal gut-derived sepsis, the authors have defined many of these cues; they include endogenous opioids, immune elements, and end products of ischemia.

An interesting aspect of this work was the identification by the authors' laboratory that bacteria also have membrane sensors that assess the abundance of resources present in the local microenvironment. One highly conserved sensor system is the system that senses phosphate abundance. Most bacteria possess a membrane-based phosphosensory, phosphoregulatory 2-component system that is connected to their core virulence mechanism, such as the quorum sensing signaling system. When phosphate is abundant, incoming cues, such as opioids, do not transduce virulence; however, when phosphate is low, opioid responsiveness and, hence, virulence is enhanced. From an evolutionary perspective, these results indicate that when microbes sense abundant resources within the local microenvironment that support their growth and proliferation (ie, phosphate), they do not waist energy expressing virulence, unless predation is sensed. As this plays out in the gut during critical illness, both host-derived cues and depleted local resources create conditions associated with virulence activation. The authors tested whether embedding phosphate in the local intestinal microenvironment of mice during surgical stress would prevent pathogen virulence activation and lethal sepsis. The authors intestinally inoculated mice with health care–acquired pathogens (ie, *Candida albicans*, *Enterococcui faecalis*, *Serratia marcescens*, *Klebsiella oxytoca*) and performed a surgical injury (30% hepatectomy), a model that results in lethal gut-derived sepsis. When phosphate was embedded into the host pathogen interaction in the gut by locally applying it as a covalently bonded polymer carrier, the microbiota proliferated, the pathogens were attenuated in expressing virulence, and mortality was prevented.[44] Thus provision of key resources within the host pathogen interaction in the gut, using compounds that do not kill but attenuate microbes, may be an approach to consider in a clinical trial. Unlike SDD or the addition of a probiotics, this approach may leverage the strength of the microbiota to suppress virulence while also suppressing virulence directly by triggering phosphosensory and phosphoregulatory pathways.

Wound Infection

During the process of investigating the human microbiome and its association with the authors' patients, they recognized that many traditional aspects of surgical care have a detrimental impact on the state of the innate microbiome and, thus, can affect clinical outcomes.[1] One example of the detrimental effects on the innate microbiome is the administration of antibiotics. The administration of perioperative antibiotics is known to be the standard of care in certain circumstances. In accordance with national entities, such as the Surgical Care Improvement Project, the proper timing, regimen, and duration of therapy are viewed as important quality measures.[45] The motivation behind the administration of prophylactic antibiotics before surgery is to reduce the preoperative bacterial burden and, as a result, decrease the rate of surgical site infections, a complication that costs an estimated $3.5 to $10 billion annually in the United States.[46] However, the use of prophylactic antibiotics should be further evaluated because inappropriate overuse leads to the emergence of resistant organisms; on the other hand, inadequate antibiotic use may adversely affect patient outcomes. This point has been shown to be true in patients with pneumonia, bacteremia, and also surgical site infections as measured by end points ranging from length of stay to death.[47–49] The application of genomic and metagenomic analysis to studies of wound infection has the potential to provide a more high-resolution readout of the microbial community structure, taxa, and function that assembles in a wound over time and may better calibrate our use, choice, and dose of antibiotics to prevent wound infections.

SUMMARY

The way we view surgical infection and our interaction with microbes both beneficial and pathogenic has changed immensely over the past couple of decades. Technological advances have fueled these advances as the time and cost to sequence whole genomes and to measure whole preoteomes and metabolomes has been significantly reduced. Understanding and demonstrating the information within these mega datasets is becoming a reality as computational scientists, mathematicians, physicists, and bioinformatics experts work together. However, there are still limitations of these advances. We must be cautious not to ascribe causality to data that are purely descriptive. Rather we must correlate this new data with disease states and inform the system's biology. Armed with new approaches to examine the microbiome and its correlation to varying states of health and disease, new treatment strategies may emerge and antibiotic use may even diminish.

REFERENCES

1. Morowitz MJ, Babrowski T, Carlisle EM, et al. The human microbiome and surgical disease. Ann Surg 2011;253(6):1094–101. http://dx.doi.org/10.1097/SLA.0b013e31821175d7.
2. Viaud S, Saccheri F, Mignot G, et al. The intestinal microbiota modulates the anticancer immune effects of cyclophosphamide. Science 2013;342(6161):971–6. http://dx.doi.org/10.1126/science.1240537.
3. Iida N, Dzutsev A, Stewart CA, et al. Commensal bacteria control cancer response to therapy by modulating the tumor microenvironment. Science 2013;342(6161):967–70. http://dx.doi.org/10.1126/science.1240527.
4. Mangram AJ, Horan TC, Pearson ML, et al. Guideline for prevention of surgical sit infection, 1999. Surg Outcomes 1999;27(2):98–134.

5. Alexander J. The contributions of infection control to a century of surgical progress. Ann Surg 1985;201:423–8.
6. Wangensteen O, Wandensteen S, Klinger C. Surgical cleanliness, hospital salubrity, and surgical statistics, historically considered. Surgery 1972;71:477–93.
7. Burke J. The effective period of preventive antibiotic action in experimental incision and dermal lesions. Surgery 1960;50:161–8.
8. Bernard H, Cole W. The prophylaxis of surgical infection: the effect of prophylactic antimicrobial drugs on the incidence of infection following potentially contaminated operations. Surgery 2014;56:151–9.
9. Nichols R. Surgery annual. Nyhus LM, editor. Vol 13. New York: Appleton-Century-Crofts; 1981.
10. Antimicrobial prophylaxis in surgery. Med Lett Drugs Ther 2014;41:75–80.
11. Guenaga KF, Matos D, Wille-Jorgensen P. Mechanical bowel preparation for elective colorectal surgery. Cochrane Database Syst Rev 2009;(1):CD001544.
12. Contant CM, Hop WC, van Sant HP, et al. Mechanical bowel preparation for elective colorectal surgery: a multicentre randomised trial. The Lancet 2007; 370(9605):2112–7. http://dx.doi.org/10.1016/S0140-6736(07)61905-9.
13. Platell C, Hall J. What is the role of mechanical bowel preparation in patients undergoing colorectal surgery. Dis Colon Rectum 1998;41(7):882–3.
14. Slim K, Vicaut E, Panis Y, et al. Meta-analysis of randomized clinical trials of colorectal surgery with or without mechanical bowel preparation. Br J Surg 2004; 91(9):1125–30. http://dx.doi.org/10.1002/bjs.4651.
15. van den Bogaard A, Weidema W, van Boven C, et al. Recolonization and colonization resistance of the large bowel after three methods of preoperative preparation of the gastrointestinal tract for elective colorectal surgery. J Hyg 1986;97: 49–59.
16. Jung B, Matthiessen P, Smedh K, et al. Mechanical bowel preparation does not affect the intramucosal bacterial colony count. Int J Colorectal Dis 2010;25(4): 439–42. http://dx.doi.org/10.1007/s00384-009-0863-3.
17. Arabi Y, Dimock F, Burdon D, et al. Influence of bowel preparation and antimicrobials on colonic microflora. Br J Surg 1978;65(8):555–8.
18. Clarke J, Condon R, Barlett J. Preoperative oral antibiotics reduce septic complications of colon operations: results of prospective, randomized, double-blind clinical study. Ann Surg 1977;186(3):251–9.
19. Blumetti J, Luu M, Sarosi G, et al. Surgical site infections after colorectal surgery: do risk factors vary depending on the type of infection considered? Surgery 2007;142(5):704–11. http://dx.doi.org/10.1016/j.surg.2007.05.012.
20. Khan AA, Wheeler JM, Cunningham C, et al. The management and outcome of anastomotic leaks in colorectal surgery. Colorectal Dis 2008;10(6):587–92. http://dx.doi.org/10.1111/j.1463-1318.2007.01417.x.
21. Tytherleigh MG, Bokey L, Chapuis PH, et al. Is a minor clinical anastomotic leak clinically significant after resection of colorectal cancer? J Am Coll Surg 2007; 205(5):648–53. http://dx.doi.org/10.1016/j.jamcollsurg.2007.05.031.
22. Kirkland KB, Meriwether RA, MacKenzie WR, et al. Clinician judgment as a tool for targeting HIV counseling and testing in North Carolina state mental hospitals, 1994. AIDS Patient Care STDS 1999;13(8):473–9.
23. Sears CL. A dynamic partnership: celebrating our gut flora. Anaerobe 2005; 11(5):247–51. http://dx.doi.org/10.1016/j.anaerobe.2005.05.001.
24. Turnbaugh PJ, Ley RE, Mahowald MA, et al. An obesity-associated gut microbiome with increased capacity for energy harvest. Nature 2006;444(7122): 1027–131. http://dx.doi.org/10.1038/nature05414.

25. das UN. Obesity: genes, brain, gut, and environment. Nutrition 2010;26(5): 459–73. http://dx.doi.org/10.1016/j.nut.2009.09.020.

26. Backhed F, Manchester JK, Semenkovich CF, et al. Mechanisms underlying the resistance to diet-induced obesity in germ-free mice. Proc Natl Acad Sci U S A 2007;104(3):979–84. http://dx.doi.org/10.1073/pnas.0605374104.

27. Backhed F, Ding H, Wang T, et al. The gut microbiota as an environmental factor that regulates fat storage. Proc Natl Acad Sci U S A 2004;101(44):15718–23. http://dx.doi.org/10.1073/pnas.0407076101.

28. Wostmann B, Larkin C, Moriarty A, et al. Dietary intake, energy metabolism, and excretory losses of adult male germfree Wistar rats. Lab Anim Sci 1983;33(1): 46–50.

29. Ley R, Turnbaugh PJ, Klein S, et al. Microbial ecology: human gut microbes associated with obesity. Nature 2006;444(21):1–2. http://dx.doi.org/10.1038/nature 4441021a.

30. Zhang H, DiBaise JK, Zuccolo A, et al. Human gut microbiota in obesity and after gastric bypass. Proc Natl Acad Sci U S A 2009;106(7):2365–70. http://dx.doi.org/10.1073/pnas.0812600106.

31. Vaishnava S, Behrendt C, Ismail A, et al. Paneth cells directly sense gut commensals and maintain homeostasis at the intestinal host-microbial interface. Proc Natl Acad Sci U S A 2008;105:20858–63.

32. Littman D, Pamer E. Role of the commensal microbiota in normal and pathogenic host immune responses. Cell Host Microbe 2011;10(4):311–23. http://dx.doi.org/10.1016/j.chom.2011.10.004.

33. Peterson J, Garges S, Giovanni M, et al. The NIH human microbiome project. Genome Res 2009;19(12):2317–23. http://dx.doi.org/10.1101/gr.096651.109.

34. Zoetendal EG, Rajilic-Stojanovic M, de Vos WM. High-throughput diversity and functionality analysis of the gastrointestinal tract microbiota. Gut 2008;57(11): 1605–15. http://dx.doi.org/10.1136/gut.2007.133603.

35. Gosalbes MJ, Durbán A, Pignatelli M, et al. Metatranscriptomic approach to analyze the functional human gut microbiota. PLoS One 2011;6(3):e17447. http://dx.doi.org/10.1371/journal.pone.0017447.

36. Jansson J, Willing B, Lucio M, et al. Metabolomics reveals metabolic biomarkers of Crohn's disease. PLoS One 2009;4(7):e6386. http://dx.doi.org/10.1371/journal.pone.0006386.

37. Kolmeder CA, Vos WM, de Vos WM. Metaproteomics of our microbiome — developing insight in function and activity in man and model systems. J Proteomics 2014;97:3–16. http://dx.doi.org/10.1016/j.jprot.2013.05.018.

38. Cohn I, Rives J Jr. Antibiotic protection of colon anastomosis. Ann Surg 1955; 141(5):707–17.

39. Cohen S, Cornell C, Collins M, et al. Healing of ischemic colonic anastomoses in the rat: role of antibiotic preparation. Surgery 1985;97(4):443–6.

40. Shimizu K, Ogura H, Asahara T, et al. Probiotic symbiotic therapy for treating critically ill patients from a gut microbiota perspective. Dig Dis Sci 2012;58:23–32.

41. Jones R. Microbial etiologies of hospital-acquired bacterial pneumonia and ventilator-associated bacterial pneumonia. Clin Infect Dis 2010;51(Suppl 1):S81–7.

42. Fenandez-Guerrero M, Verdejo C, Azofra J, et al. Hospital-acquired infectious endocarditis not associated with cardiac surgery: an emerging problem. Clin Infect Dis 1995;20:16–23.

43. Hussein K, Raz-Pasteur A, Finkelztein R, et al. Impact of carbapenem resistance on the outcome of patients' hospital acquired bacteraemia caused by Klebsiella pneumoniae. J Hosp Infect 2013;83:307–13.

44. Zaborin A, Defazio JR, Kade M, et al. Phosphate-containing polyethylene glycol polymers prevent lethal sepsis by multidrug-resistant pathogens. Antimicrobial Agents Chemother 2014;58(2):966–77. http://dx.doi.org/10.1128/AAC.02183-13.

45. Nhien YS, Kaloostian C, Abbas MA, et al. The surgical care improvement project (SCIP) initiative to reduce infection in elective colorectal surgery: which performance measures affect outcome? Am Surg 2008;74(10):1012–6.

46. Thompson KM, Oldenburg WA, Deschamps C, et al. Chasing zero. Ann Surg 2011;254(3):430–7. http://dx.doi.org/10.1097/SLA.0b013e31822cc0ad.

47. Kardas P, Devine S, Golembesky A, et al. A systematic review and meta-analysis of misuse of antibiotic therapies in the community. Int J Antimicrob Agents 2005; 26(2):106–13. http://dx.doi.org/10.1016/j.ijantimicag.2005.04.017.

48. Falagas M, Barefoot L, Griffith J. Risk factors leading to clinical failure in the treatment of intra-abdominal or skin/soft tissue infections. Eur J Clin Microbiol Infect Dis 1996;15(12):913–21.

49. Eagye KJ, Kim A, Laohavaleeson S, et al. Surgical site infections: does inadequate antibiotic therapy affect patient outcomes? Surg Infect (Larchmt) 2009; 10(4):323–31. http://dx.doi.org/10.1089/sur.2008.053.

Advancing Technologies for the Diagnosis and Management of Infections

 CrossMark

Daithi S. Heffernan, MD, AFRCSI[a],*, Elizabeth D. Fox, MD[b]

KEYWORDS

• Infections • Diagnosis • Management • Advancing technologies

KEY POINTS

- No longer limited to culture-based methods of pathogen detection and characterization, or standard antimicrobial therapies, surgeons now have exciting new options for the diagnosis, treatment, and prophylaxis of surgical infections.
- Infections remain a significant problem among surgical patients. As technological advances continue, our understanding of the host pathogen interaction, especially in the era of computer-based modeling, will grow exponentially, expediting many research endeavors.

INTRODUCTION

The history of surgical infections spans the ages from the tenets of the ancients encompassing tumor, rubor, dolor, and calor, through the beginnings of germ theory in the sixteenth century, into Fleming's earliest days of penicillin, arriving at the gates of Hades with the current epidemic of antimicrobial resistance. As the field has changed over the centuries, so too have diagnostic and therapeutic modalities. Technologies once exclusively found in cutting-edge laboratories are now being used as point-of-care testing and have expanded our ability to identify resistant organisms. Furthermore, although oral and parenteral antibiotics remain a mainstay of antimicrobial therapy for infections, novel technologies are expanding the therapeutic and prophylactic options available to clinicians. Enhanced delivery of antibiotics, local release of immunomodulatory and antimicrobial substances, and alterations in local physical and chemical properties are emerging as attractive alternatives to standard antibiotic therapy. Herein, the authors explore the emerging technologies that are poised to change surgical infections.

[a] Division of Trauma and Surgical Critical Care, Department of Surgery, Alpert Medical School Brown University, Rhode Island Hospital, 435 APC Building, 593 Eddy Street, Providence, RI 02903, USA; [b] Department of Surgery, Alpert Medical School Brown University, Rhode Island Hospital, 429 APC Building, 593 Eddy Street, Providence, RI 02903, USA
* Corresponding author.
E-mail address: Dheffernan@Brown.edu

Surg Clin N Am 94 (2014) 1163–1174
http://dx.doi.org/10.1016/j.suc.2014.08.013
0039-6109/14/$ – see front matter © 2014 Elsevier Inc. All rights reserved.

surgical.theclinics.com

DIAGNOSIS

Microbial culture has long been the leading method of pathogen isolation and identification. However, it relies on highly skilled technicians and significant expenditures of time and money. Culture techniques may require up to 72 hours of incubation. Subsequent antibiotic susceptibility requires an additional 24 to 48 hours. Despite advances in culture techniques, there are still several critical shortcomings. In the context of multidrug-resistant organisms, the prolonged time to detect these resistance profiles leaves patients with prolonged durations of inappropriate antimicrobial coverage. Further, many of the current techniques fail to detect fastidious organisms or, in the case of a patient with recent exposure to antibiotics, results are reported as negative despite the presence of a virulent organism. Furthermore, there is an increasing need for rapid testing. Any delay in diagnosis and initiation of appropriate antimicrobial agents for an infection is well known to negatively affect outcomes. Kumar and colleagues[1] reported a 7.6% decrease in survival for every hour effective antibiotic therapy is delayed following the onset of sepsis shock. New diagnostic technologies have the potential to address many of the limitations of current culture-based technology with high automatization potential, low cost, and rapid return of results.

Polymerase Chain Reaction

Polymerase chain reaction (PCR) is one of the earliest modern techniques for diagnosing infection, and its use in infections was first described in 1987.[2] PCR has been used in the diagnosis of infections, such as human immunodeficiency virus, *Clostridium difficile*, and in screening for methicillin-resistant *Staphylococcus aureus* (MRSA) carriage.[3] PCR relies on the amplification of nucleic acids. In the case of universal PCR, the 16S ribosomal RNA, common to all bacteria, is amplified. This amplification is then followed by DNA sequencing of the amplification products, probe hybridization techniques, or immunoassays. Specific PCR, however, relies on primers complementary to known DNA sequences of predefined bacteria to verify its presence. When compared with conventional culture techniques, PCR has been shown capable of diagnosing bacterial endophthalmitis in patients with prior exposure to antibiotics.[4] PCR processing times continue to shorten, including assays, such as SeptiFast (Roche Diagnostics, Indianapolis, IN), allowing for rapid adjustment of antimicrobial therapy.[5,6]

Next-Generation Sequencing

Next-generation sequencing (NGS) integrates a variety of technologies to identify microbial DNA. First-generation (Sanger) genomic sequencing uses nucleotide chain termination and requires specific primers. NGS creates a variety of DNA fragments that then undergo parallel sequencing, massive parallel sequencing. This sequencing typically involves *whole-genome sequencing* of bacterial isolates permitting sequencing of an entire genome in less than a day. Organisms relevant to surgical practice, such as MRSA, *Escherichia coli, C difficile*, and carbapenem-resistant *Klebsiella pneumoniae* have been identified using this technology.[7] Despite the complexity and the ability to achieve higher throughput with greater characterization, the cost of NSG is comparable with the Sanger method.[8] PathoQuest and Pathogenica are currently involved in clinical trials to evaluate NGS in clinical microbiologic diagnostics. Beyond pathogen identification, this technique can assess for antibiotic resistance traits,[9,10] virulence factors, and genetically distinct isolates of tuberculosis.[11]

Microarray Analysis

Microarray analysis offers high yield on a large scale allowing the detection and analysis of a large number of microbial genes, including specific strains of a bacterium with their virulence and resistance genes. Oligonucleotide probes are bound and immobilized on a microchip in a predefined array. A pathogen's nucleic acids are labeled with a fluorescent. These labeled nucleic acids are hybridized to the complementary immobilized probe on the array. This hybridization is then measured with a fluorescent scanner or cytometer. Advances in array techniques include the use of in situ synthesis on a quartz wafer surface, high- versus low-density arrays, or liquid-based suspensions. Microbial diagnostic microarrays have been used to characterize various *E coli, S aureus,* and *Pseudomonas aeruginosa* isolates[12] as well as to identify specific functional genes responsible for toxin production, virulence, and resistance.[13,14] Microarray analysis has further been able to detect subtle differences in coagulase profile among these *S aureus* isolates.[15]

Bacteriophages

Bacteriophages are bacterial viruses that recognize their target host bacteria and inject their genetic material into them. Following this, the bacteriophage uses the bacteria to rapidly reproduce within the host bacteria, which ultimately kills the host bacteria releasing large quantities of bacteriophage progeny. This production of large numbers of rapidly produced bacteriophage progeny is thereby used as a secondary detector of the presence of the offending bacteria. Advances to this technology use the reporter labeling or luciferase assay.

Because bacteriophages are specific to a particular organism, bacteriophage diagnostics use this specificity to secondarily detect the presence of a bacterium. The speed of reproduction allows for near real-time detection of the infecting bacteria. Unlike PCR, which cannot distinguish between live and dead cells, bacteriophage technology relies on the presence of a live host bacterium capable of reproduction. If used in the presence of an antimicrobial agent, reproduction and, therefore, detection of the bacteriophage is possible only if the bacterium is resistant to the antimicrobial agent. The speed of production of bacteriophage progeny in a resistant organism, therefore, allows for earlier detection of a resistant bacterium. Advances in phage technology in multidrug-resistant tuberculosis[16] are now being applied across a variety of surgically relevant resistant organisms, including the KeyPath assay (MicroPhage, Longmont, CO),[17,18] in multidrug-resistant *S aureus* infections. Incubation with cefoxitin (a methicillin surrogate) provides further information about the presence of MRSA. The MicroPhage system yielded results 30 hours sooner than conventional microbiological methods. Bacteriophage technology has been used for both treatment and diagnostic applications *(see later discussion)*.

Microfluidics

Microfluidics technology involves microscopic analysis of droplets of fluid, often incorporating a variety of techniques, including microscale PCR,[19] flow cytometry, and immunoassays.[20] Bacteria that are difficult to culture are particularly attractive targets for this technology. Difficult-to-culture microbes, including *Mycoplasma pneumoniae,* can be detected with equal sensitivity using Microfluidics-based techniques but in less than half the time of conventional PCR-based methods.[21] This microscale technology is particularly attractive for detection of infections in resource-limited developing countries.[20]

Matrix-Assisted Laser Desorption/Ionization Time-of-Flight Mass Spectrometry

Matrix-assisted laser desorption/ionization time-of-flight mass spectrometry compares a pathogen's mass spectrometry against a database of spectrometry profiles from known pathogens.[10,22] Several groups have shown that the combination of PCR with mass spectrometry can accurately identify pathogens from whole blood and surgical site cultures. Examples include gene analysis for resistance profiles (MRSA) with results as quickly as 6 to 8 hours.[23,24] Using combination mass spectrometry/PCR techniques, Jacovides and colleagues[24] detected pathogens in revision arthroplasties from patients in whom the hardware failure was originally thought to be aseptic. The investigators proposed that this combination technology has the potential to identify previously undiagnosed and subclinical infections.

On the Horizon

In vivo testing would allow for either pathogen detection or exclusion without the need for removal of such potentially noninfected devices. Paredes and colleagues[25] reported a "smart central venous catheter" prototype that uses a microelectrode to assess electrical impedance characteristics related to bacterial biofilm formation. The device is capable of detecting biofilm-related bioimpedance changes within 10 hours of the appearance of bacteria. A promising application of in vivo detection would be in immune-compromised patients who do not develop the typical infected profile of fever or leukocytosis.

TREATMENT AND NANOTECHNOLOGY

Nanotechnology is the study and application of nanoscale particles. By definition, nanoparticles measure in the 1- to 100-nm range. Nanoscale substances potentially exhibit properties that differ chemically and biologically from the properties seen at the macroscale level. Nanotechnology in medicine uses these specific nanoscale-related alterations in properties to significantly improve drug delivery, overcome antibiotic resistance, and decrease the rates of implantable device-related infections. The antibacterial properties of silver are well recognized. However, decreasing the size of silver particles to nanoparticle range, the antibacterial activity is significantly increased. Several other metals, including magnesium and iron, exhibit bactericidal activity against E coli or S aureus when in nanoparticle size.

A vast number of compounds have been explored under the umbrella of nanotechnology. These compounds include liposomes (vesicles composed of a lipid bilayer), polymeric microspheres, and metal ion compounds, such as silver, zinc, and gold.[26] The surface of implantable devices as diverse as endotracheal tubes and prosthetic joints can undergo nanoscale modifications, leading to alterations in characteristics such as roughness, hydrophobicity, and charge. These changes are largely targeted toward achieving a particular concentration, bioactivity, or conformation of a compound that is needed to be adsorbed onto a material surface.[27]

Drug Design

Antimicrobial therapeutics often belonged to limited categories: agents affecting bacterial cell wall synthesis, protein synthesis, and nucleic acid synthesis and modification. The epidemic of antimicrobial resistance drives technological advances in drug design and delivery.

The pore-forming toxins, drivers of the pathogenesis of S aureus, Streptococcus pneumoniae, and E coli infections, offer a potential therapeutic target. Nanosponges have been shown to effectively bind alpha-toxin (S aureus) and streptolysin O (S pyogenes), reducing cellular exposure to the toxins.[28] In these sponges, the polymeric core is coated with a red blood cell bilayer. This combination is capable of nonspecifically absorbing a wide variety of toxins. Prior immunologic approaches to toxins rely on individualized knowledge of, and isolation of antisera from, a specific infecting organism. The Nanosponge could obviate the diagnosis of the exact infecting organism.

Photodynamic antimicrobial therapy, which synergizes visible light and photosensitizing drugs, has apparent effects independent of the specific infecting organism and has shown promise in localized skin and soft tissue infections. Diverse bacteria and fungi often colonize chronic lower extremity wounds, and treatment is limited by poor tissue penetration of antibiotics. Morley and colleagues[29] applied PPA904, a phenothiazine photosensitizer, coupled with phototherapy to chronic leg wounds in a placebo-controlled study. Immediate bacterial count reduction was noted in the treatment arm. This effect, however, was lost at 24 hours. Further studies are underway to determine if sustained eradication can be achieved with repeated dosing. Intriguingly, despite the lack of bacterial eradication, improved wound healing was noted in the PPA904 group at 3 months, indicating a potential immunomodulatory role beyond an antimicrobial effect.

Naturally occurring host defense peptides (HSPs), also called *antimicrobial peptides*, are components of the innate immune response in humans that have direct broad-spectrum antimicrobial effects.[30] They are also capable of activity against viruses and even cancer cells. These small naturally produced molecules are also capable of immunomodulation via their chemotactic properties, ability to alter gene expression, and modulation of inflammatory cytokines release.[31] The two most studied are α- and β-defensins. Two such peptides, LL-37 and human beta-defensin, demonstrate antimicrobial activity against numerous gram-positive and gram-negative bacterial as well as fungi. Ongoing work is aimed at creating antimicrobial peptide elicitors, which are chemical or biological agents that enhance HSP expression.[31,32] A recently completed clinical trial (NCT01211470) found that the defensin peptide mimetic PMX 30063 (Poly-Medix) showed high clinical response rates in the treatment of methicillin sensitive *Staphylococcus aureus* and MRSA-related acute skin and soft tissue infections.

Pleuromutilins represent a new class of antimicrobial agents. First discovered in 1959,[33] pleuromutilins exhibit unique bacterial protein synthesis inhibition by selectively binding to peptidyl transferase center of the 50S ribosome subunit. Retapamulin was the first approved topical pleuromutilin, and BC-3781 recently completed a phase II trial demonstrating systemic efficacy. Pleuromutilins demonstrate potency against methicillin-sensitive and methicillin-resistant *S aureus*, beta-hemolytic *Streptococci*, and *Haemophilus influenzae*.[34,35]

Treatment

Bioavailability of antimicrobial agents can be increased through variations in nanoparticle formulations, including solid lipid nanoparticle formulations, nanosuspensions, and liposomal-mediated drug delivery. Directing nanoparticles to specific sites of infection reduces exposure of normal tissues and flora to the antimicrobial agent. Nanoparticle modification has improved isoniazid and rifampin delivery decreasing systemic toxicity.[36] Many of these processes require nanoparticle recognition of an epitope (a part of molecule or protein) found in the bacterial biofilm. Suci and colleagues[37] demonstrated that viral nanoparticles coated with antibodies to staphylococcal protein A (a surface protein and virulence factor) were markedly better able to target *S aureus* biofilms.

Nanotechnology offers potential in overcoming antimicrobial resistance.[38] Fayaz and colleagues[39] demonstrated that gold nanoparticles coated with vancomycin were capable of inhibiting vancomycin-resistant *S aureus*. Intriguingly, gold-vancomycin nanoparticles also exerted antibacterial activity against *E coli*, an organism not normally susceptible to vancomycin given the drug's inability to penetrate gram-negative bacteria.[39,40] Gold particles are hypothesized to alter binding properties leading to the antimicrobial efficacy, a process called polyvalent inhibition.[41]

Beyond diagnostic applications (see later discussion), bacteriophages demonstrate antimicrobial properties. Phages may have lytic properties wherein products of phages replication are capable of bacterial cell wall destruction, leading to bacteriolysis. Phages are further capable of producing large quantities of antimicrobial molecules or toxins, thereby potentially rapidly controlling microbial growth without the use of antibiotics. Biofilm formation reduction was noted within several hours of incubation with a bacteriophage directed against uropathogenic E coli.[42]

Bacteriophages have also been used for infection prophylaxis when conjugated to polymeric surfaces, such as polytetrafluoroethylene, preventing the growth of bacteria. The targeted specificity of each bacteriophage to a specific bacterium limits the activity spectrum to individual organisms, unlike the broad-spectrum activity of many currently available antibiotics.[43]

PROPHYLAXIS

Indwelling device-related infections, such as those associated with Foley catheters and central lines, greatly contribute to hospital-associated morbidity. A recent survey from the Centers for Disease Control and Prevention found that pneumonia, urinary tract infections (UTIs), and bloodstream infections are among the most common nosocomial infections, accounting for 44.6% of all health care–associated infections.[44] A total of 39.1% of pneumoniae were associated with endotracheal tubes, 67.7% of UTIs were associated with catheter use, and 84% of bloodstream infections were associated with central venous line usage. These infections can be particularly difficult to treat because of biofilm formation. Nanoparticles incorporating a variety of molecules, including metals, peptides, and immunoglobulins, are able to alter biofilm physical characteristics, such as charge and surface topography.[27,45] Additionally, some nanoparticles can cause production of antimicrobial reactive oxygen and nitrogen species by leukocytes in response to an infection.[46]

Antimicrobial-coated indwelling devices are gaining acceptance, with up to 45% of hospitals using such technology.[47] Endotracheal (ET) tubes remain an important target for prevention of hospital-acquired pneumonia. In the NASCENT (North American Silver-Coated Endotracheal Tube) trial, patients with silver-coated ET tubes had a 36% relative risk reduction for development of ventilator-associated pneumonia.[48] Machado and colleagues[49] demonstrated that nanomodification of ET tubes, undertaken by enzymatically roughened ET tubes, was associated with a 1.5 log reduction in colony-forming units of S aureus compared with standard ET tubes.

Central venous catheters (CVCs) similarly are often causatively associated with nosocomial infections. Aggregate analyses of multiple randomized control trials of CVCs impregnated with silver sulfadiazine and chlorhexidine note a 40% reduction in CVC-related blood stream infections.[50–52] Using DNA subtyping to confirm infection, Maki and colleagues[53] noted a 5-fold reduction in blood stream infections with the use of silver sulfadiazine– and chlorhexidine-coated CVCs. Antimicrobial coating of CVCs with minocycline-rifampin has also been shown to reduce catheter colonization and blood stream infection.[54] Roe and colleagues[55] demonstrated that silver coating of central venous catheters can inhibit growth of a variety of common pathogenic bacteria, including S aureus, E coli, and Candida albicans, and reduce biofilm formation. Advances in this technology include the addition of platinum into the catheter facilitating local release of silver ions.

Indwelling urinary catheters account for most of the nosocomial UTIs. Silicon quaternary ammonium salt can form a positively charged film on urinary catheters. When applied to catheters before insertion followed by twice-daily application to both the urethral orifice and catheter, rates of UTIs are significantly lowered.[56] In a preclinical study, urinary catheters modified with a nitric oxide and acetic acid impeded bacterial growth and biofilms formation from clinically significant organisms, including *P aeruginosa, K pneumoniae,* and *Enterococcus faecalis.*[46]

Orthopedic implant infections are associated with significant morbidity. Nanotechnology has been used to alter the surfaces of joint prostheses by means such as impregnation of chlorhexidine or covalently immobilizing antibiotics, such as vancomycin.[57] Further, the use of immunomodulatory molecules has been reported.[58] Nanoscale coating of implants with the macrophage migration and activation modulators monocyte chemoattractant protein-1 and interleukin-12 has been demonstrated to lower infection rates and improve bone healing.[58] Bone grafting, which involves implanting devitalized bone, is associated with infection rates of up to 15%.[59] A fibrin gel mix can be created by impregnating the bone graft with vancomycin-alginate beads. Chang and colleagues[60] demonstrated that this antibiotic-impregnated bone graft was capable of bactericidal activity.

Surgical site infections (SSIs) represent a particular challenge for the surgeon. Technological advances aimed at this problem range from antimicrobial-coated sutures to skin sealants and biological dressings. Data from meta-analyses on antimicrobial-impregnated sutures remain discordant, with Edmiston and colleagues[61] demonstrating a reduction and Chang and colleagues[62] showing no significant benefit in superficial SSIs. Topical sealants achieve antimicrobial effects by preventing migration of skin flora into the incision and preventing recolonization of these spaces. Dohmen and colleagues[63] demonstrated a 76% relative risk reduction in cardiac surgery SSIs using a cyanoacrylate-based polymers (InteguSeal, Kimberly-Clark Health Care, Roswell, GA). A Cochrane review found a significant reduction in the rates of SSIs using antimicrobial sealants, although enthusiasm for this technology remains limited.[64] Fowler and colleagues[65] assessed preoperative vaccination against *S aureus*. Not only did vaccines not reduce rates of wound infections but rather, among those who did develop an *S aureus* infection, mortality was higher among those who had been vaccinated.

COMPUTATIONAL MODELING

Many surgical infection dicta tend to be linear and sequential. Patient factors such as being immunocompromised may allow nonvirulent organisms to prove fatal. Conversely in immunocompetent patients, intrinsic organism factors, such as virulence or antimicrobial resistance, dictate outcomes. However, this sequential thinking does not take into account the multidimensionality and complexity of the biological systems that are truly occurring in both patients and the microbe. Patients are not genetically identical; treatments vary widely by practitioner, and inflammatory responses to bacteria range from local wound infections to profound inflammatory responses, tissue destruction, and organ failure. These changes in host cells and tissues may induce changes in the bacteria during the course of an infection. Hypophosphatemia can induce gene transcription for motility and virulence factors in pseudomonas, potentially leading to a necrotizing infection. Replete phosphorus will stop such gene transcription.[66] Such complexity quickly outstrips our traditional modeling used to analyze these findings.[67]

Dynamic computational modeling and simulation has been demonstrated to be a useful approach in integrating mechanistic knowledge and bridging different scales of biological organization (genes → molecules → cells → cell population/tissue → organs → entire patient). The resulting models can aid in the analysis of overall system behavior as well as serve as experimental objects to be used alongside traditional biological models.[68] Advances in technology have created virtual bench spaces and computer-simulated experiments. Agent-based modeling (ABM)[69] uses computer simulation to allow repeated alteration and manipulation of the complex biological systems. Computer-based models are built on our existing understanding of how either the pathogen or the patients change in response to small and incremental changes in the environment.

Many traditional experimental approaches follow a standard logistic of altering only one factor at a time and following a limited number of measurable outcomes in a linear fashion. However, ABM allows for very rapid simultaneous manipulation of multiple facets of an experiment, creating the complex reality that exists wherein the pathogen may alter the host, which in turn feeds back to alter the pathogen. These experiments include alterations in microbe virulence,[70] tissue environment including electrolyte disturbances, alterations in circulation or nutrient flow and patient immune response, both cytokine and cellular alterations,[71] as well as a better understanding of the mechanisms of antimicrobial resistance.[72] Key findings from these computer-generated experiments can then be confirmed with traditional bench-based experimentation in a much more time- and resource-efficient manner.

ABM and computational modeling have led to fresh insights into the role bacteria play in enteric anastomotic breakdown[73] as well as improved delineation of the pathogenesis of necrotizing enterocolitis. Arciero and colleagues[74] assessed the optimal time to administer probiotics by varying a wide range of factors spanning from organism virulence, the infant's potential cytokine responses, type of feeding administered, and even the route of birth of the infant. Kim and colleagues[75] used ABM to assess the complex interaction between oxidative stress, toll-like receptor-4 activation, and mucus barrier dysfunction in the pathogenesis of necrotizing enterocolitis.

In essence, advances in technology have connected complex biological patterns with clinical outcomes through the use of advanced computing and analytical methods. It is potentially possible that all animal-based experimentation will need to be grounded in ABM to circumvent the need for exhaustive animal or human experimentation.

SUMMARY

Infections remain a significant problem among surgical patients. As technological advances continue, our understanding of the host-pathogen interaction, especially in the era of computer-based modeling, will grow exponentially, expediting many research endeavors. No longer limited to culture-based methods of pathogen detection and characterization, or standard antimicrobial therapies, surgeons now have exciting new options for the diagnosis, treatment, and prophylaxis of surgical infections.

REFERENCES

1. Kumar A, Roberts D, Wood K, et al. Duration of hypotension before initiation of effective antimicrobial therapy is the critical determinant of survival in human septic shock. Crit Care Med 2006;34(6):1589–96.
2. Mullins K, Faloona F. Specific synthesis of DNA in vitro via a polymerase catalyzed chain reaction. Methods 1987;155:335–50.
3. Aydiner A, Lusebrink J, Schildgen V, et al. Comparison of two commercial PCR methods for methicillin resistant staphylococcus aureus (MRSA) screening in a tertiary care hospital. PLoS One 2012;7(9):e43935.

4. Cornut P, Boisset S, Romanet J, et al. Principles and applications of molecular biology techniques for the microbiological diagnosis of acute post-operative endophthalmitis. Surv Ophthalmol 2014;59(3):286–303.

5. Chaidaroglou A, Manoli E, Marathias E, et al. Use of a multiplex polymerase chain reaction system for enhanced bloodstream pathogen detection in thoracic transplantation. J Heart Lung Transplant 2013;32(7):707–13.

6. Lodes U, Bohmeier B, Lippert H, et al. PCR-based rapid sepsis diagnosis effectively guides clinical treatment in patients with new onset of SIRS. Langenbecks Arch Surg 2012;397(3):447–55.

7. Reuter S, Ellington M, Cartwright E, et al. Rapid bacterial whole-genome sequencing to enhance diagnostic and public health microbiology. JAMA Intern Med 2013;173(15):1397–404.

8. Sabat A, Budimir A, Nashev D, et al. Overview of molecular typing methods for outbreak detection and epidemiological surveillance. Euro Surveill 2013;18(4): 20380.

9. Rishishwar L, Petit RA 3rd, Kraft C, et al. Genome sequence based discriminator for vancomycin intermediate staphylococcus aureus. J Bacteriol 2014;196(5): 940–8.

10. Fournier P, Drancourt M, Colson P, et al. Modern clinical microbiology: new challenges and solutions. Nat Rev Microbiol 2013;11(8):574–85.

11. Clark T, Mallard K, Coll F, et al. Elucidating emergence and transmission of multidrug resistant tuberculosis in treatment experienced patients by whole genome sequencing. PLoS One 2013;8(12):e83012.

12. Snyder L, Loman N, Faraj L, et al. Epidemiological investigation of Pseudomonas aeruginosa isolates from a six-year long hospital outbreak using high-throughput whole genome sequencing. Euro Surveill 2013;18(42):20611.

13. Strommenger B, Schmidt C, Werner G, et al. DNA microarray for the detection of therapeutically relevant antibiotic resistance determinants in clinical isolates of Staphylococcus aureus. Mol Cell Probes 2007;21(3):161–70.

14. Schrenzel J. Clinical relevance of new diagnostic methods for bloodstream infections. Int J Antimicrob Agents 2007;30(Suppl 1):S2–6.

15. Otsuka J, Kondoh Y, Amemiya T, et al. Development and validation of microarray based assay for epidemiological study of MRSA. Mol Cell Probes 2008;22(1): 1–13.

16. Minion J, Pai M. Bacteriophage assays for rifampicin resistance detection in mycobacterium tuberculosis: updated meta-analysis. Int J Tuberc Lung Dis 2010;14(8):941–51.

17. Bhowmick T, Mirrett S, Reller L, et al. Controlled multicenter evaluation of a bacteriophage-based method for rapid detection of staphylococcus aureus in positive blood cultures. J Clin Microbiol 2013;51(4):1226–30.

18. Sullivan K, Turner N, Roundtree S, et al. Rapid detection of methicillin-resistant staphylococcus aureus (MRSA) and methicillin-susceptible staphylococcus aureus (MSSA) using the KeyPath MRSA/MSSA blood culture and the BacT/ALERT system in a pediatric population. Arch Pathol Lab Med 2013;137(8): 1103–5.

19. Park S, Zhang Y, Lin S, et al. Advances in microfluidic PCR for point of care infectious disease diagnosis. Biotechnol Adv 2011;29(6):830–9.

20. Lee W, Kim Y, Chung B, et al. Nano/microfluidics for diagnosis of infectious diseases in developing countries. Adv Drug Deliv Rev 2010;62(4–5):449–58.

21. Wulff-Burchfield E, Schell W, Eckhardt A, et al. Microfluidic platform versus conventional real time polymerase chain reaction for the detection of Mycoplasma

pneumoniae in respiratory specimens. Diagn Microbiol Infect Dis 2010;67(1): 22–9.

22. Mancini N, De Carolis E, Infurnari L, et al. Comparative evaluation of the Bruker Biotyper and Vitek MS matrix-assisted laser desorption ionization time of flight (MALDI-TOF) mass spectrometry systems for identification of yeasts of medical importance. J Clin Microbiol 2013;51(7):2453–7.

23. Jordana-Lluch E, Carolan H, Gimenez M, et al. Rapid diagnosis of bloodstream infections with PCR followed by mass spectrometry. PLoS One 2013;8(4):e62108.

24. Jacovides C, Kreft R, Adeli B, et al. Successful identification of pathogens by polymerase chain reaction (PCR) based electron spray ionization time-of-flight mass spectrometry (ESI-TOF-MS) in culture negative peri-prosthetic joint infection. J Bone Joint Surg Am 2012;94(24):2247–54.

25. Paredes T, Alonso-Arce M, Schmidt C, et al. Smart central venous port for early detection of bacterial biofilm related infections. Biomed Microdevices 2014; 16(3):365–74.

26. Zhang L, Keogh S, Rickard C. Reducing the risk of infection associated with vascular access devices through nanotechnology: a perspective. Int J Nanomedicine 2013;8:4453–66.

27. Liu H, Webster T. Mechanical properties of dispersed ceramic nanoparticles in polymer composites for orthopedic applications. Int J Nanomedicine 2010;5: 299–313.

28. Hu C, Fang R, Copp J, et al. A biomimetic nanosponge that absorbs poreforming toxins. Nat Nanotechnol 2013;8(5):336–40.

29. Morley S, Griffiths J, Philips G, et al. Phase IIa randomized, placebo-controlled study of antimicrobial photodynamic therapy in bacterially colonized, chronic leg ulcers and diabetic foot ulcers: a new approach to antimicrobial therapy. Br J Dermatol 2013;168(3):617–24.

30. Prado Montes de Oca E. Antimicrobial peptide elicitors: a new hope for the post-antibiotic era. Innate Immun 2013;19(3):227–41.

31. Fitzgerald-Hughes D, Devocelle M, Humphreys H. Beyond conventional antibiotics for the future treatment of methicillin resistant staphylococcus aureus infections: two novel alternatives. FEMS Immunol Med Microbiol 2012;65(3):399–412.

32. van der Does A, Bergman P, Agerberth B, et al. Induction of the human cathelicidin LL-37 as a novel treatment against bacterial infections. J Leukoc Biol 2012;92(4):735–42.

33. Novak R, Shales D. The pleuromutilin antibiotics: a new class for human use. Curr Opin Investig Drugs 2010;11(2):182–91.

34. Paukner S, Sader H, Ivezic-Schoenfeld Z, et al. Antimicrobial activity of the pleuromutilin antibiotic BC-3781 against bacterial pathogens isolated in the SENTRY antimicrobial surveillance program in 2010. Antimicrob Agents Chemother 2013; 57(9):4489–95.

35. Prince W, Ivezic-Schoenfeld Z, Lell C, et al. Phase II clinical study of BC-3781, a pleuromutilin antibiotic, in treatment of patients with acute bacterial skin and skin structure infection. Antimicrob Agents Chemother 2013;57(5):2087–94.

36. Banyal S, Malik P, Tuli H, et al. Advances in nanotechnology for diagnosis and treatment of tuberculosis. Curr Opin Pulm Med 2013;19(3):289–97.

37. Suci P, Berglund D, Liepold L, et al. High-density targeting of a viral multifunctional nanoplatform to a pathogenic, biofilm-forming bacterium. Chem Biol 2007; 14(4):387–98.

38. Taylor E, Webster T. Reducing infections through nanotechnology and nanoparticles. Int J Nanomedicine 2011;6:1463–73.

39. Fayaz A, Girilal M, Mahdy S, et al. Vancomycin bound biogenic gold nanoparticles: a different perspective for development of anti-VRSA agents. Process Biochem 2011;46:636–41.
40. Gu H, Ho P, Tong E, et al. Presenting vancomycin on nanoparticles to enhance antimicrobial activities. Nano Lett 2003;3(9):1261–3.
41. Xing B, Ho P, Yu C, et al. Self-assembled multivalent vancomycin on cell surfaces against vancomycin-resistant enterococci (VRE). Chem Commun (Camb) 2003;17:2224–5.
42. Chibeu A, Lingohr E, Masson L, et al. Bacteriophages with the ability to degrade uropathogenic Escherichia coli biofilms. Viruses 2012;4(4):471–87.
43. Pearson H, Sahukhal G, Elasri M, et al. Phage-bacterium war on polymeric surfaces: can surface-anchored bacteriophages eliminate microbial infections? Biomacromolecules 2013;14(5):1257–61.
44. Magill S, Edwards J, Bamberg W, et al. Multistate point prevalence survey of health care associated infection. N Engl J Med 2014;370(12):1198–208.
45. Davies D. Understanding biofilm resistance to antibacterial agents. Nat Rev Drug Discov 2003;2(2):114–22.
46. Kishikawa H, Ebberyd A, Romling U, et al. Control of pathogen growth and biofilm formation using a urinary catheter that releases antimicrobial nitrogen oxides. Free Radic Biol Med 2013;65:1257–64.
47. Saint S, Greene M, Damschroder L, et al. Is the use of antimicrobial devices to prevent infection correlated across different healthcare-associated infections? Results from a national survey. Infect Control Hosp Epidemiol 2013;34(8):847–9.
48. Kollef M, Afessa B, Anzueto A, et al. Silver-coated endotracheal tubes and incidence of ventilator associated pneumonia: the NASCENT randomized trial. JAMA 2008;300(7):805–13.
49. Machado M, Tarquinio K, Webster T. Decreased Staphylococcus aureus biofilm formation on nanomodified endotracheal tubes: a dynamic airway model. Int J Nanomedicine 2012;7:3741–50.
50. Crnich C, Maki D. The promise of novel technology for the prevention of intravascular device-related bloodstream infection. I - pathogenesis and short term devices. Clin Infect Dis 2002;34(9):1232–42.
51. Mermel L. Prevention of intravascular catheter related infections. Ann Intern Med 2000;132:391–402.
52. Veenstra D, Saint S, Sahsa S, et al. Efficacy of antiseptic impregnated central venous catheters in preventing catheter related bloodstream infection: a meta-analysis. JAMA 1999;281:261–7.
53. Maki D, Stolz S, Wheeler S, et al. Prevention of central venous catheter related bloodstream infection by use of an antiseptic impregnated catheter. A randomized controlled trial. Ann Intern Med 1997;127(4):257–66.
54. Raad I, Darouiche R, Dupuis J, et al. Central venous catheters coated with minocycline and rifampin for the prevention of catheter-related colonization and bloodstream infections. A randomized double-blind trial. The Texas Medical Center Catheter Study Group. Ann Intern Med 1997;127(4):267–74.
55. Roe D, Karandikar B, Bonn-Savage N, et al. Antimicrobial surface functionalization of plastic catheters by silver nanoparticles. J Antimicrob Chemother 2008;61(4):869–76.
56. He W, Wang D, Ye Z, et al. Application of a nanotechnology antimicrobial spray to prevent lower urinary tract infection: a multicenter urology trial. J Transl Med 2012;10(Suppl 1):S14.

57. Goodman S, Yao Z, Keeney M, et al. The future of biological coatings for orthopedic implants. Biomaterials 2013;34(13):3174–83.

58. Li B, Jiang B, Dietz M, et al. Evaluation of local MCP-1 and IL-12 nanocoatings for infection prevention in open fractures. J Orthop Res 2010;28(1):48–54.

59. Ahn D, Park H, Choi D, et al. The difference of surgical site infection according to the methods of lumbar fusion surgery. J Spinal Disord Tech 2012;25(8): E230–4.

60. Chang Z, Hou T, Wu X, et al. An anti-infection tissue engineered construct delivering vancomycin: its evaluation in a goat model of femur defect. Int J Med Sci 2013;10(12):1761–70.

61. Edmiston C, Daoud F, Leaper D. Is there an evidence based argument for embracing an antimicrobial (triclosan) coated suture technology to reduce the risk of surgical site infections? A meta-analysis. Surgery 2013;154(1):89–100.

62. Chang W, Srinivasan V, Morton R, et al. Triclosan-impregnated sutures to decrease surgical site infections: systemic review and meta-analysis of randomized trials. Ann Surg 2012;255(5):845–59.

63. Dohmen P, Weymann A, Holinski S, et al. Use of an antimicrobial skin sealant reduces surgical site infection in patients undergoing routine cardiac surgery. Surg Infect (Larchmt) 2011;12(6):475–81.

64. Lipp A, Phillips C, Harris P, et al. Cyanoacrylate microbial sealants for skin preparation prior to surgery. Cochrane Database Syst Rev 2013;(8):CD008062.

65. Fowler V, Allen K, Moreira E, et al. Effect of an investigational vaccine for preventing staphylococcus aureus infections after cardiothoracic surgery: a randomized trial. JAMA 2013;309(13):1368–78.

66. Long J, Zaborina O, Halbrook C, et al. Depletion of intestinal phosphate after operative injury activates the virulence of P. aeruginosa causing lethal gut-derived sepsis. Surgery 2008;144(2):189–97.

67. An G. Agent based computer simulation and SIRS: building a bridge between science and clinical trials. Shock 2001;16(4):266–73.

68. Vodovotz Y, Constantine G, Rubin J, et al. Mechanistic simulations of inflammation: current state and future prospects. Math Biosci 2009;217(1):1–10.

69. An G, Mi Q, Dutta-Moscato J, et al. Agent based models in translational systems biology. Wiley Interdiscip Rev Syst Biol Med 2009;1(2):159–71.

70. Gopalakrishnan V, Kim M, An G. Using an agent based model to examined the role of dynamic bacterial virulence potential in the pathogenesis of surgical site infection. Adv Wound Care (New Rochelle) 2013;2(9):510–26.

71. Folcik VA, An GC, Orosz CG. The basic immune simulator: an agent based model to study the interactions between innate and adaptive immunity. Theor Biol Med Model 2007;4:39.

72. Fischer N, Raunest M, Schmidt T, et al. Efflux pump-mediated antibiotics resistance: insights from computational structural biology. Interdiscip Sci 2014;6(1): 1–12.

73. Stern J, Olivas A, Valuckaite V, et al. Agent based model of epithelial host pathogen interactions in anastomotic leak. J Surg Res 2013;184(2):730–8.

74. Arciero J, Ermentriut B, Upperman J, et al. Using a mathematical model to analyze the role of probiotics and inflammation in necrotizing enterocolitis. PLoS One 2010;5(4):e10066.

75. Kim M, Christley S, Alverdy J, et al. Immature oxidative stress management as a unifying principle in the pathogenesis of necrotizing enterocolitis: insights from an agent-based model. Surg Infect (Larchmt) 2012;13(1):18–32.

Infection Control in the Intensive Care Unit

Mohamed F. Osman, MD, Reza Askari, MD*

KEYWORDS

- Infection control • Intensive care unit • Health care personnel
- ICU-acquired infections

KEY POINTS

- It is critical for health care personnel to recognize and appreciate the detrimental impact of intensive care unit (ICU)-acquired infections.
- The economic, clinical, and social expenses to patients and hospitals are overwhelming. To limit the incidence of ICU-acquired infections, aggressive infection control measures must be implemented and enforced. Researchers and national committees have developed and continue to develop evidence-based guidelines to control infections in the ICU.
- A multifaceted approach, including infection prevention committees, antimicrobial stewardship programs, daily reassessments-intervention bundles, identifying and minimizing risk factors, and continuing staff education programs, is essential in the modern era of critical care medicine.
- Infection control in the ICU is an evolving area of critical care research and continued advancements in this field are foreseen.

INTRODUCTION

In the United States, more than 5 million patients are admitted to ICUs annually.[1,2] Although ICUs constitute less than 10% of total beds in most hospitals, more than 20% of all nosocomial infections are acquired in ICUs.[3] ICU-acquired infections account for substantial morbidity, mortality, and hospital costs. Infections and sepsis are the leading causes of death in noncardiac ICUs and account for 40% of all ICU expenditures.[4] As the number of ICU beds increases, the proportion of ICU infections is likely to increase, putting more strains on health care costs.

Patients in critical care settings are more susceptible to nosocomial infections. Overall, compared with the general hospital population, patients in ICUs have more chronic comorbid illnesses and more severe acute physiologic derangements. The

Disclosures: None.
Division of Trauma/Burns and Critical Care, Department of Surgery, Brigham and Women's Hospital, Harvard Medical School, 75 Francis St. Boston, MA 02115, USA
* Corresponding author.
E-mail address: raskari@partners.org

Surg Clin N Am 94 (2014) 1175–1194
http://dx.doi.org/10.1016/j.suc.2014.08.011
0039-6109/14/$ – see front matter © 2014 Elsevier Inc. All rights reserved.

surgical.theclinics.com

widespread use of indwelling catheters and devices among ICU patients provides a portal of entry of organisms into vital body organs and sites. The use and maintenance of these catheters necessitate frequent contact with health care personnel, predisposing patients to colonization and infection with nosocomial pathogens. In addition, equipment associated with the proper maintenance of these devices might serve as reservoirs for pathogens and be related to horizontal patient-to-patient transmission of pathogens.[5]

The focus of this review is to look at the current evidence-based standard practices of infection control in the critical care settings. General control measures are discussed separately, followed by measures specific to each of the common nosocomial infections: ventilator-associated pneumonia (VAP), catheter-related bloodstream infections (CLABSIs), catheter-associated urinary tract infections (CAUTIs), and *Clostridium difficile* infections (CDIs).

GENERAL INFECTION CONTROL MEASURES
Optimizing Nutritional Status

It's been well established that poor nutritional status is causally related to impaired immune function and susceptibility to infections.[6–10] Malnutrition is an independent risk factor for surgical site infections.[11] Low serum albumin level in cardiac surgery patients correlates with increased risk of postoperative infectious complications.[12] Medical ICU patients who receive suboptimal caloric supply have significantly increased risk of nosocomial bloodstream infections.[13] Parenteral nutrition necessitates long-term central venous catheters (CVCs), which are a potential cause of CLABSI. Enteral feeding, on the other hand, especially in the supine position, has been shown to increase the risk of VAP.[14–17] Compared with parenteral feeding, enteral feeding of critically ill adult patients significantly decreases the risk of overall infections.[14,18] Early enteral nutrition, when possible, is associated with lower incidence of sepsis or septic shock and improved ICU mortality.[16,19]

Glycemic Control

Hyperglycemia and insulin resistance are common in critically ill patients and are associated with adverse outcomes in diabetics, even more so in stress-induced hyperglycemia patients.[20–23] In a randomized, controlled study conducted in surgical ICU patients, strict control of blood glucose levels with insulin reduced morbidity and mortality.[24,25] Diabetic patients undergoing cardiovascular surgery develop more postoperative wound infections than nondiabetics.[26] Trauma patients admitted to an ICU with hyperglycemia have increased risk of infections, in particular respiratory infections and bloodstream infections.[27,28] The optimal blood glucose level is fluctuating and the optimal glucose level has yet to be determined and needs future studies.

Staff Education and System-Based Practices

Checklists and interventions targeting communication efficiency among all ICU staff and daily multidisciplinary rounds with discussions of mechanical ventilator, CVC, and urinary catheter protocols can significantly decrease the rate of VAP and CLABSI, with a downward trend in CAUTI.[29–31] Periodic educational programs for ICU staff with reminders of infection prevention strategies have also been shown to decrease hospital-acquired infection rate.[32–36] In addition, adequate nursing and support staff is necessary for infection control. A lower nurse-to-patient ratio increases the risk of nosocomial infection, including late-onset VAP and CLABSI.[37–39]

Intensive Care Unit Environment

The ICU environment plays an important role in exposing patients to various pathogenic organisms. These organisms may be found almost anywhere: on the hands of caretakers, on laboratory coats, on knobs of doors, on keyboards, or in the structure and environment of the room itself, increasing the chances of acquiring infections.[40–47] Measures to decrease the environmental burden of pathogens and subsequently lower the rates of hospital-acquired infections are being heavily studied. Still, experimental techniques for environmental cleansing include UV light sterilization lamps and hydrogen peroxide vapor decontamination devices, which might contribute to future attempts at reducing colonization pressure. Combining environmental cleaning with hand hygiene educational campaign can significantly decrease both environmental and hand contamination rates.[48]

Hand Hygiene

Compliance with appropriate hand hygiene is vital to patient care in ICUs and is extremely cost effective.[49] Continuous encouragement and monitoring with reinforcement of hand hygiene policies are important to maintain and improve compliance rates and reduce the ICU-acquired infection rate.[50,51]

The Hand Hygiene Task Force compiled the trials comparing soap to alcohol-based foam and determined that alcohol-based foams/gel are more effective in decreasing bacterial colony counts and in decreasing the number of multidrug-resistant pathogens than traditional hand washing with soap and water. This proves to be true with the exception of hands that are visibly soiled and for health care personnel caring for patients with CDIs (or other spores-forming organisms), because the foam does not inactivate *C difficile* toxins and does not kill the spores themselves.[52–54] Studies have shown no significant difference in bacterial colony counts on hands of ICU staff who used a chlorhexidine-containing antiseptic wash versus alcohol-based foam; however, the latter produces less skin irritation and is more cost effective.[51,53]

Patient Screening

Patients newly admitted to an ICU who are colonized with multidrug-resistant pathogens are a constant reservoir for transmission and subsequent infection. Surveillance cultures to detect methicillin-resistant *Staphylococcus aureus* (MRSA) and vancomycin-resistant enterococci (VRE) have been implemented at many hospitals, with significant success in decreasing the rate of colonization and infection with these organisms.[55–69] Cost-benefit analyses of VRE and MRSA surveillance seem to favor surveillance as a cost-saving measure.[70–72]

Isolation Measures

Both the Healthcare Infection Control Practices Advisory Committee and the Society for Healthcare Epidemiology of America guidelines encourage both gown and glove use on entering rooms of patients colonized with antibiotic-resistant pathogens.[62,73] A study of glove use by 50 health care workers who care for VRE-positive patients found the use of gloves decreased the risk of the health care workers acquiring VRE by 71%. Recent studies have found advantages in using both gowns and gloves to decrease the risk of transmitting both MRSA and VRE.[55,59,74,75] In addition, cost-benefit analyses of gown use show a temporary increase in costs, but the long-term decrease in VRE or MRSA colonization and infections overall decreases hospital costs.[75–77]

Patient Decolonization

Use of 2% chlorhexidine cloths to daily bathe ICU patients has been shown an effective method of decreasing both hospital-acquired infections (ie, bloodstream infections, surgical-site infections, and VAP) and colonization with drug-resistant organisms (ie, VRE and MRSA).[78–84] Despite the controversy about the methodology of some of these studies, given the apparent benefits, the low rate of associated adverse effects, and the ease of implementation, daily chlorhexidine bathing for all ICU patients is recommended and is currently the standard practice in most ICUs.

SPECIFIC INFECTIONS
Ventilator-Associated Pneumonia

The 2005 American Thoracic Society/Infectious Diseases Society of America guidelines defined hospital-acquired pneumonia (HAP) as pneumonia that occurs at least 48 hours after admission to the hospital. VAP is a type of HAP that develops more than 48 hours after endotracheal intubation.[85] Intubation increases the risk of pneumonia 6- to 21-fold, and VAP occurs in 9% to 27% of all intubated patients with 2.1 to 10.7 episodes of VAP per 1000 ventilator days. VAP is the leading cause of mortality from ICU-acquired infections. Patients with VAP are twice as likely to die compared with those without VAP, with a crude mortality rate that exceeds 30% if a high-risk pathogen is involved.[86,87] Several reports have shown that patients who develop VAP have an increase in ICU stay of 4.3 to 13 extra days and an increase in costs with each case of VAP ($12,000 to $40,000).[86–90]

Risk Factors

The most significant risk factor for HAP is mechanical ventilation, which is an inherent component to the development of VAP. A risk factors review by Safdar and colleagues[86] revealed that postsurgical patients, presence of multiple organ failure, age greater than 60 years, supine patient positioning, decreased gastric pH, cardiopulmonary resuscitation, continuous sedation, reintubation, presence of nasogastric tube, enteral feeding, sinusitis, and patients transported out of the ICU had increased risk of developing VAP.

Prevention

Owing to the high morbidity and mortality and economic impact of this condition, the implementation of preventive measures is paramount in the care of mechanically ventilated patients. There is clear evidence that these measures decrease the incidence of VAP and improve outcomes in ICUs. A multidisciplinary approach, continued education, and ventilator protocols ensure the implementation and compliance with these measures. The current evidence-based preventative measures are as follows.

Nonpharmacologic strategies

- Avoiding intubation and reintubation when possible. Early extubation when appropriate is the most effective preventive intervention for VAP.[91–95]
- Noninvasive ventilation should be used whenever appropriate in selected patients with respiratory failure. Patients with chronic obstructive pulmonary disease and congestive heart failure are more likely to benefit from noninvasive ventilation as a temporary support measure.[96–100]
- Use of oral endotracheal and orogastric tubes, rather than nasotracheal and nasogastric tubes. Nasotracheal intubation has been associated with

nosocomial sinusitis and high incidence of VAP. The oropharyngeal route is recommended.[91,94,95,101,102]

- Continuous aspiration of subglottic secretions. The endotracheal tube stents the epiglottis open and prevents its closure. Oropharyngeal secretions accumulate above the endotracheal tube cuff, below the glottis. Microorganisms can grow in this protected environment. Suction removal of these fluids can reduce the risk of aspiration. Suctioning prior to repositioning or extubation should be standard protocol.[103,104]
- Postural drainage, standardized endotracheal suctioning, and use of closed suction system (CSS). Standardized endotracheal suction protocols, in which everyone suctions effectively in the same way, have been shown to reduce colonization and the incidence of VAP. CSS provides a barrier to separate the contaminated catheter from the caregiver, hence other patients, as well as reducing the environmental exposure of the patient being suctioned. Moreover, closed suctioning also permits continuous ventilation, reducing respiratory stress and vulnerability.[103–106]
- Maintaining endotracheal cuff pressure at greater than 20 cm H_2O. A cuff that is underinflated forms creases that can readily allow contaminated secretions to migrate past the cuff and aspirate into the lungs. On the other hand, excessive inflation and too much pressure can prevent adequate perfusion of contacted mucosa and damage tissue. The optimal pressure for all situations has not been conclusively established but is generally held to be 20 mm Hg. Cuff pressure should be monitored and recorded routinely.[105,106]
- Semirecumbent positioning of the patients, especially when they are enterally fed. The supine position increases the accumulation of secretions in the subglottic area. Elevating the head 30° to 45° reduces this pooling and thus the microbial load and contamination pressure and has been shown to decrease the VAP rate.[17,107–109]
- Alcohol-based hand disinfection and use of protective gowns and gloves prevents horizontal patient-to-patient contamination and acquiring VAP and infections in general.[91,95]
- Staff education and compliance with isolation procedures has been shown to reduce cross-infection with multidrug resistance and VAP incidence rate.[91,94]

Pharmacologic strategies

- Chlorhexidine oral rinse. Routine oral decontamination is an effective method for reducing VAP by decreasing the contamination pressure and microbial load in the oropharyngeal cavity. It has been found that the incorporation of routine oral hygiene into standard practice reduced VAP by 57.6%. Oral hygiene programs should consist of frequent tooth brushing, oral suctioning and swabbing of the mouth with chlorhexidine antiseptic agents.[110]
- Limiting the use of sedative and neuromuscular blockers. The use of the least amount of sedation possible has been shown to decrease the duration of delirium in the ICU, number of ventilated days, and mortality.[111]

CATHETER-RELATED BLOODSTREAM INFECTIONS

Intravascular catheters are indispensable in modern-day medical practice, particularly in ICU settings. In the United States, 15 million CVC days occur in ICUs each year (ie, the total number of days of exposure to CVCs by all patients in the selected population during the selected time period).[112] Although these catheters are useful a clinical tool, their use puts patients at risk for local and systemic infectious complications, including local site infections, CLABSIs, and distant metastatic infections. CLABSIs are important cause of morbidity and attributable mortality, estimated to be 12% to 25% for each infection episode. The prevalence of CLABSIs in the ICU has yet to be determined, but in the United States, it has been estimated that there are approximately 80,000 CLABSIs per year in ICUs.[113] This number has been declining, however, with the widespread efforts of prevention. In United States ICUs, CLABSI incidence has decreased from 3.64 to 1.65 infections per 1000 central line days between 2001 and 2009.[114,115] The total cost of CLABSIs per year in the United States has been estimated at between $0.67 and $2.68 billion.[116]

Risk Factors

The incidence of CLABSIs varies considerably by catheter-related factors and patient-related factors.
Patient-related factors[117,118]

- Malnutrition
- Total parenteral nutrition administration
- Previous bloodstream infection
- Extremes of age
- Loss of skin integrity, as with burns
- Immune deficiency, especially neutropenia
- Chronic illness
- Bone marrow transplantation

Catheter-related factors

- Location of catheter insertion (higher risk with femoral or internal jugular more than subclavian)[119–122]
- Insertion technique (higher risk with nontunneled compared with tunneled insertion, and tunneled insertion compared with a totally implantable device)[123–127]
- Long duration of catheterization (the older the line the higher the risk, although there is no indication for routine line changing based on number of catheter days)[114–116,119,120]
- Conditions of insertion (higher risk with submaximal compared with maximal barrier precautions during insertion [ie, mask, cap, sterile gloves, gown, large drape])[128,129]
- Catheter-site care (emergency compared with elective, unskilled compared wtih skilled inserter)[119,120,124,125,129,130]
- Indication and use (higher risk with catheters used for hyperalimentation or hemodialysis compared with other indications)[117,118,130]
- Catheter material type (higher risk with bare catheters compared with antibiotic impregnated catheters)[131]

Prevention

- Compliance with hand hygiene measures. It is critical to observe proper hand-hygiene procedures either by washing hands with conventional antiseptic-containing soap and water or with waterless alcohol-based gels or foams. This should be maintained before and after palpating catheter insertion sites as well as before and after inserting, replacing, accessing, repairing, or dressing an intravascular catheter. Use of gloves does not obviate hand hygiene.[132–134]

- Use an all-inclusive catheter cart or kit.[135]
- Use maximal sterile barrier precautions during CVC insertion, including a full-body drape over the patient, mask, cap, sterile gloves, and gown.[119,128,133,136,137]
- Use a 2% chlorhexidine-based antiseptic for skin preparation in patients older than 2 months. In adults, although a 2% chlorhexidine-based preparation is preferred, tincture of iodine, an iodophor, or 70% alcohol can be used.[138–142]
- In adults, referentially use the subclavian vein for placement of CVC, unless contraindicated.[119,143,144] Studies in children have demonstrated that femoral catheters have a low incidence of mechanical complications and might have an infection rate similar to that of nonfemoral catheters.[145–147]
- The type of catheter selected should depend on its intended purpose and duration of use, risks and benefits of the particular catheter, and experience of the catheter operators.
- The use of dynamic 2-D ultrasound for the placement of CVCs has been shown in 2 meta-analyses to substantially reduce mechanical complications and decrease the number of attempts required to successfully cannulate the vein.[148,149]
- Disinfect catheter hubs, needleless connectors, and injection ports before accessing the catheter. Cap all stopcocks when not in use.[150–152]
- Frequently assess the need to keep intravascular catheters and promptly remove any catheter that is no longer essential. Do not routinely replace CVCs, peripherally inserted central catheters (PICCs), hemodialysis catheters, or pulmonary artery catheters to prevent catheter-related infections. Do not remove CVCs or PICCs on the basis of fever alone. Use clinical judgment regarding the appropriateness of removing the catheter if infection is evidenced elsewhere or if a noninfectious cause of fever is suspected.[114,115,119,120,153,154]
- Replace administration sets not used for blood, blood products, or lipids at intervals not longer than 96 hours.[155]
- Topical antibiotic ointment or creams should not be used on the insertion site, except for dialysis catheters, because of their potential to promote fungal infection and antimicrobial resistance.[156,157]
- Systemic antibiotics should not be administered as prophylaxis either before insertion or during use on an intravascular catheter to prevent catheter colonization or RBSI.[158]

Last but not least, it is essential to educate and periodically assess adherence of all ICU staff with the indications for intravascular catheter use, proper procedures for the insertion and maintenance of intravascular catheters, and appropriate infection control measures to prevent intravascular catheter-related infections.

CLOSTRIDIUM DIFFICILE COLITIS

Since 1978, when it was first identified as the cause of pseudomembranous colitis, C difficile has become the most common cause of nosocomial infectious diarrhea.[159–161] CDI is also the most frequent cause of ICU-acquired infectious diarrhea.[151] The incidence and severity of CDI are increasing prompting more admissions to ICUs for management of CDI-related complications.[162,163] CDI has been associated with an attributable mortality rate of 6.9% at 30 days and 16.7% at 1 year after diagnosis.[164,165]

Risk Factors

ICU stay has been commonly cited as a risk factor for CDI.[166–168] The other risk factors that are most consistently identified in the literature include antibiotic exposure, age greater than 60 years, longer duration of hospital stay, severe underlying disease, and gastric acid suppression.[167] Exposure to antimicrobials is the most important risk factor for the development of CDI with broad-spectrum antibiotics the most common offenders.[168]

Prevention

Pathogen transmission between patients and health care professionals is a major source of CDI infection in the ICU. Therefore, the most essential aspect of CDI prevention is protecting patients from initial acquisition of the organism in the health care setting. The prevention strategies are divided into 4 categories: (1) measures for health care workers, patients, and visitors; (2) environmental cleaning and disinfection; (3) antimicrobial use restrictions; and (4) use of probiotics.[168]

1. Measures for health care workers, patients, and visitors
   - Strict use of gowns and gloves on entry into room of patient infected with *C difficile* is the most effective single preventive measure.[169]
   - All health care workers must follow meticulous hand hygiene protocols. In non-outbreak settings, hand hygiene with alcohol-based hand sanitizers, in addition to wearing gloves as a component of contact precautions, is considered an acceptable method of hand hygiene after caring for patients with CDI.[168,170] In outbreak settings, however, preferential use of soap and water is recommended after caring for a patient with CDI because of the theoretic increase in risk of *C difficile* transmission.[168]
   - Educate health care personnel, housekeeping personnel, and hospital administration about CDI.
   - Educate patients and their families about CDI and contact precautions.
2. Environmental cleaning and disinfection
   - Patients with CDI should be accommodated in private rooms with contact precautions.[168]
   - Chlorine-containing cleaning agents or other sporicidal agents should be used in cleaning ICU rooms.[168]
   - Each patient in isolation should have dedicated equipment, such as stethoscopes and blood pressure cuffs.[168]
3. Antimicrobial use restrictions
   - Minimize the frequency and duration of antimicrobial therapy and the number of antimicrobial agents prescribed, to reduce CDI risk.[168]
   - Implement an antimicrobial stewardship program. Antimicrobials to be targeted should be based on the local epidemiology and the *C difficile* strains present, but restricting the use of cephalosporin and clindamycin (except for surgical antibiotic prophylaxis) may be particularly useful.[168,171]
4. Use of probiotics
   - There are few data to support the use of probiotics and currently it is not recommended as a prevention measure.[168]

CATHETER-ASSOCIATED URINARY TRACT INFECTIONS

Nosocomial urinary tract infections (UTIs) account for up to 40% of infections in hospitals and 23% of nosocomial infections in ICUs.[172–174] A vast majority of UTIs are related to indwelling urinary catheters, with 95% of UTIs occurring in ICUs developing in patients with urinary catheters. Nosocomial UTIs have been associated with a 3-fold increased risk for mortality in hospital-based studies, with estimates of more than 50,000 excess deaths occurring per year in the United

States as a result of these infections.[175] CAUTIs result in as much as $131 million excess direct medical costs nationwide annually.[176] Since October 2008, the Centers for Medicare and Medicaid Services no longer reimburses hospitals for the extra costs of managing patients with hospital-acquired CAUTI.[177] Prevention has become a priority for most hospitals, because 65% to 70% of CAUTIs are estimated to be preventable.[178]

Risk Factors

Duration of catheterization is the most important risk factor for CAUTIs. Up to 95% of UTIs in ICUs are associated with an indwelling urinary catheter.[179] Bacteriuria, the precursor to CAUTI, develops quickly at an average daily rate of 3% to 10% per day of catheterization. Almost 26% of patients with a catheter in place for 2 to 10 days develop bacteriuria, and virtually all patients catheterized for 1 month develop bacteriuria.[172] Nonmodifiable patient-related risk factors include female gender, severe underlying illness, nonsurgical disease, age greater than 50 years, diabetes mellitus, and serum creatinine level greater than 2 mg/dL. The modifiable risk factors are duration of catheterization, adherence to aseptic catheter care, catheter insertion after the sixth day of hospitalization, and catheter insertion outside the operating room.[172,174]

Prevention Strategies

- Avoid insertion of indwelling urinary catheters when possible.[179–181] The most effective strategy for CAUTI prevention is limitation or avoidance of catheterization as appropriate. The first step toward achieving this goal is through restricting urinary catheter placement to appropriate indications and activating institutional protocols that reinforces this procedure.[172–174]
- Early removal of indwelling catheters. Checklists, daily plans, nurse-based interventions, and electronic reminders were all found effective at reducing duration of catheterization and hence the rate of UTI per 10,000 patient-days.[182–187]
- Seek alternatives to indwelling catheterization when appropriate. Intermittent catheterization and condom catheter are good alternatives. Compared with indwelling urinary catheterization, intermittent urinary catheterization reduces the risk of bacteriuria and UTI. Moreover, condom catheters can be considered in appropriately selected male patients without urinary retention, dementia, or bladder outlet obstruction. A randomized trial demonstrated a decrease in bacteriuria, symptomatic UTI, and death in patients with condom catheters compared with those with indwelling catheter.[180,188–191]
- Proper techniques for insertion and maintenance of catheters are essential preventative measures. All urinary catheters should be inserted by a trained health care professional using aseptic technique and connected to a closed drainage system.[180,192]
- Avoidance of routine bladder irrigation. Prophylactic instillation of antiseptic agents or irrigation of the bladder with antimicrobial or antiseptic agents has been shown to increase infection and is not recommended.[180]

SUMMARY

It is critical for health care personnel to recognize and appreciate the detrimental impact of ICU-acquired infections. The economic, clinical, and social expenses to patients and hospitals are overwhelming. To limit the incidence of ICU-acquired infections, aggressive infection control measures must be implemented and enforced. Researchers and national committees have developed and continue to develop evidence-based guidelines to control infections in the ICU. A multifaceted approach, including infection prevention committees, antimicrobial stewardship programs, daily reassessments-intervention bundles, identifying and minimizing risk factors, and continuing staff education programs, is essential in the modern era of critical care medicine. Infection control in the ICU is an evolving area of critical care research and continued advancements in this field are foreseen.

REFERENCES

1. Society of Critical Care Medicine: evaluating ICU care in your community. 2008. Available at: http://www.myicu.org/Support_Brochures/Pages/EvaluatingICUin YourCommunity.aspx. Accessed on January 28, 2014.
2. Society of Critical Care Medicine. Critical care units: a descriptive analysis. 1st edition. Des Plaines (IL): Society of Critical Care Medicine; 2005.
3. Fridkin SK, Welbel SF, Weinstein RA. Magnitude and prevention of nosocomial infections in the intensive care unit. Infect Dis Clin North Am 1997;11:479.
4. Vincent JL, Rello J, Marshall J, et al. International study of the prevalence and outcomes of infection in intensive care units. JAMA 2009;302:2323.
5. Kaye KS, Marchaim D, Smialowicz C, et al. Suction regulators: a potential vector for hospital-acquired pathogens. Infect Control Hosp Epidemiol 2010;31:772.
6. Dempsey DT, Mullen JL, Buzby GP. The link between nutritional status and clinical outcome: can nutritional intervention modify it? Am J Clin Nutr 1988;47:352–6.
7. Bistrian BR, Blackburn GL, Scrimshaw NS, et al. Cellular immunited in semi-starved states in hospitalized adults. Am J Clin Nutr 1975;28:1148–55.
8. Cunningham-Rundles S. Analytical methods for evaluation of immune response in nutrient intervention. Nutr Rev 1998;56(1 Pt 2):S27–37.
9. Scrimshaw NS. Historical concepts of interactions, synergism and antagonism between nutrition and infection. J Nutr 2003;133(1):316S–21S.
10. Keusch GT. The history of nutrition: malnutrition, infection and immunity. J Nutr 2003;133(1):336S–40S.
11. Kaya E, Yetim I, Dervisoglu A, et al. Risk factors for and effect of a one-year surveillance program on a surgical site infection at a university hospital in Turkey. Surg Infect (Larchmt) 2006;7(6):519–26.
12. Rapp-Kesek D, Ståhle E, Karlsson T. Body mass index and albumin in the preoperative evaluation of cardiac surgery patients. Clin Nutr 2004;23:1398–404.
13. Rubinson L, Diette GB, Song X, et al. Low caloric intake is associated with nosocomial bloodstream infections in patients in the medial intensive care unit. Crit Care Med 2004;32(2):350–7.
14. Simpson F, Doig GS. Parenteral vs enteral nutrition in the critically ill patient: a meta-analysis of trials using the intention to treat principle. Intensive Care Med 2005;31(1):12–23.
15. Bonten MJ, Kollef MH, Hall JB. Risk factors for ventilator-associated pneumonia: from epidemiology to patient management. Clin Infect Dis 2004;38:1141–9.
16. Vasken A, Krayem H, DiGiovine B. Effects of early enteral feeding on the outcome of critically ill mechanically ventilated medical patients. Chest 2006;129:960–7.
17. Drakulovic MB, Torres A, Bauer TT, et al. Supine body position as a risk factor for nosocomial pneumonia in mechanically ventilated patients: a randomized trial. Lancet 1999;354:1851–8.
18. Gramlich L, Kichian K, Pinilla J, et al. Does enteral nutrition compared to parenteral nutrition result in better outcomes in critically ill adult patients? A systematic review of the literature. Nutrition 2004;20(10):843–8.

19. Radrizzani D, Bertolini G, Facchini R, et al. Early enteral immunonutrition vs. parenteral nutrition in critically ill patients without severe sepsis: a randomized clinical trial. Intensive Care Med 2006;32:1191–8.
20. Mizock BA. Alterations in carbohydrate metabolism during stress: a review of the literature. Am J Med 1995;98:75–84.
21. McCowen KC, Malhotra A, Bistrian BR. Stress-induced hyperglycemia. Crit Care Clin 2001;17:107–24.
22. Capes SE, Hunt D, Malmberg K, et al. Stress hyperglycaemia and increased risk of death after myocardial infarction in patients with and without diabetes: a systematic overview. Lancet 2000;355:773–8.
23. Cely CM, Arora P, Quartin AA, et al. Relationship of baseline glucose homeostasis to hyperglycemia during medical critical illness. Chest 2004;126:879–87.
24. Van den Berghe G, Wouters P, Weekers F, et al. Intensive insulin therapy in critically ill patients. N Engl J Med 2001;345:1359–67.
25. Van den Berghe G, Wouters PJ, Bouillon R, et al. Outcome benefit of intensive insulin therapy in the critically ill: insulin dose versus glycemic control. Crit Care Med 2003;31:359–66.
26. Latham R, Lancaster AD, Covington JF, et al. The association of diabetes and glucose control with surgical-site infections among cardiothoracic surgery patients. Infect Control Hosp Epidemiol 2001;22(10):607–12.
27. Bochicchio GV, Sung J, Joshi M, et al. Persistent hyperglycemia is predictive of outcome in critically ill trauma patients. J Trauma 2005;58(5):921–4.
28. Grey NJ, Perdrizet GA. Reduction of nosocomial infections in the surgical intensive- care unit by strict glycemic control. Endocr Pract 2004;10(Suppl 2):46–52.
29. Jain M, Miller L, Belt D, et al. Decline in ICU adverse events, nosocomial infections and cost through a quality improvement initiative focusing on teamwork and culture change. Qual Saf Health Care 2006;15(4):235–9.
30. Berriel-Cass D, Adkins FW, Jones P, et al. Eliminating nosocomial infections at Ascension health. Jt Comm J Qual Patient Saf 2006;32(11):612–20.
31. Harrigan S, Hurst D, Lee C, et al. Developing and implementing quality initiatives in the ICU: strategies and outcomes. Crit Care Nurs Clin North Am 2006; 18(4):469–79.
32. Misset B, Timsit JF, Dumay MF, et al. A continuous quality-improvement program reduces nosocomial infection rates in the ICU. Intensive Care Med 2004;30(3): 395–400.
33. Apisarnthanarak A, Pinitchai U, Thongphubeth K, et al. Effectiveness of an educational program to reduce ventilator-associated pneumonia in a tertiary care center in Thailand: a 4-year study. Clin Infect Dis 2007;45(6):704–11.
34. Zack JE, Garrison T, Trovillion E, et al. Effect of an education program aimed at reducing the occurrence of ventilator-associated pneumonia. Crit Care Med 2002;30(11):2407–12.
35. Pronovost P, Needham D, Berenholtz S, et al. An intervention to decrease catheter- related bloodstream infections in the ICU. N Engl J Med 2006;355(26): 2725–32.
36. Lobo RD, Levin AS, Gomes LM, et al. Impact of an educational program and policy changes on decreasing catheter-associated bloodstream infections in a medical intensive care unit in Brazil. Am J Infect Control 2005;33(2):83–7.
37. Hugonnet S, Chevrolet J, Pittet D. The effect of workload on infection risk in critically ill patients. Crit Care Med 2007;35(1):76–81.
38. Hugonnet S, Uc kay I, Pittet D. Staffing level: a determinant of late-onset ventilator- associated pneumonia. Crit Care 2007;11(4):R80.

39. Fridkin SK, Pear SM, Williamson TH, et al. The role of understaffing in central venous catheter-associated bloodstream infections. Infect Control Hosp Epidemiol 1996;17(3):150–8.
40. Pittet D, Dharan S, Touveneau S, et al. Bacterial contamination of the hands of hospital staff during routine patient care. Arch Intern Med 1999;159(8):821–6.
41. Markogiannakis A, Fildisis G, Tsiplakou S, et al. Cross-transmission of multidrugresistant Acinetobacter baumannii clonal strains causing episodes of sepsis in a trauma intensive care unit. Infect Control Hosp Epidemiol 2008;29(5):410–7.
42. Ojajärvi J. Effectiveness of hand washing and disinfection methods in removing transient bacteria after patient nursing. J Hyg (Lond) 1980;85(2):193–203.
43. Oelberg DG, Joyner SE, Jiang X, et al. Detection of pathogen transmission in neonatal nurseries using DNA markers as surrogate indicators. Pediatrics 2000;105(2):311–5.
44. Bures S, Fishbain JT, Uyehara CF, et al. Computer keyboards and faucet handles as reservoirs of nosocomial pathogens in the intensive care unit. Am J Infect Control 2000;28(6):465–71.
45. Hartmann B, Benson M, Junger A, et al. Computer keyboard and mouse as a reservoir of pathogens in an intensive care unit. J Clin Monit Comput 2004; 18(1):7–12.
46. Curtis L, Cali S, Conroy L, et al. Aspergillus surveillance project at a large tertiary-care hospital. J Hosp Infect 2005;59(3):188–96.
47. Lee LD, Berkheiser M, Jiang Y, et al. Risk of bioaerosol contamination with Aspergillus species before and after cleaning in rooms filtered with high-efficiency particulate air filters that house patients with hematologic malignancy. Infect Control Hosp Epidemiol 2007;28(9):1066–70.
48. Hayden MK, Bonten MJ, Blom DW, et al. Reduction in acquisition of vancoycin-resistant Enterococcus after enforcement of routine environmental cleaning measures. Clin Infect Dis 2006;42(11):1552–60.
49. Pittet D, Sax H, Hugonnet S, et al. Cost implications of successful hand hygiene promotion. Infect Control Hosp Epidemiol 2004;25(3):264–6.
50. Eldridge NE, Woods SS, Bonello RS, et al. Using the six sigma process to implement the Centers for Disease Control and Prevention Guideline for hand hygiene in 4 intensive care units. J Gen Intern Med 2006;21(Suppl 2):S35–42.
51. Boyce JM, Pittet D, Healthcare Infection Control Practices Advisory Committee, Society for Healthcare Epidemiology of America, Association for Professionals in Infection Control, Infectious Diseases Society of America, Hand Hygiene Task Force. Guideline for hand hygiene in health-care settings: recommendations of the Healthcare Infection Control Practices Advisory Committee and the HICPAC/SHEA/APIC/IDSA Hand Hygiene Task Force. Infect Control Hosp Epidemiol 2002;23(12 Suppl):S3–40.
52. Rupp ME, Fitzgerald T, Puumala S, et al. Prospective, controlled, cross-over trial of alcohol-based hand gel in critical care units. Infect Control Hosp Epidemiol 2008;29(1):8–15.
53. Girou E, Loyeau S, Legrand P, et al. Efficacy of handrubbing with alcohol based solution versus standard handwashing with antiseptic soap: randomized clinical trial. BMJ 2002;325(7360):362–6.
54. Larson EL, Aiello AE, Bastyr J, et al. Assessment of two hand hygiene regimens for intensive care unit personnel. Crit Care Med 2001;29(5):944–51.
55. Jernigan JA, Titus MG, Gröschel DH, et al. Effectiveness of contact isolation during a hospital outbreak of methicillin-resistant Staphylococcus aureus. Am J Epidemiol 1996;143(5):496–504.

56. Haley RW, Cushion NB, Tenover FC, et al. Eradication of endemic methicillinresistant Staphylococcus aureus infections from a neonatal intensive care unit. J Infect Dis 1995;171(3):614–24.

57. Safdar N, Marx J, Meyer NA, et al. Effectiveness of preemptive barrier precautions in controlling nosocomial colonization and infection by methicillin-resistant Staphylococcus aureus in a burn unit. Am J Infect Control 2006;34(8): 476–83.

58. Mangini E, Segal-Maurer S, Burns J, et al. Impact of contact and droplet precautions on the incidence of hospital-acquired methicillin-resistant Staphylococcus aureus infection. Infect Control Hosp Epidemiol 2007;28(11):1261–6.

59. Rubinovitch B, Pittet D. Screening for methicillin-resistant Staphylococcus aureus in the endemic hospital: what have we learned? J Hosp Infect 2001; 47(1):9–18.

60. Lucet JC, Paoletti X, Lolom I, et al. Successful long-term program for controlling methicillin-resistant Staphylococcus aureus in intensive care units. Intensive Care Med 2005;31(8):1051–7.

61. Huang SS, Yokoe DS, Hinrichsen VL, et al. Impact of routine intensive care unit surveillance cultures and resultant barrier precautions on hospital-wide methicillin- resistant Staphylococcus aureus bacteremia. Clin Infect Dis 2006;43(8): 971–8.

62. Muto CA, Jernigan JA, Ostrowsky BE, et al. SHEA guideline for preventing nosocomial transmission of multidrug-resistant strains of Staphylococcus aureus and Enterococcus. Infect Control Hosp Epidemiol 2003;24(5):362–86.

63. Calfee DP, Giannetta ET, Durbin LJ, et al. Control of endemic vancomycin-resistant Enterococcus among inpatients at a university hospital. Clin Infect Dis 2003;37(3):326–32.

64. Boyce JM, Mermel LA, Zervos MJ, et al. Controlling vancomycin-resistant Enterococci. Infect Control Hosp Epidemiol 1995;16(11):634–7.

65. Ostrowsky BE, Trick WE, Sohn AH, et al. Control of vancomycin-resistant Enterococcus in health care facilities in a region. N Engl J Med 2001; 344(19):1427–33.

66. Perencevich EN, Fisman DN, Lipsitch M, et al. Projected benefits of active surveillance for vancomycin-resistant Enterococci in intensive care units. Clin Infect Dis 2004;38(8):1108–15.

67. Kurup A, Chlebicki MP, Ling ML, et al. Control of a hospital-wide vancomycinresistant Enterococci outbreak. Am J Infect Control 2008;36(3):206–11.

68. Mascini EM, Troelstra A, Beitsma M, et al. Genotyping and preemptive isolation to control an outbreak of vancomycin-resistant Enterococcus faecium. Clin Infect Dis 2006;42(6):739–46.

69. Byers KE, Anglim AM, Anneski CJ, et al. A hospital epidemic of vancomycinresistant Enterococcus: risk factors and control. Infect Control Hosp Epidemiol 2001;22(3):140–7.

70. Karchmer TB, Durbin LJ, Simonton BM, et al. Cost-effectiveness of active surveillance cultures and contact/droplet precautions for control of methicillinresistant Staphylococcus aureus. J Hosp Infect 2002;51(2):126–32.

71. Muto CA, Giannetta ET, Durbin LJ, et al. Cost-effectiveness of perirectal surveillance cultures for controlling vancomycin-resistant Enterococcus. Infect Control Hosp Epidemiol 2002;23(8):429–35.

72. Tenorio A, Badri S, Sahgal N, et al. Effectiveness of gloves in the prevention of hand carriage of vancomycin-resistant Enterococcus species by health care workers after patient care. Clin Infect Dis 2001;32:826–9.

73. Siegel JD, Rhinehart E, Jackson M, et al. 2007 guideline for isolation precautions: preventing transmission of infectious agents in healthcare settings. Available at: http://www.cdc.gov/ncidod/dhqp/pdf/isolation2007.pdf. Accessed January 13, 2009.

74. Srinivasan A, Song X, Ross T, et al. A prospective study to determine whether cover gowns in addition to gloves decrease nosocomial transmission of vancomycin-resistant Enterococci in an intensive care unit. Infect Control Hosp Epidemiol 2002;23(8):424–8.

75. Puzniak LA, Gillespie KN, Leet T, et al. A cost-benefit analysis of gown use in controlling vancomycin-resistant Enterococcus transmission: is it worth the price? Infect Control Hosp Epidemiol 2004;25(5):418–24.

76. Montecalvo MA, Jarvis WR, Uman J, et al. Costs and savings associated with infection control measures that reduced transmission of vancomycin-resistant Enterococci in an endemic setting. Infect Control Hosp Epidemiol 2001;22(7):437–42.

77. Harbarth S, Fankhauser C, Schrenzel J, et al. Universal screening for methicillinresistant Staphylococcus aureus at hospital admission and nosocomial infection in surgical patients. JAMA 2008;299(10):1149–57.

78. Vernon MO, Hayden MK, Trick WE, et al. Chlorhexidine gluconate to cleanse patients in a medical intensive care unit: the effectiveness of source control to reduce the bioburden of vancomycin-resistant Enterococci. Arch Intern Med 2006;166(3):306–12.

79. Bleasdale SC, Trick WE, Gonzalez IM, et al. Effectiveness of chlorhexidine bathing to reduce catheter-associated bloodstream infections in medical intensive care unit patients. Arch Intern Med 2007;167(19):2073–9.

80. Huang SS, Septimus E, Kleinman K, et al. Targeted versus universal decolonization to prevent ICU infection. N Engl J Med 2013;368:2255.

81. Climo MW, Sepkowitz KA, Zuccotti G, et al. The effect of daily bathing with chlorhexidine on the acquisition of methicillin-resistant Staphylococcus aureus, vancomycin-resistant Enterococcus, and healthcare-associated bloodstream infections: results of a quasi-experimental multicenter trial. Crit Care Med 2009;37:1858.

82. Munoz-Price LS, Hota B, Stemer A, et al. Prevention of bloodstream infections by use of daily chlorhexidine baths for patients at a long-term acute care hospital. Infect Control Hosp Epidemiol 2009;30:1031.

83. Borer A, Gilad J, Porat N, et al. Impact of 4% chlorhexidine whole-body washing on multidrug-resistant Acinetobacter baumannii skin colonisation among patients in a medical intensive care unit. J Hosp Infect 2007;67:149.

84. O'Horo JC, Silva GL, Munoz-Price LS, et al. The efficacy of daily bathing with chlorhexidine for reducing healthcare-associated bloodstream infections: a meta-analysis. Infect Control Hosp Epidemiol 2012;33:257.

85. American Thoracic Society, Infectious Diseases Society of America. Guidelines for the management of adults with hospital-acquired, ventilator-associated, and healthcare-associated pneumonia. Am J Respir Crit Care Med 2005;171:388.

86. Safdar N, Dezfulian C, Collard HR, et al. Clinical and economic consequences of ventilator associated pneumonia: a systematic review. Crit Care Med 2005; 33(10):2184–93.

87. Rello J, Ollendorf DA, Oster G, et al. Epidemiology and outcomes of ventilator associated pneumonia in a large US database. Chest 2002;122(6):2115–21.

88. Heyland DK, Cook DJ, Griffith L, et al. The attributable morbidity and mortality of ventilator-associated pneumonia in the critically ill patient. Am J Respir Crit Care Med 1999;159:1249–56.

89. Kappstein I, Schulgen G, Beyer U, et al. Prolongation of hospital stay and extra costs due to ventilator-associated pneumonia in an intensive care unit. Eur J Clin Microbiol Infect Dis 1992;11:504–8.

90. Fagon JY, Chastre J, Hance AJ, et al. Nosocomial pneumonia in ventilated patients: a cohort study evaluating attributable mortality and hospital stay. Am J Med 1993b;94:281–8.

91. Tablan OC, Anderson LJ, Besser R, et al, Healthcare Infection Control Practices Advisory Committee, Centers for Disease Control and Prevention. Guidelines for preventing health-care–associated pneumonia, 2003: recommendations of the CDC and the Healthcare Infection Control Practices Advisory Committee. MMWR Recomm Rep 2004;53(RR-3):1–36.

92. Celis R, Torres A, Gatell JM, et al. Nosocomial pneumonia: a multivariate analysis of risk and prognosis. Chest 1988;93:318–24.

93. Torres A, Gatell JM, Aznar E, et al. Re-intubation increases the risk of nosocomial pneumonia in patients needing mechanical ventilation. Am J Respir Crit Care Med 1995;152:137–41.

94. Kollef MH. The prevention of ventilator-associated pneumonia. N Engl J Med 1999;340:627–34.

95. Craven DE, Steger KA. Nosocomial pneumonia in mechanically ventilated adult patients: epidemiology and prevention in 1996. Semin Respir Infect 1996;11:32–53.

96. Esteban A, Frutos-Vivar F, Ferguson ND, et al. Noninvasive positive-pressure ventilation for respiratory failure after extubation. N Engl J Med 2004;350:2452–60.

97. Nava S, Ambrosino N, Clini E, et al. Noninvasive mechanical ventilation in the weaning of patients with respiratory failure due to chronic obstructive pulmonary disease: a randomized, controlled trial. Ann Intern Med 1998;128:721–8.

98. Carlucci A, Richard JC, Wysocki M, et al. Noninvasive versus conventional mechanical ventilation: an epidemiologic survey. Am J Respir Crit Care Med 2001;163:874–80.

99. Nourdine K, Combes P, Carton MJ, et al. Does noninvasive ventilation reduce the ICU nosocomial infection risk? A prospective clinical survey. Intensive Care Med 1999;25:567–73.

100. Keenan SP. Noninvasive positive pressure ventilation in acute respiratory failure. JAMA 2000;284:2376–8.

101. Holzapfel L, Chastang C, Demingeon G, et al. A randomized study assessing the systematic search for maxillary sinusitis in nasotracheally mechanically ventilated patients. Influence of nosocomial maxillary sinusitis on the occurrence of ventilator associated pneumonia. Am J Respir Crit Care Med 1999;159:695–701.

102. Valles J, Artigas A, Rello J, et al. Continuous aspiration of subglottic secretions in preventing ventilator-associated pneumonia. Ann Intern Med 1995;122:179–86.

103. Mahul P, Auboyer C, Jospe R, et al. Prevention of nosocomial pneumonia in intubated patients: respective role of mechanical subglottic secretions drainage and stress ulcer prophylaxis. Intensive Care Med 1992;18:20–5.

104. Kollef MH, Skubas NJ, Sundt TM. A randomized clinical trial of continuous aspiration of subglottic secretions in cardiac surgery patients. Chest 1999;116:1339–46.

105. Cook D, De Jonghe B, Brochard L, et al. Influence of airway management on ventilator-associated pneumonia: evidence from randomized trials. JAMA 1998;279:781–7.

106. Rello J, Sonora R, Jubert P, et al. Pneumonia in intubated patients: role of respiratory airway care. Am J Respir Crit Care Med 1996;154:111–5.

107. Torres A, Serra-Batlles J, Ros E, et al. Pulmonary aspiration of gastric contents in patients receiving mechanical ventilation: the effect of body position. Ann Intern Med 1992;116:540–3.

108. Orozco-Levi M, Torres A, Ferrer M, et al. Semirecumbent position protects from pulmonary aspiration but not completely from gastroesophageal reflux in mechanically ventilated patients. Am J Respir Crit Care Med 1995;152:1387–90.

109. Davis K Jr, Johannigman JA, Campbell RS, et al. The acute effects of body position strategies and respiratory therapy in paralyzed patients with acute lung injury. Crit Care 2001;5:81–7.

110. DeRiso AJ II, Ladowski JS, Dillon TA, et al. Chlorhexidine gluconate 0.12% oral rinse reduces the incidence of total nosocomial respiratory infection and non-prophylactic systemic antibiotic use in patients undergoing heart surgery. Chest 1996;109:1556–61.

111. Kress JP, Pohlman AS, O'Connor MF, et al. Daily interruption of sedative infusions in critically ill patients undergoing mechanical ventilation. N Engl J Med 2000;342:1471–7.

112. Mermel LA. Prevention of intravascular catheter-related infections. Ann Intern Med 2000;132:391–402 [Erratum appears in Ann Intern Med 2000;133:395].

113. Mermel LA. Prevention of central venous catheter-related infections: what works other than impregnated or coated catheters? J Hosp Infect 2007;65:30–3.

114. Centers for Disease Control and Prevention (CDC). Vital signs: central line-associated blood stream infections–United States, 2001, 2008, and 2009. MMWR Morb Mortal Wkly Rep 2011;60:243.

115. Fagan RP, Edwards JR, Park BJ, et al. Incidence trends in pathogen-specific central line-associated bloodstream infections in US intensive care units, 1990-2010. Infect Control Hosp Epidemiol 2013;34:893.

116. Scott RD. The direct medical costs of healthcare-associated infections in U.S. hospitals and the benefits of prevention. Available at: http://www.cdc.gov/hai/pdfs/hai/scott_costpaper.pdf. Accessed on January 28, 2014.

117. Tokars JI, Cookson ST, McArthur MA, et al. Prospective evaluation of risk factors for bloodstream infection in patients receiving home infusion therapy. Ann Intern Med 1999;131:340.

118. Reunes S, Rombaut V, Vogelaers D, et al. Risk factors and mortality for nosocomial bloodstream infections in elderly patients. Eur J Intern Med 2011; 22:e39.

119. Mermel LA, McCormick RD, Springman SR, et al. The pathogenesis and epidemiology of catheter-related infection with pulmonary artery Swan-Ganz catheters: a prospective study utilizing molecular subtyping. Am J Med 1991; 91(3B):197S–205S.

120. Richet H, Hubert B, Nitemberg G, et al. Prospective multicenter study of vascular-catheter-related complications and risk factors for positive central-catheter cultures in intensive care unit patients. J Clin Microbiol 1990;28:2520.

121. Merrer J, De Jonghe B, Golliot F, et al. Complications of femoral and subclavian venous catheterization in critically ill patients: a randomized controlled trial. JAMA 2001;286:700.

122. Ronco C. The place of early haemoperfusion with polymyxin B fibre column in the treatment of sepsis. Crit Care 2005;9:631.

123. Pessa ME, Howard RJ. Complications of Hickman-Broviac catheters. Surg Gynecol Obstet 1985;161:257.

124. Darbyshire PJ, Weightman NC, Speller DC. Problems associated with indwelling central venous catheters. Arch Dis Child 1985;60:129.
125. Groeger JS, Lucas AB, Thaler HT, et al. Infectious morbidity associated with long-term use of venous access devices in patients with cancer. Ann Intern Med 1993;119:1168.
126. Ross MN, Haase GM, Poole MA, et al. Comparison of totally implanted reservoirs with external catheters as venous access devices in pediatric oncologic patients. Surg Gynecol Obstet 1988;167:141.
127. Carde P, Cosset-Delaigue MF, Laplanche A, et al. Classical external indwelling central venous catheter versus totally implanted venous access systems for chemotherapy administration: a randomized trial in 100 patients with solid tumors. Eur J Cancer Clin Oncol 1989;25:939.
128. Raad II, Hohn DC, Gilbreath BJ, et al. Prevention of central venous catheter-related infections by using maximal sterile barrier precautions during insertion. Infect Control Hosp Epidemiol 1994;15:231–8.
129. Maki DG. Yes, Virginia, aseptic technique is very important: maximal barrier precautions during insertion reduce the risk of central venous catheter-related bacteremia. Infect Control Hosp Epidemiol 1994;15:227.
130. Wilcox TA. Catheter-related bloodstream infections. Semin Intervent Radiol 2009;26:139.
131. Veenstra DL, Saint S, Saha S, et al. Efficacy of antiseptic-impregnated central venous catheters in preventing catheter-related bloodstream infection: a meta-analysis. JAMA 1999;281:261.
132. Goede MR, Coopersmith CM. Catheter-related bloodstream infection. Surg Clin North Am 2009;89:463–74.
133. Centers for Disease Control and Prevention. Guideline for hand hygiene in health-care settings: recommendations of the Healthcare Infection Control Practices Advisory Committee and the HICPAC/SHEA/APIC/IDSA Hand Hygiene Task Force. MMWR Recomm Rep 2002;51(RR–16):1–45.
134. Rosenthal VD, Guzman S, Safdar N. Reduction in nosocomial infection with improved hand hygiene in intensive care units of a tertiary care hospital in Argentina. Am J Infect Control 2005;33:392–7.
135. Berenholtz SM, Pronovost PJ, Lipsett PA, et al. Eliminating catheter-related bloodstream infections in the intensive care unit. Crit Care Med 2004;32:2014–20.
136. Hu KK, Lipsky BA, Veenstra DL, et al. Using maximal sterile barriers to prevent central venous catheter-related infection: a systematic evidence-based review. Am J Infect Control 2004;32:142–6.
137. Young EM, Commiskey ML, Wilson SJ. Translating evidence into practice to prevent central-venous catheter-associated bloodstream infections: a systems based intervention. Am J Infect Control 2006;34:503–6.
138. Maki DG, Ringer M, Alvarado CJ. Prospective randomized trial of povidoneiodine, alcohol, and chlorhexidine for prevention of infection associated with central venous and arterial catheters. Lancet 1991;338:339–43.
139. Humar A, Ostromecki A, Direnfeld J, et al. Prospective randomized trial of 10% povidone-iodine versus 0.5% tincture of chlorhexidine as cutaneous antisepsis for prevention of central venous catheter infection. Clin Infect Dis 2000;31:1001–7.
140. Chaiyakunapruk N, Veenstra DL, Lipsky BA, et al. Chlorhexidine compared with povidone-iodine solution for vascular catheter-side care: a meta-analysis. Ann Intern Med 2002;136:792–801.

141. Chaiyakunapruk N, Veenstra DL, Lipsky BA, et al. Vascular catheter site care; the clinical and economic benefits of chlorhexidine gluconate compared with povidone iodine. Clin Infect Dis 2003;37:764–71.

142. Valles J, Fernandez I, Alcaraz D, et al. Prospective randomized trial of 3 anti-septic solutions for prevention of catheter colonization in an intensive care unit for adult patients. Infect Control Hosp Epidemiol 2008;29:847–53.

143. Goetz AM, Wagener MM, Muder RR. Risk of infection due to central venous catheters: effect of site of placement and catheter type. Infect Control Hosp Epidemiol 1998;19:842–5.

144. Hamilton HC, Foxcroft D. Central venous access sites for the prevention of venous thrombosis, stenosis and infection in patients requiring long-term intravenous therapy [review]. Cochrane Database Syst Rev 2007;(3):CD004084. http://dx.doi.org/10.1002/14651858.pub2:CD004084.

145. Hind D, Calvert N, McWiliams R, et al. Ultrasonic location devices for central venous cannulation: meta-analysis. BMJ 2003;327:361.

146. Venkataraman ST, Thompson AE. Femoral vascular catheterization in critically ill infants and children. Clin Pediatr (Phila) 1997;36:311–9.

147. Sheridan RL, Weber JM. Mechanical and infectious complications of central venous cannulation in children: lessons learned from a 10-year experience placing more than 1000 catheters. J Burn Care Res 2006;27:713–8.

148. Stenzel JP, Green TP, Fuhrman RP, et al. Percutaneous central venous catheterization in a pediatric intensive care unit: a survival analysis of complications. Crit Care Med 1989;17:984–8.

149. Randolph AG, Cook DJ, Gonzales CA, et al. Tunneling short-term central venous catheters to prevent catheter-related infection: a meta-analysis of randomized, controlled trials. Crit Care Med 1998;26:1452–7.

150. Salzman MB, Isenberg HD, Rubin LG. Use of disinfectants to reduce microbial contamination of hubs of vascular catheters. J Clin Microbiol 1993;31:475–9.

151. Luebke MA, Arduino MJ, Duda DL, et al. Comparison of the microbial barrier properties of a needleless and a conventional needle-based intravenous access system. Am J Infect Control 1998;26:437–41.

152. Casey AL, Worthington T, Lambert PA, et al. A randomized, prospective clinical trial to access the potential infection risk associated with the PosiFlow needle-less connector. J Hosp Infect 2003;54:288–93.

153. Lederle FA, Parenti CM, Berskow LC, et al. The idle intravenous catheter. Ann Intern Med 1992;116:737–8.

154. Parenti CM, Lederle FA, Impola CL, et al. Reduction of unnecessary intravenous catheter use. Arch Intern Med 1994;154:1829–32.

155. Gillies D, Walen NM, Morrison AL, et al. Optimal timing for intravenous administration set replacements. Cochrane Database Syst Rev 2005;(4):CD003588. http://dx.doi.org/10.1002/14651858.pub2:CD003588.

156. Zakrzewska-Bode A, Muytjens HL, Liem KD, et al. Mupirocin resistance in coagulase- negative staphylococci, after topical prophylaxis for the reduction of colonization of central venous catheters. J Hosp Infect 1995;31:189–93.

157. Flowers RH, Schwenzer KJ, Kopel RF, et al. Efficacy of an attachable subcutaneous cuff for the prevention of intravascular catheter-related infection. A randomized, controlled trial. JAMA 1989;10:878–83.

158. van de Wetering MD, van Woensel JB. Prophylactic antibiotics for preventing early central venous catheter gram positive infections among oncology patients. Cochrane Database Syst Rev 2007;(24):CD003295.

159. Bartlett JG, Chang TW, Gurwith M, et al. Antibiotic-associated pseudomembranous colitis due to toxin-producing clostridia. N Engl J Med 1978;298:531–4.
160. Barbut F, Corthier G, Charpak Y, et al. Prevalence and pathogenicity of Clostridium difficile in hospitalized patients. A French multicenter study. Arch Intern Med 1996;156:1449–54.
161. Wiesen P, Van Gossum A, Preiser JC. Diarrhoea in the critically ill. Curr Opin Crit Care 2006;12:149–54.
162. Zilberberg MD. Clostridium difficile-related hospitalizations among US adults, 2006. Emerg Infect Dis 2009;15:122–4.
163. Labbe AC, Poirier L, Maccannell D, et al. Clostridium difficile infections in a Canadian tertiary care hospital before and during a regional epidemic associated with the BI/NAP1/027 strain. Antimicrob Agents Chemother 2008;52:3180–7.
164. Loo VG, Poirier L, Miller MA, et al. A predominantly clonal multiinstitutional outbreak of *Clostridium difficile*-associated diarrhea with high morbidity and mortality. N Engl J Med 2005;353:2442–9.
165. Pepin J, Valiquette L, Cossette B. Mortality attributable to nosocomial *Clostridium difficile*-associated disease during an epidemic caused by a hypervirulent strain in Quebec. CMAJ 2005;173:1037–42.
166. Bignardi GE. Risk factors for Clostridium difficile infection. J Hosp Infect 1998; 40:1–15.
167. Dubberke ER, Reske KA, Yan Y, et al. Clostridium difficile–associated disease in a setting of endemicity: identification of novel risk factors. Clin Infect Dis 2007; 45:1543–9.
168. Cohen SH, Gerding DN, Johnson S, et al. Clinical practice guidelines for clostridium difficile infection in adults: 2010 update by the Society for Healthcare Epidemiology of America (SHEA) and the Infectious Diseases Society of America (IDSA). Infect Control Hosp Epidemiol 2010;31:431–55.
169. Johnson S, Samore MH, Farrow KA, et al. Epidemics of diarrhea caused by clindamycin-resistant strain of Clostridium difficile in four hospitals. N Engl J Med 1999;341(22):1645–51.
170. Gerding DM, Muto CA, Owens RC. Measures to control and prevent Clostridium difficile infection. Clin Infect Dis 2008;46(Suppl 1):S43–9.
171. Valiquette L, Cossette B, Garant MP, et al. Impact of a reduction in the use of high-risk antibiotics on the course of an epidemic of Clostridium difficile-associated disease caused by the hypervirulent NAP1/027 strain. Clin Infect Dis 2007;45(Suppl 2):S112–21.
172. Chenoweth CE, Saint S. Urinary tract infections. Infect Dis Clin North Am 2011; 25:103–17.
173. Nicolle LE. Urinary catheter-associated infections. Infect Dis Clin North Am 2012;26:13–27.
174. Shuman K, Chenoweth CE. Recognition and prevention of healthcare-associated urinary tract infections in the intensive care unit. Crit Care Med 2010;38:S373–9.
175. Platt R, Polk BF, Murdock B, et al. Mortality associated with nosocomial urinary-tract infection. N Engl J Med 1982;307:637–42.
176. Burton DC, Edwards JR, Srinivasan A, et al. Trends in catheter-associated urinary tract infections in adult intensive care units-United States, 1990-2007. Infect Control Hosp Epidemiol 2011;32:748–56.
177. Saint S, Meddings JA, Calfee D, et al. Catheter-associated urinary tract infection and the medicare rule changes. Ann Intern Med 2009;150:877–84.

178. Umsheid CA, Mitchell MD, Doshi JA, et al. Estimating the proportion of healthcare-associated infections that are reasonably preventable and the related mortality and costs. Infect Control Hosp Epidemiol 2011;32:101–14.

179. Rebmann T, Greene LR. Preventing catheter-associated urinary tract infections: an executive summary of the Association for Professionals in Infection Control and Epidemiol. Am J Infect Control 2010;38:644–6.

180. Gould CV, Umscheid CA, Agarwal RK, et al, Healthcare Infection Control Practices Advisory Committee (HICPAC). CDC guideline for prevention of catheter-associated urinary tract infections 2009. Infect Control Hosp Epidemiol 2010;31:319–26.

181. Lo E, Nicolle L, Classen D, et al. Strategies to prevent catheter-associated urinary tract infections in acute care hospitals. Infect Control Hosp Epidemiol 2008;29(Suppl 1):S41–50.

182. Fakih MG, Dueweke C, Meisner S, et al. Effect of nurse-led multidisciplinary rounds on reducing the unnecessary use of urinary catheterization in hospitalized patients. Infect Control Hosp Epidemiol 2008;29:815–9.

183. Saint S, Kaufman SR, Thompson M, et al. A reminder reduces urinary catheterization in hospitalized patients. Jt Comm J Qual Patient Saf 2005;31:455–62.

184. Huang WC, Wann SR, Lin SL, et al. Catheter-associated urinary tract infections in intensive care units can be reduced by prompting physicians to remove unnecessary catheters. Infect Control Hosp Epidemiol 2004;25:974–8.

185. Cornia PB, Amory JK, Fraser S, et al. Computer-based order entry decreases duration of indwelling urinary catheterization in hospitalized patients. Am J Med 2003;114:404–7.

186. Meddings J, Rogers MA, Macy M, et al. Systematic review and metaanalysis: reminder systems to reduce catheter-associated urinary tract infections and urinary catheter use in hospitalized patients. Clin Infect Dis 2010;51:550–60.

187. Wright MO, Kharasch M, Beaumont JL, et al. Reporting catheter-associated urinary tract infections: denominator matters. Infect Control Hosp Epidemiol 2011; 32:635–40.

188. Niel-Weise BS, van den Broek PJ. Urinary catheter policies for short-term bladder drainage in adults. Cochrane Database Syst Rev 2005;(3):CD004203.

189. Stevens E. Bladder ultrasound: avoiding unnecessary catheterizations. Medsurg Nurs 2005;14:249–53.

190. Saint S, Kaufman SR, Rogers MA, et al. Condom versus indwelling urinary catheters: a randomized trial. J Am Geriatr Soc 2006;54:1055–61.

191. Saint S, Lipsky BA, Baker PD, et al. Urinary catheters: what type do men and their nurses prefer? J Am Geriatr Soc 1999;47:1453–7.

192. Pratt RJ, Pellowe C, Loveday HP, et al. Guidelines for preventing infections associated with the insertion and management of short term indwelling urethral catheters in acute care. J Hosp Infect 2001;47(Suppl):S39–46.

Resistant Pathogens, Fungi, and Viruses

Christopher A. Guidry, MD[a,1], Sara A. Mansfield, MD[b,1], Robert G. Sawyer, MD[a], Charles H. Cook, MD[c,*]

KEYWORDS

- Surgery • Resistance • Bacteria • Fungi • Viruses

KEY POINTS

- The complexity of patients managed by surgeons continues to increase. With this complexity comes the unique host susceptibility to infections with microbes that were unknown pathogens even 50 years ago, including antimicrobial-resistant bacteria, fungi, and viruses.
- Although most surgeons will not primarily manage these organisms, it will be important for them to maintain a working knowledge of them to be able to provide optimum care for their most vulnerable patients.

RESISTANT PATHOGENS AND FUNGI

Introduction

Infections of all kinds are an unfortunate and common condition among the surgical population. Management of these infections often requires multiple treatment modalities but usually involves some form of antimicrobial therapy. Over the years, antimicrobial resistance has become increasingly common across a wide range of pathogens. This section discusses some of the more common resistant pathogens the surgeon is likely to encounter.

Disclosure Statement: The authors have no conflicts of interest to report.
Funding: The National Institutes of Health Awards T32-AI078875, T32-CA090223 & RO1-GM 066115 supported research reported in this publication. The content is solely the responsibility of the authors and does not necessarily represent the official views of the National Institutes of Health.
[a] Division of Acute Care Surgery and Outcomes Research, Department of Surgery, University of Virginia, Charlottesville, VA 22908, USA; [b] Division of Trauma, Critical Care, and Burn, Department of Surgery, The Ohio State University College of Medicine, Columbus, OH 43210, USA; [c] Division of Acute Care Surgery, Trauma and Surgical Critical Care, Department of Surgery, Beth Israel Deaconess Medical Center, Harvard Medical School, 110 Francis Street, Lowry 2G, Boston, MA 02215, USA
[1] The first 2 authors contributed equally to the article.
* Corresponding author.
E-mail address: chcook@bidmc.harvard.edu

Hospital-Associated Methicillin-Resistant Staphylococcus aureus

Staphylococcus aureus is the most commonly isolated bacterial pathogen.[1] It is therefore not surprising that methicillin-resistant *Staphylococcus aureus* (both community-acquired [CA-MRSA] and hospital-acquired [HA-MRSA]) is one of the most common resistant pathogens encountered by surgeons. Since its discovery in 1960, the incidence of nosocomial infection caused by MRSA has increased steadily. Today, *S aureus* is the predominate isolate in intensive care units (ICUs) in the United States.[2] Resistance to methicillin, and other β-lactams, results from the acquisition of the *mec*A gene cassette, which modifies the penicillin-binding protein in the cell wall.[3]

Risk factors for hospital-acquired methicillin-resistant S aureus

- Any of the following within the last year[1,4]:
  ○ Hospitalization
  ○ Surgery
  ○ Intubation
  ○ Dialysis
  ○ Residence in long-term care facility
- Indwelling catheter or other percutaneous device
- Prior exposure to antibiotics
- Prior history of MRSA infection
- Pressure ulcer
- Colonization

The clinical spectrum of all MRSA infections ranges from asymptomatic colonization to severe invasive disease. Compared with CA-MRSA, HA-MRSA is less likely to cause skin and soft-tissue infections (SSTI). SSTI accounts for only 37% of HA-MRSA infections.[4] Uncomplicated abscesses 5 cm or less in diameter may be managed with incision and drainage alone. However, systemic signs or evidence of invasive disease such as cellulitis, pneumonia, endocarditis, and bone or joint infection require systemic antibiotics. Vancomycin is the empiric treatment of choice if MRSA is suspected. Other agents such as linezolid, daptomycin, quinupristin/dalfopristin, and tigecycline may also be considered.[4] Local susceptibility patterns should be reviewed when choosing the appropriate antibiotic. A recent study surprisingly demonstrated no difference in outcomes between hospital-associated and community-associated MRSA infections.[5]

Although the prevalence of MRSA colonization varies widely in the literature, it is an important risk factor for subsequent clinical MRSA infection.[6–9] In a recent study, 40% of all patients with a clinical MRSA infection were known to be previously colonized within the prior 1-year period.[9] Efforts to decolonize patients of MRSA, particularly on admission or before surgery, have met with some success.[10–15] These strategies typically consist of chlorhexidine bathing or intranasal mupirocin either alone or in combination. A recent multicenter randomized trial demonstrated a marked decline in clinical MRSA infections after the implementation of a universal decolonization strategy for ICU patients.[15]

Community-Associated Methicillin-Resistant S aureus

In the early 1990s, reports began to emerge of infections caused by MRSA in populations that did not exhibit traditional risk factors for MRSA colonization or infection. Typically, these patients were younger and healthier than the usual population susceptible to MRSA.[1] Eventually these infections were identified as a new strain of MRSA, dubbed CA-MRSA. CA-MRSA varies molecularly from HA-MRSA by having a smaller *mec* chromosomal cassette (type IV or V compared with I, II, or III for HA-MRSA).[1,16,17] In the United States, USA300 and USA400 are the dominant clonal isolates, with USA300 being the most common.[18] Despite its name, CA-MRSA is often encountered in the hospital setting. One recent study demonstrated that 52% of all MRSA isolates from the ICU were CA-MRSA.[19]

CA-MRSA has become an increasingly common pathogen; however, evaluating its true epidemiology is difficult given inconsistencies in the definition.[20] The definition by the Centers for Disease Control and Prevention (CDC) underestimates the proportion of CA-MRSA in the population. Genetic testing is not routinely performed, and is therefore not practical in defining CA-MRSA for the average physician. Others advocate a practical definition based on either temporal patterns or antimicrobial suscep-tibility.[1] The authors suggest using all of these factors in evaluating patients for potential CA-MRSA infection.

Various definitions of community-acquired methicillin-resistant S aureus

CDC definition[1]:
- Outpatient diagnosis
- Diagnosis within 48 hours of admission if no other risk factors for HA-MRSA (see the section on HA-MRSA)

Temporal definition:
- Outpatient diagnosis
- Diagnosis within 48 hours of admission

Antimicrobial susceptibility definition:
- No or limited resistance to non-β-lactam antimicrobials (particularly clindamycin)

Risk factors for community-acquired methicillin-resistant S aureus infection

- Children (neonates in particular)[1,4,9]
- Adults age 65 years or older
- Women (pregnant and postpartum)
- Athletes
- Household contacts of MRSA SSTI patients
- Emergency department patients
- Urban and/or low socioeconomic status
- Indigenous populations
- Populations living in close proximity (military, jail, or prison)
- Cystic fibrosis patients
- Men who have sex with men (MSM)
- Human immunodeficiency virus (HIV) patients
- Veterinarians, livestock handlers, and pet owners
- History of endocarditis
- Antibiotic exposure within the last year
- Chronic skin disorder
- Tobacco use
- Tattoo recipients

SSTI represent 90% of CA-MRSA infections.[21] Typically these infections present as a superficial abscess often mistaken for a spider bite. The presence of an abscess with surrounding erythema with a central black eschar is 94% predictive of some form of MRSA isolate. Unfortunately, CA-MRSA cannot be distinguished from HA-MRSA, methicillin-sensitive *S aureus*, or other causes of SSTI on physical characteristics alone.[1] However, one study of 137 patients presenting with cellulitis identified the presence of abscesses (odds ratio [OR] 2.7; 95% confidence interval [CI] 1.3–5.8) and a body mass index greater than 30 kg/m^2 (OR 2.3; 95% CI 1.1–5.0) to be independently associated with the presence of CA-MRSA.

Uncomplicated SSTI, presenting as an abscess (without systemic signs), may be managed with incision and drainage alone.[1,17] If antibiotics are indicated (cellulitis), clindamycin or trimethoprim-sulfamethoxazole (TMP-SMX) are the empiric antibiotics of choice, because USA300 is typically sensitive to these antimicrobials.[17,18] However, as clindamycin use has increased, so has clindamycin resistance.[17] Doxycycline and minocycline may also be considered. Linezolid is also an effective choice but is limited by its high cost.[1] Resistance to fluoroquinolones (particularly ciprofloxacin) may be high in certain populations (MSM).[4,18] Caution should be urged when choosing antimicrobials for cellulitis, as doxycycline and TMP-SMX may not be effective against group A streptococci.[17] Local susceptibility patterns should always be considered when selecting appropriate antimicrobials.

Invasive infections, particularly pneumonia, can be rapidly fatal (mortality 50%–63%). Patients with necrotizing CA-MRSA pneumonia present with hemoptysis, leukopenia, high fever, and cavitary lung lesions.[22] These patients have an OR of dying of 11.3 (95% CI 5.6–23) compared with other severe CA-MRSA infections.[1,23] One study reported a 56% mortality rate for CA-MRSA pneumonia with a median age of 14.5 years.[1,24]

Regardless of the site of infection, vancomycin remains the mainstay of severe MRSA-related infections. Linezolid may be considered in cases of a high vancomycin minimum inhibitory concentration (MIC), whereas clindamycin may be considered (for CA-MRSA only) as an adjunctive antimicrobial to reduce toxin production. Linezolid may also be considered in necrotizing CA-MRSA pneumonia given the relatively low lung penetration of vancomycin.[1]

Vancomycin-Resistant Enterococcus spp

Enterococcus faecalis and *Enterococcus faecium* are a normal part of human intestinal flora. Combined, these account for most *Enterococcus* infections in humans. These pathogens are notoriously difficult to treat, as they are intrinsically resistant to most penicillins, cephalosporins, and TMP-SMX. Furthermore, they easily acquire resistance to many other antibiotic classes. Whereas some strains of *E faecalis* may be susceptible to some penicillins, cephalosporins, and fluoroquinolones, this is not the case for *E faecium*. Resistance to vancomycin is mediated through the acquisition of a group of genes collectively known as the *van* gene complex. These genes encode an alteration in the cell wall with reduced affinity for vancomycin.[25]

Risk factors for vancomycin-resistant Enterococcus spp infection

- VRE colonization, generally required for infection[25,26]
- Advanced age
- Severe underlying illness
- Interhospital transfer
- Residence in long-term care facility
- Nutritional support (total parenteral nutrition [TPN])
- Central venous catheterization
- Hematologic malignancies
- Surgery for inflammatory bowel disease
- Biliary tract or liver abnormality
- Transplant patients
- Hemodialysis

- Previous antibiotic exposure, particularly:
  - Vancomycin
  - Third-generation cephalosporins
  - Antianaerobic antibiotics (metronidazole)
  - Antibiotic combinations
  - Long-term antibiotic use

Colonized patients develop VRE infections that are similar in scope to vancomycin-susceptible isolates: intra-abdominal, skin and soft tissue, urinary tract, bloodstream, and endocarditis. VRE pneumonia or central nervous system infections are rare.[25] Approximately 8% of colonized patients develop a VRE infection either during or shortly after hospital admission.[26] The associated mortality for these infections remains high (13%–46%).[27]

Linezolid or daptomycin are the drugs of choice for most VRE infections. Daptomycin's rapid bactericidal activity makes it the preferred agent in bloodstream infections and endocarditis. Some strains of *E faecalis* may be susceptible to ampicillin or pipericillin, but this is becoming uncommon. Quinupristin/dalfopristin has some use against *E faecium* only.[25,28] Resistance to linezolid has been reported and is an emerging problem.[28]

Susceptible patients while undergoing medical care easily acquire VRE. A recent study found that 12.3% of patients who were initially VRE negative were colonized before leaving the ICU.[29] VRE transmission often occurs via health care workers, and once acquired may be lifelong. Therefore, methods to reduce transmission such as active screening and isolation have been instituted in some locations. Screening and isolation for VRE-positive patients, however, remains controversial, with no consensus criteria for the removal of patients from isolation.[25]

Extended-Spectrum β-Lactamase–Producing Bacteria

Many organisms have acquired, either through point mutation or plasmid acquisition, the ability to produce a group of enzymes collectively known as extended-spectrum β-lactamases (ESBL). Carbapenem-resistant Enterobacteriaceae (CRE; see later discussion) actually represent a special case of this phenomenon. These enzymes were originally described as a point mutation in the classic TEM and SHV β-lactamases, thereby conferring expanded activity. Soon other plasmid mediated ESBL enzymes were also discovered. Unlike CRE, ESBL enzymes are not limited to the Enterobacteriaceae family and are commonly found in *Pseudomonas* species. In 2007, a survey identified that up to 17% of *Klebsiella pneumoniae* and 10% of *Escherichia coli* demonstrated ESBL activity. Most of these (65%) produce members of the CTX-M class of β-lactamases.[30]

ESBL transmission between pathogens generally occurs via a large plasmid, which often encodes resistance to other antibiotic classes, particularly fluoroquinolones, aminoglycosides, and TMP-SMX. The high likelihood of concomitant resistance among ESBL-producing pathogens limits therapeutic options. For this reason cephalosporins, fluoroquinolones, and TMP-SMX are not appropriate options for treating most ESBL infections. Unless CRE is suspected, carbapenems remain the antibiotic class of choice for treating these infections.[30,31] Although the data are limited, β-lactam/β-lactamase inhibitor combinations, such as pipericillin/tazobactam, have also demonstrated efficacy in treating these infections, particularly in the urinary tract.[30–32] Among the β-lactamase inhibitors, tazobactam is the most potent and is active against many ESBL classes (TEM, SHV, and CTX-M).[30] Tigecycline, colistin, and fosfomycin are additional therapeutic options.[30,32] The wide range of ESBL activities, along with associated resistances, highlight the need to perform appropriate antibiotic sensitivity assays, and to consult local antibiotic susceptibility patterns when choosing the appropriate therapeutic agent.

Carbapenem-Resistant Enterobacteriaceae

Enterobacteriaceae is a large family of gram-negative rods that contains many common human pathogens, including *E coli*, *Klebsiella* species, *Enterobacter* species, and more than 70 other genera. Resistance to many broad-spectrum antibiotics is common among members of this family, and until recently physicians could depend on the carbapenem antimicrobial class to reliably treat these pathogens. However, since 2000 carbapenem resistance has been growing. While still uncommon, the percentage of Enterobacteriaceae in the United States that were CRE increased from 1.2% in 2001% to 4.2% in 2011. The largest increase was among *Klebsiella* species, particularly *K pneumoniae*.[33] Another report describes carbapenem resistance in *E coli* at 4.0% and at 10.8% among *K pneumoniae*.[34]

CRE produce ESBL with the largest spectrum of activity. Unlike MRSA or VRE, carbapenem resistance is not mediated by a single set of genes within a single species. Instead, CRE is mediated through multiple plasmid-encoded enzymes across an entire family of organisms.[33,35] The most common resistance gene is the highly transmissible *K pneumoniae* carbapenemase (*kpc*), so named because of its initial discovery in that species.[33] The metallo-β-lactamases (MBL) VIM (Verona integrin-encoded MBL) and IMP (active on imipenem) are also common.[34]

Risk factors for carbapenem-resistant enterobacteriaceae

- Advanced age[35,36]
- ICU stay in previous 3 months
- Central venous catheterization
- Receipt of antibiotics (particularly fluoroquinolones) in previous 3 months
- Diabetes mellitus
- Recent invasive procedure in the last 6 months
- Isolation of resistant bacteria in previous 6 months
- Dependent functional status
- Permanent residency in institution
- Charlson comorbidity index greater than or equal to 3

CRE infection and colonization have been managed with strict cohorting and isolation.[37] A recent study suggests that, unlike VRE, asymptomatic colonization may not be lifelong. This study found that at 1 year following the index admission with CRE, only 39% of patients remained positive. A lack of hospitalization during this time increased the likelihood of becoming CRE negative.[38]

CRE infections carry a high mortality rate of between 40% and 50%, which is increased to 72% in CRE bloodstream infections.[33,39] The current mainstays of treatment include colistin, tigecycline, and aminoglycosides. Fosfomycin and polymyxin are additional options. Some investigators advocate prolonged profusion carbapenem or double carbapenem therapy for CRE with an MIC less than or equal to 4 mg/L.[39]

Candida

Candida species are the most common invasive fungal pathogens in humans. It is the third most common cause of infection overall and is the second most common pathogen in North American ICUs.[40] Although *Candida albicans* remains the most common individual isolate in the United States and Canada, non-*albicans* species make up 57.1% of all cases of candidemia.[40] When all forms of candidiasis are considered, including hair, skin, and nail infections, *C albicans* is the causative pathogen in 80% of cases.[41] The incidence of invasive candidiasis is increasing. Between 2003 and 2005, the incidence of candidemia increased from 3.65 to 5.56 per 100,000 persons.[42]

Risk factors for invasive candidiasis

- Colonization of several body sites[40–42]
- Extremes of age
- Exposure to broad-spectrum antibiotics
- Immunocompromised
  - Cytotoxic chemotherapy
  - Corticosteroids
  - Transplant
  - Neutropenia
  - HIV
- Disruption of the physiologic barriers of the gastrointestinal tract
- Major abdominal surgery
- Other surgery during hospitalization
- Surgery on the urinary system in the setting of candiduria
- Major trauma (Injury Severity Score >20)
- APACHE II score greater than 20
- Candiduria greater than 10^5 cfu/mL
- Diabetes
- Hemodialysis
- Mechanical ventilation
- Central venous catheterization
- Enterocutaneous fistula
- TPN
- ICU stay longer than 7 days
- Multiple transfusions

Colonization by *Candida* species is a key risk factor for invasive candidiasis. Alteration of normal host flora via broad-spectrum antibiotic exposure allows for fungal overgrowth. Increasing burden of *Candida* as demonstrated by semiquantitative cultures from multiple sites at multiple time points has been associated with the development of invasive candidiasis. Some view the identification of Candida from more than 2 body sites as a justification for antifungal therapy.[42] Eggimann and colleagues[43] describe criteria for "preemptive" antifungal therapy as substantial colonization in the presence of multiple risk factors. Likewise, "prophylactic" antifungal therapy is justified for certain subgroups at particularly high risk for infection: organ transplant recipients or immunocompromised patients with expected or long-term neutropenia.

Selective pressure from the frequent use of prophylactic fluconazole has contributed to the increase in azole-resistant *Candida* species, particularly *Candida glabrata* and *Candida krusei*.[40,42,44] *C glabrata* is the most common of the non-*albicans* species and tends to occur in patients with prior antifungal therapy, older patients, and transplant recipients (both solid organ and hematopoietic stem cell transplants). It is uncommon in younger patients and neonates.[40,41] Risk factors for *Candida parapsilosis* infection include recent surgery, younger age, transplant patients, and those receiving TPN. It is also a frequent pathogen in the neonatal ICU.[40,41] *Candida tropicalis* is common in patients with hematologic malignancies and neutropenia.[40,41]

Most patients with *C krusei* candidemia have had prior antifungal exposure, are neutropenic, or have received a hematopoietic stem cell transplant.[40]

Overall, mortality following fungal infection remains high but varies somewhat based on the individual pathogen. Ninety-day mortality following candidemia ranged from 30% for *C parapsilosis* to 46.4% for *C krusei*.[40] Overall mortality for invasive candidiasis ranges between 40% and 60%, but can be as high as 80% in selected populations (immunocompromised).[42,43]

Azole class antifungals, particularly fluconazole, are the most commonly prescribed antifungals in the surgical population. This usage is probably appropriate in many cases, particularly for proven *C albicans* infection or empirically in an otherwise low-risk patient. However, in critically ill patients or those with previous azole exposure, echinocandins (caspofungin, micafungin, anidulafungin) should be considered first-line agents. Amphotericin B is another option for azole-resistant strains but comes with a significant side-effect profile. Lipid formulations have lowered, but not eliminated, the risks of nephrotoxicity and infusion-related reactions. Therefore, amphotericin B should be reserved for salvage therapy.[45]

VIRUSES
Human Herpes Viruses in Surgical Patients

Introduction to human herpes viruses
There are 8 human herpes viruses (HHV), including herpes simplex virus 1 (HSV-1/ HHV-1), herpes simplex 2 (HSV-2/HHV-2), varicella zoster virus (VZV/HHV-3), Epstein-Barr virus (EBV/HHV-4), cytomegalovirus (CMV/HHV-5), roseola virus (HHV-6 and HHV-7), and Kaposi sarcoma–associated virus (KSHV/HHV-8). As summarized in (**Table 1**), these viruses are highly prevalent in humans.[46–51] These viruses share a similar life cycle of primary infection, often inducing mononucleosis or flu-like symptoms, followed by control and disease resolution in immune-competent hosts. Following resolution these viruses then enter a state of latency, characterized as relative dormancy with little if any appreciable viral replication during most of the host's life. Although these viruses are known to reactivate in immunosuppressed individuals, sometimes causing devastating disease, until recently little attention has been given to these viruses in immune-competent hosts. During the last 3 decades, there has been increasing awareness of reactivation of latent herpes viruses in immune-competent hosts with surgical disease.

Latency and reactivation
To better understand reactivation, it is important to first define latency. In general, herpes viruses become quiescent after infection, with viral DNA present in host cells with very little (if any) transcriptional activity. Such latency seems to be maintained by a combination of host immunity and epigenetic regulation. Following primary infections, the host mounts concomitant innate and adaptive immune responses to control viral spread, but control typically occurs well after full dissemination of virus to its target cells/tissues. Thus, in addition to inducing nonspecific innate antiviral responses, all HHV induce epitope-specific immunoglobulin and CD4/CD8 T-cell responses. It must be borne in mind that most of what is known about latency and reactivation mechanisms comes from animal models of CMV and HSV, with less known about VZV, EBV, or HHV-6/-7/-8 because of a lack of good animal models for these infections.

The importance of epigenetics in herpesvirus latency is becoming increasingly clear. Herpesvirus DNA are not typically integrated into host DNA, but are maintained as episomes in infected cells. Like other eukaryotic DNA, HHV-DNA become wrapped

Table 1
Overview and epidemiology of herpes viruses

Common Name	Formal Name	Prevalence (%)	Primary Targets	Transmission	Sites of Latency	Primary Disease
Herpes simplex virus 1	HHV-1	50–80	Mucoepithelia	Oropharyngeal contact	Sensory and cranial nerve ganglia	Cold sores
Herpes simplex virus 2	HHV-2	20–25	Mucoepithelia	Sexual contact, congenital	Sensory nerve ganglia	Genital lesions
Varicella zoster virus	HHV-3	>90 (prevaccine)	Mucoepithelia	Airborne	Dorsal root ganglia	Chicken pox
Epstein-Barr virus	HHV-4	95	Epithelial, oral lymphoid cells	Saliva	B lymphocytes	Infectious mononucleosis
Cytomegalovirus	HHV-5	50–80	Monocytes, lymphocytes, and epithelia	Saliva, sexual contact, congenital, blood transfusions, transplant	Monocytes, lymphocytes	Asymptomatic, mononucleosis-like symptoms
Roseola virus	HHV-6, HHV-7	100	T cells	Saliva	Various leukocytes	Asymptomatic (90%), roseola infantum (10%)
Kaposi sarcoma–associated virus	HHV-8	Varies	Lymphocytes and epithelia	Sexual contact, saliva	B cells	Asymptomatic, oncogenic in immunosuppressed

around histone proteins in a repeating nucleosome pattern (reviewed in Ref.[52]). This process leaves most of the viral genomes inaccessible to transcription and replication. It is clear that most viral genomes in host tissues are thereby epigenetically regulated and are quiescent at any given time.[53–55] This "chromatinization" of viral DNA occurs very rapidly after infection, thereby contributing to development of latency.[56]

Most likely as a viral survival advantage, this epigenetic regulation can be interrupted, leading to localized reactivation events.[57] Such reactivation events likely lead to transient viral replication and shedding, thus allowing perpetuation of virus within communities. In immune-competent hosts, however, these reactivation episodes are quickly controlled by memory T-cell and B-cell responses, leading to resumption of latency. By contrast, hosts with impaired immunity often have reactivation episodes that progress to viral disease, with shedding and transmission of live virus. Unlike HHV with cutaneous manifestations, such as HSV-1/-2 and VZV, whose reactivation episodes are obvious, it is unknown how frequently the other HHV may reactivate in immune-competent hosts. It does seem clear, however, that transient compromise in host immunity will allow transcriptional reactivation of these viruses.[58,59] For the purposes of this article, immune-competent hosts are defined as those not undergoing canonical immune suppression or that have disease-related immune compromise (such as AIDS), understanding that following surgery, trauma, or critical illness there may well be transient compromise in host immunity.[60]

Diagnosis of human herpes virus infection/reactivation

One of the major obstacles in our understanding of HHV infection and reactivation is that with the exception of HSV and VZV, there are no cutaneous manifestations of reactivation. For most, it is difficult not to notice a perioral cold sore, or the painful outbreak of VZV/HHV-3 in the form of herpes zoster, making diagnosis of reactivation episodes for these viruses a simple matter. The other herpes viruses do not typically have cutaneous manifestations, thus requiring serologic or tissue diagnosis. Before the introduction of the monospot test, Paul-Bunnell testing for EBV infection was the method used to detect EBV-associated infectious mononucleosis.[61] Although immune-globulin monitoring remains one of the best ways to diagnose acute or previous HHV infection, for monitoring/diagnosing reactivation it has far less accuracy and utility. Immune-globulin monitoring has therefore been mostly replaced by DNA-based molecular methods to diagnose HHV reactivation in immune-competent hosts.

Triggers of human herpes virus reactivation

There are myriad triggers for reactivation of latent HHV, and one of the best studied in healthy hosts is stress. Glaser and colleagues[62] were among the first to show that the social stress during academic examinations can induce reactivation of HHV in healthy medical students. These findings were supported further by an animal model of HSV-1/HHV-1 reactivation following social stress.[63] Certainly among the most healthy immune-competent hosts are astronauts, and numerous studies have shown that preflight stress and the stress of spaceflight can stimulate reactivation of CMV, HSV, VZV, and EBV.[64–67] It should therefore come as no surprise in the sections that follow that more aggressive stressors, such as surgical disease or infections that induce critical illness, are also triggers for viral reactivation.

Human herpes viruses following cardiac surgery Herpes viruses were first associated with surgical disease in immune-competent patients in the late 1950s. Battele and Hewlett, and subsequently others, described a peculiar viral illness that befell 4% to 30% of patients undergoing cardiac surgery with extracorporeal bypass.[68–73] These cases usually occurred 3 to 6 weeks after surgery and had symptoms consistent with viral mononucleosis, but most were EBV negative (by Paul-Bunnell testing). Ultimately, Kääriäinen and colleagues[74] made the first connection between these febrile illnesses and CMV, and it was later concluded that many cases were likely a consequence of blood transfusion practices during extracorporeal circulation in that era. Because of limitations in diagnostics at that time, it remained unclear whether postpump CMV was a primary infection or reactivation of latent virus, until later work suggested that most were reactivations.[75]

The consequences of CMV reactivation in patients undergoing cardiac surgery remain unclear. Although the early observations of CMV activity were not linked with worsened outcomes, later work in patients with complications after cardiac surgery suggested otherwise.[76] It was observed that patients with CMV infection concomitant to bacterial infections often had far worse outcomes.[77] For example, in patients with mediastinitis following cardiac surgery, CMV viremia or viruria was associated with higher mortality and impaired clearance of local infection.[76] This finding was hypothesized to be related to impaired neutrophil function.[78] Likewise, Rand and Merigan[79] observed that mice given primary CMV plus bacterial infection had experienced 80% to 100% mortality, compared with none in control groups.

Less is known about EBV-associated and HSV-associated disease in cardiac surgery. VZV has been reported to reactivate as herpes zoster following cardiac surgeries.[80–82] Prompt diagnosis and treatment is important, as misdiagnosis can lead to short-term and long-term pain control issues or other related sequelae.

HHV have also been associated with other cardiac diseases. CMV viremia correlates with disease severity in patients admitted with acute heart failure ($P<.001$), and this is thought to be secondary to the proinflammatory state associated with progression of heart failure.[83] HHV have also been implicated in atherosclerosis, and biopsy of the major arteries in young trauma patients identified HSV and CMV in atherosclerotic lesions and foam cells of the intimal layer.[84,85] Acute infection with CMV in rats causes endothelial injury,[86] and some have postulated that this contributes to hypertension.[87] Later studies evaluating mechanisms indicate that presence of lifelong, latent herpes viruses in atherosclerotic plaque may exert pathogenic effects by penetrating the arterial wall, modifying lipid metabolism, and stimulating the production of proinflammatory cytokines and growth factors.[88]

Human herpes viruses after trauma/burn injury   Although HHV have likely been reactivating in humans since their acquaintance hundreds of thousands of years ago,[89] description of reactivation events did not become common until the twentieth century. It is perhaps not surprising that the first described trauma-associated HHV reactivation was a case of VZV/HHV-3 herpes zoster, although its association with a lightning strike makes somewhat remarkable.[90] The association between herpes zoster and trauma has been subsequently elaborated in case reports and series, and was recently confirmed in a large case-control study of Medicare patients.[91] The first report of CMV/HHV-5 related to trauma followed some years after recognition of CMV reactivation in patients undergoing cardiac surgery, and occurred in a man who died of disseminated CMV disease following severe facial fractures.[92] Soon after this, the first case of HSV/HHV-1 was reported after oral trauma.[93] It was several years later that the first confirmed case of EBV/HHV-4 was reported in a patient who had suffered trauma requiring splenectomy and transfusions.[94]

HHVs also have a long-standing association with burn injury, beginning with the observations of systemic CMV[95] and herpes simplex activity in burn wounds.[95] Some years later other reports emerged describing CMV infections in patients with burn injuries.[96–98] Subsequent studies suggested high rates of reactivation (>50%) in addition to primary infections (12%–15%) following burn injury.[99,100] Major burns have subsequently been shown to be one of the strongest CMV reactivation stimuli in humans, with incidence as high as approximately 70%.[101,102] There are only case reports of VZV in adult burn patients,[103] and pediatric burn patients with primary VZV have higher likelihoods for pneumonitis.[104] It seems that the editors of the *British Medical Journal* were prescient when they observed that "…there seems to be at least as much for virologists to do in the surgical wards as in the medical ones."[105] Unfortunately, at least for burns, little attention is being paid in the United States to this entity.[106]

This lack of attention may be because it is unclear what impact HHV may have on outcomes in burns. Reactivation of CMV in burn patients has not been associated with worsened mortality,[98,99,107] although it has been associated with longer ICU stays and duration of mechanical ventilation.[101] Primary infection in burn patients is also of concern, as CMV can be detected in cadaveric skin grafts[108] and transmission by seropositive skin grafts can cause severe disease.[109] Cutaneous HSV reactivation, seen in up to 25% of burns, presents 1 to 3 weeks postburn as a cluster of vesicles around the margins of a healing burn.[110] Areas of active epidermal regeneration appear to be the most commonly affected,[100] but progression to visceral HSV involvement has been described, manifesting as necrotizing adrenal and hepatic lesions.[95] HSV reactivation of the respiratory tract is seen in up to 50% of burn patients.[110,111] The impact of pulmonary HSV reactivation on mortality has been mixed, with larger prospective studies still needed.[107,112,113]

Human herpes viruses in critical care/sepsis Similarly to trauma patients, there have been numerous reports of HHV eruptions/cutaneous manifestations during critical illness, but those HHVs without obvious outward signs have taken much longer to recognize as an entity. During the mid- to late 1990s, several different investigators began reporting herpesvirus infections/reactivations in previously immune-competent patients during critical illness. These first reports included both HSV and CMV, and since then more limited work has evaluated the other viruses in the herpes family during critical illness. There is a growing body of knowledge in this area that includes both medical and surgical patients, and the use of animal models has contributed significantly to our understanding of mechanisms and consequences of such reactivation events. Although it has not been confirmed for all HHV, because of the similarities in infection, control, and development of latency between the HHVs, it seems likely that each HHV follows a pattern of reactivation similar to that of CMV. The following paragraphs review each of the viruses in the herpes family and their associations with critical illness in previously immune-competent patients.

It has become clear that CMV can reactivate during critical illness, with sensitive polymerase chain reaction–based methods showing that approximately one-third of latently infected patients have CMV reactivation during critical illness.[114] These reactivation events can lead to live virus shed in the blood and pulmonary secretions of affected hosts.[115,116] It seems likely that these reactivation events are consequent to inflammatory insults that trigger the release of cytokines, epigenetic deregulation of viral genomes, and, possibly, immune compromise.[58,67,117–119] It remains unclear, however, whether CMV is a true pathogen or merely an indicator of severity of illness. When considering all of the currently available studies,[76,101,115,116,120–129] reactivation is associated with roughly doubled risks of hospital mortality and duration of mechanical ventilation (**Fig. 1**). When one considers the potential pathogenic mechanisms associated with CMV, including pulmonary injury[117] and immune modulation,[130] the

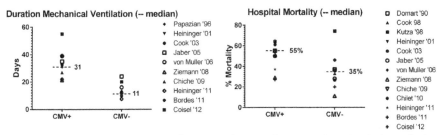

Fig. 1. Summary of clinical studies of cytomegalovirus: duration of mechanical ventilation and hospital mortality. *Data from* Refs.[76,101,115,116,120–129]

possibility that CMV actually contributes to poor outcomes in immune-competent patients is intriguing.

HSV-1/HHV-1 is the second best studied HHV that reactivates during critical illness. In mechanically ventilated patients, HSV-1 can be detected in tracheal aspirates and lower respiratory tract secretions of ICU patients in 22% to 54% and 16% to 32% of cases, respectively.[131] However, this is confused by the observation that asymptomatic shedding of HSV can occur in up to 5% to 10% of healthy individuals.[132,133] Furthermore, HSV haplotypes isolated from lower respiratory tracts of intubated patients have been shown to be identical to those isolated from the oropharynx, suggesting possible spread down the tracheobronchial tree through secretions.[134] The lack of association of HSV reactivation with worsened outcomes in numerous studies casts further doubt on its importance as a possible pathogen.[116,128,135–138] Nonetheless, there are reports that link HSV reactivation with prolonged mechanical ventilation,[136,138] prolonged ICU stays,[136] and even increased mortality.[131,139,140] One possible explanation is that viral load is important, as suggested by worsened mortality in patients with high viral loads.[141] For now, however, the preponderance of data suggests that HSV activity during critical illness is simply an indicator of disease severity.

To date there are very few data for the other HHV in critically ill patients. EBV has been thought to reactivate during times of stress as detected by elevated antibody levels, which has since been confirmed by data showing EBV reactivation in 61% of ICU patients.[142,143] The lack of in vivo models has impeded progress in understanding EBV reactivation, and therefore there are no published data on mechanisms or consequences of EBV reactivation in immune-competent hosts. Similarly there are very few data for VZV/HHV-3 and HHV-6/-7/-8 during critical illness. VZV has been reported following spinal surgery, but otherwise remains understudied in critically ill patients.[81,144–147] As with other HHV, aberrations in cell-mediated immunity are thought to be one of the causes of VZV reactivation.[148,149] HHV-6 and HHV-7 have been shown to reactivate during critical illness, but the consequence of this is unknown.[150] Finally, like CMV, KSHV/HHV-8 has been associated with lung disease (idiopathic pulmonary fibrosis), but has not yet been reported in critically ill immune-competent hosts.[151]

Human herpes viruses in gastrointestinal disease HHV can cause a variety of gastrointestinal diseases, many of which have surgical implications. One example is the relatively long-standing relationship between HHV and gastrointestinal ulcerative diseases in immunosuppressed HIV and transplant patients. It is now recognized that immune-competent trauma, critical care, and postoperative patients can also suffer from HHV-related intestinal ulceration. CMV, for example, can cause colonic mucosal ulceration sometimes leading to perforation in immune-competent hosts.[152–154]

Because this presentation can mimic other infectious colitides, CMV colitis should be considered when an infectious causes is suspected but cannot be identified. Severe inflammation and ulcerative lesions have primarily been noted in areas of predominant endothelial distribution of CMV inclusion bodies,[155] and ischemia from narrowing of the capillary circulation has been postulated in ulcer/perforation pathogenesis. CMV enteritis has been suggested to have higher mortality in immune-competent patients than in immune-compromised populations, possibly because of a lower index of suspicion.[156,157] Although CMV is a common cause of upper gastrointestinal ulceration in transplant and AIDS patients, it does not seem to play a meaningful role in immune-competent patients.[158] A diagnosis of HHV-associated ulceration can be made with endoscopic or surgical biopsy, but is often made in surgical specimens post hoc. Whether patients with perforation and subsequent diagnoses made by pathologic evaluation will benefit from antiviral treatment is unclear, and will require further study.

Another common disease recently associated with HHV is appendicitis. There has been a long-standing suspicion that non-HHV viral infections are associated with appendicitis, given its bimodal and seasonal occurrence.[158] The first described association of HHV with appendicitis was in an AIDS patient,[159] but a recent study of childhood appendicitis has shown periodic reactivation (21%) of CMV in lymphoid tissue of the appendix.[160] In this study, HHV-6 was also identified in approximately 8% of specimens. It is unclear whether this is a cause or simply a consequence of the appendicitis, given that sepsis can cause HHV reactivation.[161]

There is also a long-standing relationship between HHV/infectious mononucleosis and splenic disease. HHV have been known for many years to cause splenomegaly, which on occasion can lead to splenic rupture.[162] Spontaneous splenic rupture is less common in acute CMV infection than in EBV infection, despite one-third of acute CMV infections demonstrating splenomegaly.[163–165] By contrast, HHV infection after splenectomy likely represents a distinct clinicopathologic syndrome.[166] Acute CMV infection was first identified in postsplenectomy trauma patients in 1982.[167] Review of case reports shows that these infections typically occur within 2 to 4 weeks after splenectomy.[166–169] The syndrome likely results from poor control of early viremia because of the lack of both splenic function and the typical brisk immunoglobulin M response. Although it is difficult to determine acute versus reactivated CMV in these cases, one study using anti-CMV immunoglobulin G maturation indices supports acute infection in this syndrome.[170] These cases of widely disseminated postsplenectomy CMV can sometimes be fatal.[153]

Treatment of human herpes virus reactivation/infection

There are few data to support or refute treatment of HHV reactivation in surgical patients. While there are scattered reports of treatment in immune-competent patients, these all follow reactivation, likely suffer from selection bias, and perhaps not surprisingly show no benefit. The best available data come from animal models, showing that CMV reactivation events induced by sepsis can be prevented with antiviral therapy.[117,171] Unfortunately, antiviral treatment works best if administered prophylactically, which would require treating all patients, many of whom would never develop reactivation.[172] For now there are no good data to support treatment of critically ill patients with HHV reactivation outside of a clinical trial.[173] Fortunately, there is a randomized controlled trial evaluating ganciclovir for prevention of CMV reactivation and acute lung injury in immune-competent hosts (ClinicalTrials.gov #NCT01335932).

There are also no strong data for the treatment of other HHV reactivations in critical care populations. A randomized controlled trial showed that acyclovir treatment can prevent HSV reactivation, but seems to have no effect on survival or duration of mechanical ventilation.[174,175] Clinically severe or symptomatic cutaneous HSV or herpes zoster reactivations are usually treated with acyclovir once diagnosis is confirmed.[176] There are some concerns that delay in diagnosis and treatment of HSV may lead to systemic dissemination causing necrotizing hepatic and adrenal lesions, bacterial superinfection, and even death, although data supporting this are lacking.[97,177] There are no data to support or refute treatment of HHV-2, -4, -6, -7, or -8 during critical illness in immune-competent hosts.

SUMMARY

The complexity of patients managed by surgeons continues to increase. With this complexity comes the unique host susceptibility to infections with microbes that were unknown pathogens even 50 years ago, including antimicrobial-resistant bacteria, fungi, and viruses. Although most surgeons will not primarily manage these organisms, it will be important for them to maintain a working knowledge of them to be able to provide optimum care for their most vulnerable patients.

REFERENCES

1. David MZ, Daum RS. Community-associated methicillin-resistant *Staphylococcus aureus*: epidemiology and clinical consequences of an emerging epidemic. Clin Microbiol Rev 2010;23:616–87.
2. Boucher HW, Corey GR. Epidemiology of methicillin-resistant *Staphylococcus aureus*. Clin Infect Dis 2008;46(Suppl 5):S344–349.
3. Goyal N, Miller A, Tripathi M, et al. Methicillin-resistant *Staphylococcus aureus* (MRSA): colonisation and pre-operative screening. Bone Joint J 2013;95-B:4–9.
4. Hansra NK, Shinkai K. Cutaneous community-acquired and hospital-acquired methicillin-resistant *Staphylococcus aureus*. Dermatol Ther 2011;24:263–72.
5. Eells SJ, McKinnell JA, Wang AA, et al. A comparison of clinical outcomes between healthcare-associated infections due to community-associated methicillin-resistant *Staphylococcus aureus* strains and healthcare-associated methicillin-resistant S. aureus strains. Epidemiol Infect 2013;141:2140–8.
6. Jain R, Kralovic SM, Evans ME, et al. Veterans affairs initiative to prevent methicillin-resistant *Staphylococcus aureus* infections. N Engl J Med 2011;364:1419–30.
7. McKinnell JA, Huang SS, Eells SJ, et al. Quantifying the impact of extranasal testing of body sites for methicillin-resistant *Staphylococcus aureus* colonization at the time of hospital or intensive care unit admission. Infect Control Hosp Epidemiol 2013;34:161–70.
8. Edgeworth JD. Has decolonization played a central role in the decline in UK methicillin-resistant *Staphylococcus aureus* transmission? A focus on evidence from intensive care. J Antimicrob Chemother 2011;66(Suppl 2):ii41–47.
9. Otter JA, Herdman MT, Williams B, et al. Low prevalence of methicillin-resistant *Staphylococcus aureus* carriage at hospital admission: implications for risk-factor-based vs universal screening. J Hosp Infect 2013;83:114–21.
10. Kassakian SZ, Mermel LA, Jefferson JA, et al. Impact of chlorhexidine bathing on hospital-acquired infections among general medical patients. Infect Control Hosp Epidemiol 2011;32:238–43.
11. Rupp ME, Cavalieri RJ, Lyden E, et al. Effect of hospital-wide chlorhexidine patient bathing on healthcare-associated infections. Infect Control Hosp Epidemiol 2012;33:1094–100.

12. Climo MW, Yokoe DS, Warren DK, et al. Effect of daily chlorhexidine bathing on hospital-acquired infection. N Engl J Med 2013;368:533–42.

13. Evans HL, Dellit TH, Chan J, et al. Effect of chlorhexidine whole-body bathing on hospital-acquired infections among trauma patients. Arch Surg 2010;145: 240–6.

14. Ridenour G, Lampen R, Federspiel J, et al. Selective use of intranasal mupirocin and chlorhexidine bathing and the incidence of methicillin-resistant *Staphylococcus aureus* colonization and infection among intensive care unit patients. Infect Control Hosp Epidemiol 2007;28:1155–61.

15. Huang SS, Septimus E, Kleinman K, et al. Targeted versus universal decolonization to prevent ICU infection. N Engl J Med 2013;368:2255–65.

16. Maree CL, Daum RS, Boyle-Vavra S, et al. Community-associated methicillin-resistant *Staphylococcus aureus* isolates causing healthcare-associated infections. Emerg Infect Dis 2007;13:236–42.

17. Odell CA. Community-associated methicillin-resistant *Staphylococcus aureus* (CA-MRSA) skin infections. Curr Opin Pediatr 2010;22:273–7.

18. Chua K, Laurent F, Coombs G, et al. Antimicrobial resistance: not community-associated methicillin-resistant *Staphylococcus aureus* (CA-MRSA)! A clinician's guide to community MRSA—its evolving antimicrobial resistance and implications for therapy. Clin Infect Dis 2011;52:99–114.

19. Wang JT, Liao CH, Fang CT, et al. Incidence of and risk factors for community-associated methicillin-resistant *Staphylococcus aureus* acquired infection or colonization in intensive-care-unit patients. J Clin Microbiol 2010;48:4439–44.

20. Otter JA, French GL. Community-associated meticillin-resistant *Staphylococcus aureus*: the case for a genotypic definition. J Hosp Infect 2012;81:143–8.

21. Skov R, Christiansen K, Dancer SJ, et al. Update on the prevention and control of community-acquired methicillin-resistant *Staphylococcus aureus* (CA-MRSA). Int J Antimicrob Agents 2012;39:193–200.

22. Karampela I, Poulakou G, Dimopoulos G. Community acquired methicillin resistant *Staphylococcus aureus* pneumonia: an update for the emergency and intensive care physician. Minerva Anestesiol 2012;78:930–40.

23. Wiersma P, Tobin D'Angelo M, Daley WR, et al. Surveillance for severe community-associated methicillin-resistant *Staphylococcus aureus* infection. Epidemiol Infect 2009;137:1674–8.

24. Gillet Y, Vanhems P, Lina G, et al. Factors predicting mortality in necrotizing community-acquired pneumonia caused by *Staphylococcus aureus* containing Panton-Valentine leukocidin. Clin Infect Dis 2007;45:315–21.

25. Mazuski JE. Vancomycin-resistant enterococcus: risk factors, surveillance, infections, and treatment. Surg Infect (Larchmt) 2008;9:567–71.

26. Nguyen GC, Leung W, Weizman AV. Increased risk of vancomycin-resistant enterococcus (VRE) infection among patients hospitalized for inflammatory bowel disease in the United States. Inflamm Bowel Dis 2011;17:1338–42.

27. Whang DW, Miller LG, Partain NM, et al. Systematic review and meta-analysis of linezolid and daptomycin for treatment of vancomycin-resistant enterococcal bloodstream infections. Antimicrob Agents Chemother 2013;57:5013–8.

28. Napolitano LM. Emerging issues in the diagnosis and management of infections caused by multi-drug-resistant, gram-positive cocci. Surg Infect (Larchmt) 2005;6(Suppl 2):S-5–22.

29. Kim YJ, Kim SI, Kim YR, et al. Risk factors for vancomycin-resistant enterococci infection and mortality in colonized patients on intensive care unit admission. Am J Infect Control 2012;40:1018–9.

30. Kanj SS, Kanafani ZA. Current concepts in antimicrobial therapy against resistant gram-negative organisms: extended-spectrum beta-lactamase-producing Enterobacteriaceae, carbapenem-resistant Enterobacteriaceae, and multidrug-resistant *Pseudomonas aeruginosa.* Mayo Clin Proc 2011;86:250–9.
31. Vardakas KZ, Tansarli GS, Rafailidis PI, et al. Carbapenems versus alternative antibiotics for the treatment of bacteraemia due to Enterobacteriaceae producing extended-spectrum beta-lactamases: a systematic review and meta-analysis. J Antimicrob Chemother 2012;67:2793–803.
32. Pitout JD. Infections with extended-spectrum beta-lactamase-producing enterobacteriaceae: changing epidemiology and drug treatment choices. Drugs 2010;70:313–33.
33. Centers for Disease Control and Prevention (CDC). Vital signs: carbapenem-resistant Enterobacteriaceae. MMWR Morb Mortal Wkly Rep 2013;62:165–70.
34. Gupta N, Limbago BM, Patel JB, et al. Carbapenem-resistant Enterobacteriaceae: epidemiology and prevention. Clin Infect Dis 2011;53:60–7.
35. Schechner V, Kotlovsky T, Kazma M, et al. Asymptomatic rectal carriage of blaKPC producing carbapenem-resistant Enterobacteriaceae: who is prone to become clinically infected? Clin Microbiol Infect 2013;19:451–6.
36. Marchaim D, Chopra T, Bhargava A, et al. Recent exposure to antimicrobials and carbapenem-resistant Enterobacteriaceae: the role of antimicrobial stewardship. Infect Control Hosp Epidemiol 2012;33:817–30.
37. Rosenberger LH, Hranjec T, Politano AD, et al. Effective cohorting and "super-isolation" in a single intensive care unit in response to an outbreak of diverse multi-drug-resistant organisms. Surg Infect (Larchmt) 2011;12:345–50.
38. Zimmerman FS, Assous MV, Bdolah-Abram T, et al. Duration of carriage of carbapenem-resistant Enterobacteriaceae following hospital discharge. Am J Infect Control 2013;41:190–4.
39. van Duin D, Kaye KS, Neuner EA, et al. Carbapenem-resistant Enterobacteriaceae: a review of treatment and outcomes. Diagn Microbiol Infect Dis 2013;75:115–20.
40. Pfaller M, Neofytos D, Diekema D, et al. Epidemiology and outcomes of candidemia in 3648 patients: data from the Prospective Antifungal Therapy (PATH Alliance(R)) registry, 2004-2008. Diagn Microbiol Infect Dis 2012;74:323–31.
41. Silva S, Negri M, Henriques M, et al. *Candida glabrata, Candida parapsilosis* and *Candida tropicalis*: biology, epidemiology, pathogenicity and antifungal resistance. FEMS Microbiol Rev 2012;36:288–305.
42. Eggimann P, Bille J, Marchetti O. Diagnosis of invasive candidiasis in the ICU. Ann Intensive Care 2011;1:37.
43. Eggimann P, Garbino J, Pittet D. Management of Candida species infections in critically ill patients. Lancet Infect Dis 2003;3:772–85.
44. Gleason TG, May AK, Caparelli D, et al. Emerging evidence of selection of fluconazole-tolerant fungi in surgical intensive care units. Arch Surg 1997;132:1197–201.
45. Playford EG, Eggimann P, Calandra T. Antifungals in the ICU. Curr Opin Infect Dis 2008;21:610–9.
46. Whitley RJ, Roizman B. Herpes simplex virus infections. Lancet 2001;357:1513–8.
47. Stone RC, Micali GA, Schwartz RA. Roseola infantum and its causal human herpesviruses. Int J Dermatol 2014;53:397–403.

48. Butterly A, Schmidt U, Wiener-Kronish J. Methicillin-resistant *Staphylococcus aureus* colonization, its relationship to nosocomial infection, and efficacy of control methods. Anesthesiology 2010;113:1453–9.

49. Mesri EA, Cesarman E, Boshoff C. Kaposi's sarcoma and its associated herpesvirus. Nat Rev Cancer 2010;10:707–19.

50. Jenson HB. Epstein-Barr virus. Pediatr Rev 2011;32:375–83 [quiz: 384].

51. Cannon MJ, Schmid DS, Hyde TB. Review of cytomegalovirus seroprevalence and demographic characteristics associated with infection. Rev Med Virol 2010;20:202–13.

52. Bilimoria KY, Liu Y, Paruch JL, et al. Development and evaluation of the universal ACS NSQIP surgical risk calculator: a decision aid and informed consent tool for patients and surgeons. J Am Coll Surg 2013;217:833–42.e1–3.

53. Sinclair J. Human cytomegalovirus: latency and reactivation in the myeloid lineage. J Clin Virol 2008;41:180–5.

54. Duan S, Yang YC, Xiang LF, et al. Incidence and risk factors of HIV infection among sero-negative spouses of HIV patients in Dehong prefecture of Yunnan province. Zhonghua Liu Xing Bing Xue Za Zhi 2010;31:997–1000 [in Chinese].

55. Lieberman PM. Keeping it quiet: chromatin control of gammaherpesvirus latency. Nat Rev Microbiol 2013;11:863–75.

56. Nitzsche A, Paulus C, Nevels M. Temporal dynamics of cytomegalovirus chromatin assembly in productively infected human cells. J Virol 2008;82:11167–80.

57. Hummel M, Yan S, Li Z, et al. Transcriptional reactivation of murine cytomegalovirus ie gene expression by 5-aza-2'-deoxycytidine and trichostatin A in latently infected cells despite lack of methylation of the major immediate-early promoter. J Gen Virol 2007;88:1097–102.

58. Campbell J, Trgovcich J, Kincaid M, et al. Transient CD8-memory contraction: a potential contributor to latent cytomegalovirus reactivation. J Leukoc Biol 2012; 92:933–7.

59. Ogata M, Satou T, Kawano R, et al. High incidence of cytomegalovirus, human herpesvirus-6, and Epstein-Barr virus reactivation in patients receiving cytotoxic chemotherapy for adult T cell leukemia. J Med Virol 2011;83:702–9.

60. Wang H, Liu XX, Liu YX, et al. Incidence and risk factors of non-fatal injuries in Chinese children aged 0-6 years: a case-control study. Injury 2011;42:521–4.

61. Seitanidis B. A comparison of the Monospot with the Paul-Bunnell test in infectious mononucleosis and other diseases. J Clin Pathol 1969;22:321–3.

62. Glaser R, Kiecolt-Glaser JK, Speicher CE, et al. Stress, loneliness, and changes in herpesvirus latency. J Behav Med 1985;8:249–60.

63. Padgett DA, Sheridan JF, Dorne J, et al. Social stress and the reactivation of latent herpes simplex virus type 1. Proc Natl Acad Sci U S A 1998;95:7231–5 [Erratum appears in Proc Natl Acad Sci U S A 1998;95(20):12070.].

64. Mehta SK, Cohrs RJ, Forghani B, et al. Stress-induced subclinical reactivation of varicella zoster virus in astronauts. J Med Virol 2004;72:174–9.

65. Bhamidipati CM, LaPar DJ, Mehta GS, et al. Albumin is a better predictor of outcomes than body mass index following coronary artery bypass grafting. Surgery 2011;150:626–34.

66. Pierson DL, Stowe RP, Phillips TM, et al. Epstein-Barr virus shedding by astronauts during space flight. Brain Behav Immun 2005;19:235–42.

67. Mehta SK, Crucian BE, Stowe RP, et al. Reactivation of latent viruses is associated with increased plasma cytokines in astronauts. Cytokine 2013;61:205–9.

68. Battle JD Jr, Hewlett JS. Hematologic changes observed after extracorporeal circulation during open-heart operations. Cleve Clin Q 1958;25:112–5.

69. Holswade GR, Engle MA, Redo SF, et al. Development of viral diseases and a viral disease-like syndrome after extracorporeal circulation. Circulation 1963; 27:812–5.
70. Seaman AJ, Starr A. Febrile postcardiotomy lymphocytic splenomegaly: a new entity. Ann Surg 1962;156:956–60.
71. Ross BA. Pyrexia after heart surgery due to virus infection transmitted by blood transfusion. Thorax 1964;19:159–61.
72. Smith DR. A syndrome resembling infectious mononucleosis after open-heart surgery. Br Med J 1964;1:945–8.
73. Perillie PE, Glenn WW. Fever, splenomegaly, lymphocytosis and eosinophilia. Yale J Biol Med 1962;34:625–8.
74. Kääriäinen L, Klemola E, Paloheimo J. Rise of cytomegalovirus antibodies in an infectious-mononucleosis-like syndrome after transfusion. BMJ 1966;1:1270–2.
75. Adler SP, Baggett J, McVoy M. Transfusion-associated cytomegalovirus infections in seropositive cardiac surgery patients. Lancet 1985;326:743–6.
76. Domart Y, Trouillet JL, Fagon JY, et al. Incidence and morbidity of cytomegaloviral infection in patients with mediastinitis following cardiac surgery [see comments]. Chest 1990;97:18–22.
77. Abramson JS, Mills EL. Depression of neutrophil function induced by viruses and its role in secondary microbial infections. Rev Infect Dis 1988;10:326–41.
78. Hamilton JR, Overall JC, Glasgow LA. Synergistic effect on mortality in mice with murine cytomegalovirus and *Pseudomonas aeruginosa*, *Staphylococcus aureus*, or *Candida albicans* infections. Infect Immun 1976;14:982–9.
79. Rand KH, Merigan TC. Cytomegalovirus: a not so innocent bystander. JAMA 1978;240:2470–1.
80. Dirbas FM, Swain JA. Disseminated cutaneous herpes zoster following cardiac surgery. J Cardiovasc Surg (Torino) 1990;31:531–2.
81. Godfrey EK, Brown C, Stambough JL. Herpes zoster-varicella complicating anterior thoracic surgery: 2 case reports. J Spinal Disord Tech 2006;19: 299–301.
82. Sachdeva S, Prasher P. Herpes zoster following saphenous venectomy for coronary bypass surgery. J Card Surg 2010;25:28–9.
83. Nunez J, Chilet M, Sanchis J, et al. Prevalence and prognostic implications of active cytomegalovirus infection in patients with acute heart failure. Clin Sci 2010;119:443–52.
84. Yamashiroya HM, Ghosh L, Yang R, et al. Herpesviridae in the coronary arteries and aorta of young trauma victims. Am J Pathol 1988;130:71–9.
85. Fabricant CG, Fabricant J, Litrenta MM, et al. Virus-induced atherosclerosis. J Exp Med 1978;148:335–40.
86. Span AH, Van Boven CP, Bruggeman CA. The effect of cytomegalovirus infection on the adherence of polymorphonuclear leucocytes to endothelial cells. Eur J Clin Invest 1989;19:542–8.
87. Aung AK, Skinner MJ, Lee FJ, et al. Changing epidemiology of bloodstream infection pathogens over time in adult non-specialty patients at an Australian tertiary hospital. Commun Dis Intell 2012;36:E333–341.
88. Epstein SE, Zhu J, Najafi AH, et al. Insights into the role of infection in atherogenesis and in plaque rupture. Circulation 2009;119:3133–41.
89. Mukherjee S, Allen RM, Lukacs NW, et al. STAT3-mediated IL-17 production by postseptic T cells exacerbates viral immunopathology of the lung. Shock 2012; 38:515–23.
90. Parfitt DN. Herpes Zoster as a sequel to lightning trauma. Br Med J 1936;1:111.

91. Liu XF, Wang X, Yan S, et al. Epigenetic control of cytomegalovirus latency and reactivation. Viruses 2013;5:1325–45.

92. Constant E, Davis DG, Maldonado WE. Disseminated cytomegalovirus infection associated with death in a patient with severe facial injuries. Case report. Plast Reconstr Surg 1973;51:336–9.

93. Guggenheimer J, Fletcher RD. Traumatic induction of an intraoral reinfection with herpes simplex virus: report of a case. Oral Surg Oral Med Oral Pathol 1974;38:546–9.

94. Purtilo DT, Paquin LA, Sakamoto K, et al. Persistent transfusion-associated infectious mononucleosis with transient acquired immunodeficiency. Am J Med 1980;68:437–40.

95. Foley FD, Greenawald KA, Nash G, et al. Herpesvirus infection in burned patients. N Engl J Med 1970;282:652–6.

96. Deepe GS Jr, MacMillan BG, Linnemann CC Jr. Unexplained fever in burn patients due to cytomegalovirus infection. JAMA 1982;248:2299–301.

97. Kagan RJ, Naraqi S, Matsuda T, et al. Herpes simplex virus and cytomegalovirus infections in burned patients. J Trauma 1985;25:40–5.

98. Kealey GP, Bale JF, Strauss RG, et al. Cytomegalovirus infection in burn patients. J Burn Care Rehabil 1987;8:543–5.

99. Bale JF Jr, Kealey GP, Massanari RM, et al. The epidemiology of cytomegalovirus infection among patients with burns. Infect Control Hosp Epidemiol 1990;11:17–22.

100. Hayden FG, Himel HN, Heggers JP. Herpesvirus infections in burn patients. Chest 1994;106:15S–21S [discussion: 34S–5S].

101. Bordes J, Gaillard T, Maslin J, et al. Cytomegalovirus infection monitored by quantitative real-time PCR in critically ill patients. Crit Care 2011;15:412.

102. Limaye AP, Kirby KA, Rubenfeld GD, et al. Cytomegalovirus reactivation in critically ill immunocompetent patients. JAMA 2008;300:413–22.

103. Schroeder JE, Tessone A, Angel M, et al. Disseminated Varicella infection in an adult burn victim—a transfused disease? Burns 2009;35:297–9.

104. Sheridan RL, Weber JM, Pasternak MM, et al. A 15-year experience with varicella infections in a pediatric burn unit. Burns 1999;25:353–6.

105. Herpesvirus infection in burned patients [editorial]. BMJ 1970;2:618–9.

106. Tenenhaus M, Rennekampff HO, Pfau M, et al. Cytomegalovirus and burns: current perceptions, awareness, diagnosis, and management strategies in the United States and Germany. J Burn Care Res 2006;27:281–8.

107. D'Avignon LC, Hogan BK, Murray CK, et al. Contribution of bacterial and viral infections to attributable mortality in patients with severe burns: an autopsy series. Burns 2010;36:773–9.

108. Kobayashi H, Kobayashi M, McCauley RL, et al. Cadaveric skin allograft-associated cytomegalovirus transmission in a mouse model of thermal injury. Clin Immunol 1999;92:181–7.

109. Kealey GP, Aguiar J, Lewis RW 2nd, et al. Cadaver skin allografts and transmission of human cytomegalovirus to burn patients. J Am Coll Surg 1996;182:201–5.

110. Fidler PE, Mackool BT, Schoenfeld DA, et al. Incidence, outcome, and long-term consequences of herpes simplex virus type 1 reactivation presenting as a facial rash in intubated adult burn patients treated with acyclovir. J Trauma 2002;53:86–9.

111. Nash G, Asch MJ, Foley FD, et al. Disseminated cytomegalic inclusion disease in a burned adult. JAMA 1970;214:587–8.

112. Tuxen DV, Cade JF, McDonald MI, et al. Herpes simplex virus from the lower respiratory tract in adult respiratory distress syndrome. Am Rev Respir Dis 1982; 126:416–9.
113. Byers RJ, Hasleton PS, Quigley A, et al. Pulmonary herpes simplex in burns patients. Eur Respir J 1996;9:2313–7.
114. Kalil AC, Florescu DF. Prevalence and mortality associated with cytomegalovirus infections in non-immunosuppressed ICU patients. Crit Care Med 2009;37:2350–8.
115. Cook CH, Yenchar JK, Kraner TO, et al. Occult herpes family viruses may increase mortality in critically ill surgical patients. Am J Surg 1998;176:357–60.
116. Cook CH, Martin LC, Yenchar JK, et al. Occult herpes family viral infections are endemic in critically ill surgical patients. Crit Care Med 2003;31:1923–9.
117. Aarts MA, Granton J, Cook DJ, et al. Empiric antimicrobial therapy in critical illness: results of a surgical infection society survey. Surg Infect (Larchmt) 2007;8:329–36.
118. Docke WD, Prosch S, Fietze E, et al. Cytomegalovirus reactivation and tumour necrosis factor. Lancet 1994;343:268–9.
119. Seckert CK, Griessl M, Buttner JK, et al. Immune surveillance of cytomegalovirus latency and reactivation in murine models: link to memory inflation. In: Reddehase MJ, editor. Cytomegaloviruses. Norfolk (United Kingdom): Caister Academic Press; 2013. p. 374–416.
120. Kutza AS, Muhl E, Hackstein H, et al. High incidence of active cytomegalovirus infection among septic patients. Clin Infect Dis 1998;26:1076–82.
121. Heininger A, Jahn G, Engel C, et al. Human cytomegalovirus infections in nonimmunosuppressed critically ill patients. Crit Care Med 2001;29:541–7.
122. Jaber S, Chanques G, Borry J, et al. Cytomegalovirus infection in critically ill patients: associated factors and consequences. Chest 2005;127:233–41.
123. von Muller L, Klemm A, Weiss M, et al. Active cytomegalovirus infection in patients with septic shock. Emerg Infect Dis 2006;12:1517–22.
124. Ziemann M, Sedemund-Adib B, Reiland P, et al. Increased mortality in long-term intensive care patients with active cytomegalovirus infection. Crit Care Med 2008;36:3145–50.
125. Chiche L, Forel JM, Roch A, et al. Active cytomegalovirus infection is common in mechanically ventilated medical intensive care unit patients. Crit Care Med 2009;37:1850–7.
126. Chilet M, Aguilar G, Benet I, et al. Virological and immunological features of active cytomegalovirus infection in nonimmunosuppressed patients in a surgical and trauma intensive care unit. J Med Virol 2010;82:1384–91.
127. Heininger A, Haeberle H, Fischer I, et al. Cytomegalovirus reactivation and associated outcome of critically ill patients with severe sepsis. Crit Care 2011; 15:R77.
128. Coisel Y, Bousbia S, Forel JM, et al. Cytomegalovirus and herpes simplex virus effect on the prognosis of mechanically ventilated patients suspected to have ventilator-associated pneumonia. PLoS One 2012;7:e51340 [Electronic Resource].
129. Papazian L, Fraisse A, Garbe L, et al. Cytomegalovirus. An unexpected cause of ventilator-associated pneumonia. Anesthesiology 1996;84:280–7.
130. Chatterjee SN, Fiala M, Weiner J, et al. Primary cytomegalovirus and opportunistic infections. Incidence in renal transplant recipients. JAMA 1978;240:2446–9.
131. Bouza E, Giannella M, Torres MV, et al. Herpes simplex virus: a marker of severity in bacterial ventilator-associated pneumonia. J Crit Care 2011;26: 432.e1–6.

132. Schuller D. Lower respiratory tract reactivation of herpes simplex virus. Comparison of immunocompromised and immunocompetent hosts. Chest 1994;106: 3S–7S [discussion: 34S–5S].

133. Centers for Disease Control and Prevention (CDC). Vital signs: central line-associated blood stream infections—United States, 2001, 2008, and 2009. MMWR Morb Mortal Wkly Rep 2011;60:243–8.

134. Deback C, Luyt CE, Lespinats S, et al. Microsatellite analysis of HSV-1 isolates: from oropharynx reactivation toward lung infection in patients undergoing mechanical ventilation. J Clin Virol 2010;47:313–20.

135. Simoons-Smit AM, Kraan EM, Beishuizen A, et al. Herpes simplex virus type 1 and respiratory disease in critically-ill patients: Real pathogen or innocent bystander? Clin Microbiol Infect 2006;12:1050–9.

136. Luyt CE, Combes A, Deback C, et al. Herpes simplex virus lung infection in patients undergoing prolonged mechanical ventilation. Am J Respir Crit Care Med 2007;175:935–42.

137. van den Brink JW, Simoons-Smit AM, Beishuizen A, et al. Respiratory herpes simplex virus type 1 infection/colonisation in the critically ill: marker or mediator? J Clin Virol 2004;30:68–72.

138. Scheithauer S, Manemann AK, Kruger S, et al. Impact of herpes simplex virus detection in respiratory specimens of patients with suspected viral pneumonia. Infection 2010;38:401–5.

139. Engelmann I, Gottlieb J, Meier A, et al. Clinical relevance of and risk factors for HSV-related tracheobronchitis or pneumonia: results of an outbreak investigation. Crit Care 2007;11:R119.

140. Apisarnthanarak A, Holzmann-Pazgal G, Hamvas A, et al. Antimicrobial use and the influence of inadequate empiric antimicrobial therapy on the outcomes of nosocomial bloodstream infections in a neonatal intensive care unit. Infect Control Hosp Epidemiol 2004;25:735–41.

141. Linssen CF, Jacobs JA, Stelma FF, et al. Herpes simplex virus load in bronchoalveolar lavage fluid is related to poor outcome in critically ill patients. Intensive Care Med 2008;34:2202–9.

142. Glaser R, Pearson GR, Jones JF, et al. Stress-related activation of Epstein-Barr virus. Brain Behav Immun 1991;5:219–32.

143. Honda H, Krauss MJ, Coopersmith CM, et al. Staphylococcus aureus nasal colonization and subsequent infection in intensive care unit patients: does methicillin resistance matter? Infect Control Hosp Epidemiol 2010;31:584–91.

144. Drazin D, Hanna G, Shweikeh F, et al. Varicella-zoster-mediated radiculitis reactivation following cervical spine surgery: case report and review of the literature. Case Rep Infect Dis 2013;2013:647486.

145. Anderson MD, Tummala S. Herpes myelitis after thoracic spine surgery. J Neurosurg Spine 2013;18:519–23.

146. Grauvogel J, Vougioukas VI. Herpes radiculitis following surgery for symptomatic cervical foraminal stenosis. Can J Neurol Sci 2008;35:661–3.

147. Weiss R. Herpes zoster following spinal surgery. Clin Exp Dermatol 1989;14:56–7.

148. Miller AE. Selective decline in cellular immune response to varicella-zoster in the elderly. Neurology 1980;30:582–7.

149. Cohen JI, Brunell PA, Straus SE, et al. Recent advances in varicella-zoster virus infection. Ann Intern Med 1999;130:922–32.

150. Razonable RR, Fanning C, Brown RA, et al. Selective reactivation of human herpesvirus 6 variant A occurs in critically ill immunocompetent hosts [see comment]. J Infect Dis 2002;185:110–3.

151. Tang YW, Johnson JE, Browning PJ, et al. Herpesvirus DNA is consistently detected in lungs of patients with idiopathic pulmonary fibrosis. J Clin Microbiol 2003;41:2633–40.
152. Machens A, Bloechle C, Achilles EG, et al. Toxic megacolon caused by cytomegalovirus colitis in a multiply injured patient. J Trauma 1996;40:644–6.
153. Heininger A, Vogel U, Aepinus C, et al. Disseminated fatal human cytomegalovirus disease after severe trauma. Crit Care Med 2000;28:563–6.
154. Wildenauer R, Suttorp AC, Kobbe P. Cytomegalievirus-Kolitis bei einer polytraumatisierten alteren Patientin. [Cytomegalovirus colitis in an elderly polytraumatised patient]. Dtsch Med Wochenschr 2008;133:2383–6 [in German].
155. Cheung AN, Ng IO. Cytomegalovirus infection of the gastrointestinal tract in non-AIDS patients. Am J Gastroenterol 1993;88:1882–6.
156. Chamberlain RS, Atkins S, Saini N, et al. Ileal perforation caused by cytomegalovirus infection in a critically ill adult. J Clin Gastroenterol 2000;30:432–5.
157. Page MJ, Dreese JC, Poritz LS, et al. Cytomegalovirus enteritis: a highly lethal condition requiring early detection and intervention. Dis Colon Rectum 1998;41:619–23.
158. Murray RN, Parker A, Kadakia SC, et al. Cytomegalovirus in upper gastrointestinal ulcers. J Clin Gastroenterol 1994;19:198–201.
159. Blackman E, Vimadalal S, Nash G. Significance of gastrointestinal cytomegalovirus infection in homosexual males. Am J Gastroenterol 1984;79:935–40.
160. Katzoli P, Sakellaris G, Ergazaki M, et al. Detection of herpes viruses in children with acute appendicitis. J Clin Virol 2009;44:282–6.
161. Cook C, Zhang X, McGuinness B, et al. Intra-abdominal bacterial infection reactivates latent pulmonary cytomegalovirus in immunocompetent mice. J Infect Dis 2002;185:1395–400.
162. Frecentese DF, Cogbill TH. Spontaneous splenic rupture in infectious mononucleosis. Am Surg 1987;53:521–3.
163. Rogues AM, Dupon M, Cales V, et al. Spontaneous splenic rupture: an uncommon complication of cytomegalovirus infection. J Infect 1994;29:83–5.
164. Alliot C, Beets C, Besson M, et al. Spontaneous splenic rupture associated with CMV infection: report of a case and review. Scand J Infect Dis 2001;33:875–7.
165. Horwitz CA, Henle W, Henle G, et al. Clinical and laboratory evaluation of cytomegalovirus-induced mononucleosis in previously healthy individuals. Report of 82 cases. Medicine (Baltimore) 1986;65:124–34.
166. Al-Tawfiq JA, Abed MS, Al-Yami N, et al. Promoting and sustaining a hospital-wide, multifaceted hand hygiene program resulted in significant reduction in health care-associated infections. Am J Infect Control 2013;41:482–6.
167. Baumgartner JD, Glauser MP, Burgo-Black AL, et al. Severe cytomegalovirus infection in multiply transfused, splenectomized, trauma patients. Lancet 1982;2:63–6.
168. Okun DB, Tanaka KR. Profound leukemoid reaction in cytomegalovirus mononucleosis. JAMA 1978;240:1888–9.
169. Langenhuijsen MM, van Toorn DW. Splenectomy and the severity of cytomegalovirus infection. Lancet 1982;2:820.
170. Assy N, Gefen H, Schlesinger S, et al. Reactivation versus primary CMV infection after splenectomy in immunocompetent patients. Dig Dis Sci 2007;52:3477–80.
171. Forster MR, Trgovcich J, Zimmerman P, et al. Antiviral prevention of sepsis induced cytomegalovirus reactivation in immunocompetent mice. Antiviral Res 2010;85:496–503.

172. Cook C. Cytomegalovirus reactivation and mortality during critical illness: a $64,000 question. Crit Care Med 2009;37:2475–6.
173. Cook CH, Trgovcich J. Cytomegalovirus reactivation in critically ill immunocompetent hosts: a decade of progress and remaining challenges. Antiviral Res 2011;90:151–9.
174. Camps K, Jorens PG, Demey HE, et al. Clinical significance of herpes simplex virus in the lower respiratory tract of critically ill patients. Eur J Clin Microbiol Infect Dis 2002;21:758–9.
175. Tuxen DV. Prevention of lower respiratory herpes simplex virus infection with acyclovir in patients with adult respiratory distress syndrome. Chest 1994;106: 28S–33S.
176. Haik J, Weissman O, Stavrou D, et al. Is prophylactic acyclovir treatment warranted for prevention of herpes simplex virus infections in facial burns? A review of the literature. J Burn Care Res 2011;32:358–62.
177. Bourdarias B, Perro G, Cutillas M, et al. Herpes simplex virus infection in burned patients: epidemiology of 11 cases. Burns 1996;22:287–90.

Upcoming Rules and Benchmarks Concerning the Monitoring of and the Payment for Surgical Infections

Nitin Sajankila, BS, John J. Como, MD, MPH, Jeffrey A. Claridge, MD, MS*

KEYWORDS

- Pay for performance • Value-based purchasing • Surgery • SCIP
- Surgical infections

KEY POINTS

- In fiscal year (FY) 2013, the Hospital Value-Based Purchasing (VBP) program became active, introducing an incentive program into the already established Inpatient Prospective Payment System. Although this program was created to replace volume-based medicine with value-based medicine through a pay-for-value system, the Hospital VBP program is more accurately described as a not-pay-for-value or not-pay-for-services system.
- Because the stakes are high when hospitals risk losing Medicare funding, up to 2% by 2017, it is essential for health care teams to understand these complex rules. With respect to surgery-related infections, there are 8 measures that affected or will affect payment in FY 2013 to 2017; these measures include the Surgical Care Improvement Project (SCIP)–infection measures 1 to 3 and 9, pneumonia 30-day mortality rate, central line-associated blood stream infection, catheter-associated urinary tract infections, and surgical site infections.
- Although the SCIP guidelines have been assessed in great deal, the outcome measures have not been discussed or studied as thoroughly. There are still many key concerns and questions around VBP and reimbursement. First, it is unclear how these rules from the Centers for Medicare and Medicaid Services will be generalized or adopted by other insurance providers.
- A second key concern is whether or not hospitals will send out high-risk patients to larger tertiary hospitals or safety net hospitals in order to keep infections low by treating low-risk patients and conversely passing on higher-risk patients.

Continued

The authors have nothing to disclose.
Department of Surgery, MetroHealth Medical Center, Case Western Reserve University School of Medicine, Cleveland, OH 44109-1998, USA
* Corresponding author.
E-mail address: Jclaridge@metrohealth.org

Continued

- Another concern is that it is unclear how these rules will affect surgeons and other health care providers.
- Lastly, and most likely an emotional concern, is the thought that complications can happen despite high-quality care. Should reimbursement be withheld because of bad outcomes even in the face of high quality care?

INTRODUCTION

Clinicians are faced, in today's society, with the challenges of increased workload and a need for better documentation. In addition, they are appropriately asked to take on the responsibilities of patient experience,[1] improvement in quality, and monitoring of patient outcomes. A concern is that these important duties require both hospital and physician investment in time and money. Improving quality should involve a continuous and rigorous approach to the implementation of strategies that allow health care workers to both adopt best-evidence care pathways and to constantly monitor outcomes. The typical surgeon, as much as other health care workers, highly values quality improvement,[2,3] and specific issues related to surgical infections are important components of many quality-improvement projects.

There has been a large amount of dialogue between health care workers, hospital administrators, and legislators about pay for performance and linking outcomes with reimbursement, especially given the recent national health care legislation. The practical concern from the point of view of the clinician and the hospital administrator is a decrease in reimbursement for services that hospitals and health care workers provide. Many such concerns are caused by upcoming changes that have been outlined in the Affordable Care Act (ACA). This article discusses these upcoming changes and reviews some of the literature that supports them, specifically those related to surgical infection. Likewise, the lack of support for some of these changes in the academic literature is discussed. Finally, we will review some of the proposed key benchmarks and the methodologies behind the design of those benchmarks.

By demanding a shift in focus from volume-based medicine to value-based medicine, the Patient Protection and ACA, passed in 2010, inspired a host of changes in Medicare funding to hospitals. One of the most significant of these ongoing changes is the Hospital Value-Based Purchasing (VBP) initiative. This Center for Medicare and Medicaid Services' (CMS) program aims to tie the payment of Medicare patients with the patients' experience and the quality of services provided, as opposed to the volume of procedures done or the costs of those procedures.[4] Many of the rules specific to surgery and surgery-related infections are still being written or have not been completely implemented at this time. At this stage, it is important to review the history and planning of the VBP system and to understand how it will impact payment for surgical Medicare patients in the future. In this article, the authors first discuss the ACA and the exact design of the VBP system before highlighting the specific measures pertaining to surgical infections that will affect Medicare reimbursement.

THE INPATIENT PROSPECTIVE PAYMENT SYSTEM AND THE VALUE-BASED PURCHASING SYSTEM

Wishing to improve the reimbursement of hospitals for the Medicare services provided, the ACA established the Hospital VBP program, an incentive program intended to reward hospitals for achieving certain previously established benchmarks. As it is easiest to think of this program as an addition to the inpatient prospective payment system (IPPS), we will discuss IPPS before VBP.

The IPPS is a payment system mandated by Section 1886 (d) of the Social Security Act (the Act) to provide hospitals with support for treating Medicare patients. It basically defines reimbursement, based on rates that are prospectively determined, for acute care inpatient hospital stays and dictates how much Medicare Part A (hospital insurance) will fund for certain types of patients. Essentially, each inpatient stay is placed into a diagnosis-related group (DRG) that has a set payment value. This payment value is defined based on the average cost of treating patients, specifically Medicare patients, of that DRG. By categorizing patients in this manner, the IPPS offers a simplified method for funding Medicare patients.[5]

However, the passing of the ACA, specifically section 3001(a)(1), added another layer of complexity to this already established system. As a result of the ACA, Section 1886 (o) was added to the Act in an effort to introduce *pay for value* into the Medicare reimbursement system. This rule basically stated that the government is required to pay value-based incentives, through the Hospital VBP program, "to hospitals that meet or exceed performance standards for a performance period for a fiscal year."[6]

In order to justify whether a hospital has excelled or not, the CMS calculates a total performance score (TPS); as an example, we will now outline how CMS calculated the TPS for the fiscal year 2013 (FY2013). In FY2013, the first year of the Hospital VBP program, performance standards were categorized into 2 domains: clinical process-of-care measures and patient experience-of-care measures. In order to calculate a TPS, CMS utilized the FY 2013 data for each of these domains and baseline data collected from 2009 to 2010 in order to assess both current achievement and improvement. Based on the FY2013 data, hospitals earned 0–10 points for achievement depending on how their performance for a measure, within a domain, compared to both the achievement threshold and the benchmark. The achievement threshold is defined as the performance at the 50th percentile while the benchmark is defined as performance at the mean of the top decile. Furthermore, hospitals earned 0–9 points based on their improvement on a measure, within a domain, compared to the baseline period performance for that measure - CMS has made a point that hospitals should not receive a full 10 points for improving. Thus, for each measure within a domain, CMS calculated the hospital's achievement and improvement scores; however, only the highest score, either the achievement or improvement, was awarded to the hospital for that measure. The awarded score for that measure was what was used subsequently for the TPS score.[7]

Once all of the measures within each domain were assigned either an improvement or achievement score, the scores were summed within a domain to generate a domain score. The domain score was subsequently weighted as 70% for clinical process of care measures or 30% for patient experience of care measures and then summed in order to generate a TPS. This TPS was translated into a value-based incentive by using a linear exchange function.[6]

In FY2014, an outcomes domain was added, and there is a plan to add an efficiency domain in FY2015. **Table 1** shows the proposed changes over time. In summary, the clinical process-of-care measures will be decreased in weight, and the weight of the outcomes measures will be increased. At the same time, the relative weights of the efficiency and patient experience-of-care measures will remain roughly the same.[6,8]

Although this program is often described as a *pay-for-value* system, it is more appropriately described as a *not-pay-for-value* or *not-pay-for-services* system. This

Table 1 Domain weights for FY 2013 to FY 2016				
	2013 (%)	2014 (%)	2015 (%)	2016 (%)
Clinical process of care	70	45	20	10
Patient experience of care	30	30	30	25
Outcomes	—	25	30	40
Efficiency	—	—	20	25

Adapted from Hospital Value-Based Purchasing Program. 2013; Breakdown of Hospital VBP Domains and Domain Weights for FY 2013–2015. 2013. Available at: http://www.cms.gov/Outreach-and-Education/Medicare-Learning-Network-MLN/MLNProducts/downloads/Hospital_VBPurchasing_Fact_Sheet_ICN907664.pdf. Accessed June 27, 2014; and *Data from* Services CfMM. Federal Register. In: Services DoHaH, editor. vol. 78. 2013. p. 50676–705.

is because a certain fraction of funding that is provided for Medicare patients under Medicare Part A, defined by the IPPS, is withheld from participating hospitals and returned only if the hospitals achieve above-average measures of value. In other words, the total amount of funding that is available for value-based incentives within a fiscal year is exactly equal to the total amount of payment reductions (thus the phrase *not pay for value*) that occurs for all participating hospitals that FY.

In FY 2013, the percent reduction, or what the CMS defines as an incentive, was 1.00% of the Medicare funding by IPPS, and in 2014 it is 1.25%; this percent reduction will steadily increase from 1.50% in FY 2015 to 1.75% in FY 2016 and 2.00% in FY 2017. So, by FY 2017, the motivation to achieve a significant TPS will have significantly increased.[6]

It has been well documented that many surgical patients are at risk for developing postoperative infections; including those of the urinary tract, lungs, blood stream, and surgical site.[9] Of all the performance measures that CMS has proposed to base the 2013–2016 TPS, 8 are directly relevant to surgical infections: Surgical Care Improvement Project (SCIP)-Inf measures 1 to 3 and 9, pneumonia 30-day mortality rate (MORT-30 PN), central line–associated blood stream infections (CLABSIs), catheter-associated urinary tract infections (CAUTIs), and surgical site infections (SSIs). These measures are illustrated and explained more completely in **Table 2**. Moreover, all of these performance measures fall into either the clinical process-of-care-measures domain or the outcome-measures domain. As the Surgical Care Improvement Project SCIP guidelines have been the most commonly discussed, the authors begin with these measures.

SURGICAL CARE IMPROVEMENT PROJECT

Although the Hospital VBP program was only activated in 2013, its component measures have been in circulation as benchmarks for quite some time. Of the initial 13 clinical process-of-care measures that were introduced in FY 2013 and FY 2014, the SCIP guidelines are some of the most well-studied measures.[10] While SCIP originally consisted of many guidelines, the only guidelines in FY2013 and F2014 that were included in the VBP program and were relevant to surgical infections included SCIP-Inf 1–3 and 9.[4]

SCIP (an outgrowth of the Surgical Infection Project) was formed in 2002 by the CMS and a panel of experts, not immediately as a measure to be tied to VBP but as a set of publicly available performance measures. The goal of these measures was to decrease the number of infections that occur as a result of surgery. It was

Table 2
Domains and performance measures relevant to surgery-related infections

Domain	Subcategory	Description	FY Added/Removed
Clinical process of care	SCIP-Inf-1	Prophylactic antibiotic received within 1 h before surgical incision	2013/2016
	SCIP-Inf-2	Prophylactic antibiotic selection for surgical patients	2013
	SCIP-Inf-3	Prophylactic antibiotics discontinued within 24 h after surgery end time	2013
	SCIP-Inf-9	Urinary catheter removed on postoperative d 1 or postoperative d 2	2014
Patient experience of care	—	—	—
Outcome	MORT-30 PN	—	2014
	CLABSI	—	2015
	CAUTI	—	2016
	SSI	SSI: Colon + abdominal hysterectomy	2016
Efficiency	—	—	—

Note: Although CLABSI was finalized for 2015, it may not be guaranteed for 2015.
Data from Services CfMM. Federal register. In: Services DoHaH, editor. vol. 78. 2013. p. 50676–705.

hoped that by making these data publically available, hospitals would be incentivized to comply and thus improve.

Previous studies have shown that there are still compliance issues that need to be addressed for many of the core SCIP guidelines. For example, Bratzler and colleagues[11] showed that, although the choice of prophylactic antibiotic met the standards (SCIP-Inf 2), many hospitals were not compliant with the appropriate CMS-mandated start and end times for prophylactic antibiotics; starting within 1 hour of incision (SCIP-Inf 1) and stopping within 24 hours after the procedure completion (SCIP-Inf 3), respectively. Furthermore, even when compliance was controlled, not all of the SCIP guidelines were found to be relevant in controlling SSIs. One major study recently looked at 295 hospital groups from 2007 to 2010 and analyzed the significance of measures SCIP-Inf 1 to 3. This study found that as compliance increased for SCIP-Inf 1 and 2, the SSI rate decreased; however, compliance for SCIP-Inf 3 had no clear significance on infection prevention.[10] Premature cessation, however, may actually be harmful.[12] Inappropriate continuation of antibiotics may lead to increased costs, an effect, not yet clearly documented in the literature, and may have unit- and hospital-wide consequences with antibiotic resistance and antibiograms, such as with *Clostridium difficile*.[13–15]

Although there may still be compliance issues in FY 2014 with respect to SCIP-Inf 1, the CMS has already finalized plans to remove SCIP-Inf 1 from its Hospital VBP program, as this measure has been deemed topped out, or removable. Per CMS data, most hospitals by 2016 will be compliant enough that it will not be necessary to incentivize hospitals in this way; in other words, using these measures will not help the hospitals achieve a higher-than-current TPS.[6,7]

The relationship between SCIP-Inf 9 (urinary catheter removed on postoperative day 1 or postoperative day 2) and the incidence of UTIs has not been well documented. One of the reports discussing this measure concluded, after looking at 2459 patients, that although compliance to SCIP-Inf 9 increased over time, the incidence of UTIs did not change. The reasoning was that the exclusions for this measure, also a part of the SCIP guidelines, are too lax. This laxity may have allowed surgeons to avoid removing the catheter within 48 hours without being noncompliant, by documenting the necessity of leaving the catheter in. The fact that more than 70% of the patients with postoperative UTIs belonged to the excluded group shows that the exclusions for this measure need to be addressed in order to promote the timely removal of these catheters.[16] Thus, this guideline seems to have a limitation that will allow the provider to circumvent the effective goal of decreasing urinary catheter days. Again, it is important to recognize that these initial rules from the SCIP are related to clinical processes of care.

OTHER SURGICAL INFECTIONS MEASURES

Although measures SCIP-Inf 1 to 3 and 9 address improving clinical process of care, the most important component in the control of surgical infections is focused attention on outcomes. As the authors discuss earlier, as the CMS decreases the weight of the clinical process-of of-care domain, that of the outcomes-measures domain will increase. However, many of these measures will not be active or tied to VBP payment until much later; pneumonia (PN) 30-day mortality rate (MORT-30 PN) becomes active in 2014; CLABSI becomes active in 2015; and both CAUTI and SSI become active in 2016.[6]

Although there is still time before many of these measures are tied to VBP, some stakeholders have raised concerns about how outcomes will be reported and whether the guidelines provided will actually decrease the rates of surgical infection. For example, with respect to CAUTI, many are concerned that mandatory reporting will cause an increase in defensive testing of patients on admission,[17] whereas others have shown that this is not the case.[18] More attention is needed with respect to these outcome measures and CMS's reporting guidelines to understand the validity of tying them to the VBP program.

The authors have included an adapted version of the benchmarks and achievement thresholds that the CMS will be using for VBP in 2016 in **Table 3**. The CMS defines the achievement threshold as the median or 50th percentile of hospital performance during a baseline year for a specific measure; in this definition, *baseline period* refers to a specific previous year used to judge achievement or improvement with the recent fiscal year for Hospital VBP purposes. Similarly, the CMS defines *benchmarks* to be the arithmetical mean of the highest-performing hospitals, belonging to the top decile, within a baseline period. Thus, with each fiscal year, both the values for achievement threshold and benchmarks have the potential to change. As the authors had mentioned before, the benchmark and achievement thresholds are used to assign achievement points before a TPS can be calculated. The authors now define each infection type and discuss issues relating to each type of infection.

CATHETER-ASSOCIATED URINARY TRACT INFECTION

CAUTI is a specific type of UTI involving any of the components of the urinary tract (kidney, ureters, bladder, or urethra) as a result of the use of a catheter in the urinary tract. Indwelling urinary catheters are essentially drainage devices that are placed through the urethra into the urinary bladder in order to directly drain urine; these catheters are often left in place for a significant amount of time, which can result in an infection. CAUTIs occur when bacteria enter the urinary tract and subsequently cause infection, via the catheter.[19] This type of UTI, along with pneumonia, is the second leading cause of hospital-acquired infection, after SSI.[20]

Table 3
An adapted version of CMS's finalized achievement thresholds and benchmarks for the 2016 VBP program, specific to surgery-related infections

Measure ID	Description	Achievement Threshold	Benchmark
SCIP-Inf 2	Prophylactic antibiotic selection for surgical patients	0.99074	1.00000
SCIP-Inf 3	Prophylactic antibiotics discontinued within 24 h after surgery end time	0.98086	1.00000
SCIP-Inf 9	Urinary catheter removed on postoperative d 1 or postoperative d 2	0.97059	1.00000
CAUTI	—	0.801	0.000
CLABSI	—	0.465	0.000
SSI	—	0.737	0.000
MORT-30 PN	—	0.882651	0.904181

Definitions:
- Achievement threshold—The median or 50th percentile of hospital performance during a baseline year for a specific measure; in this definition, baseline period refers to a specific previous year used to judge improvement.
- Benchmarks—The arithmetic mean of the highest performing hospitals, belonging to the top decile, within a baseline period.
Adapted from Services CfMM. Federal register. In: Services DoHaH, editor. vol. 78. 2013. p. 50676–705.

The diagnosis of CAUTI is made by identifying bacteriuria in patients who are currently catheterized or have had a catheter removed within the last 48 hours and have the signs and symptoms of patients with a UTI. These signs and symptoms include fever (>38°C), unexplained suprapubic tenderness, costovertebral angle pain, leukocytosis, malaise, delirium, decrease in blood pressure, metabolic acidosis, and respiratory alkalosis. Pyuria, although not diagnostic, is also noted in many cases. The diagnosis is confirmed by culture growth as standardized by the Infectious Diseases Society of America's (IDSA) guidelines. In these guidelines, symptomatic bacteriuria is a symptomatic UTI with a culture growth of 10^3 or more colony-forming units per milliliter of uropathogenic bacteria (with no more than 2 species of microorganisms), whereas asymptomatic bacteriuria is a nonsymptomatic UTI with a culture growth of 10^5 or more colony-forming units per millimeter of uropathogenic bacteria (with no more than 2 species of microorganisms).[20,21]

Although the CMS is still actively clarifying the implementation of CAUTI in the Hospital VBP, the authors have found several issues that are still troublesome. First, the CAUTI CMS measure includes both symptomatic and asymptomatic forms of CAUTIs. This point was specifically clarified in the comments for the CAUTI measure in the 2013 *Federal Register*, where the CMS justified keeping the name of the measure as CAUTI over "symptomatic urinary tract infections due to an indwelling urinary catheter."[6] However, from a quality-control perspective, grouping both symptomatic CAUTI with asymptomatic bacteriuria, two clinically different conditions, is troubling as it may inspire overprescribing habits for antibiotics for patients with asymptomatic bacteriuria. Not only is this harmful from a societal perspective as it can cause resistant organisms and result in a great deal of monetary waste but it is also deleterious on an individual patient level as it can promote the development of *C difficile* infections. Furthermore, hospitals may be unfairly punished or have reimbursement withheld through payment reductions for CAUTI, although what is actually being described is asymptomatic bacteriuria, a condition for which treatment is unclear.[22]

Furthermore, it has already been established that certain risk factors mark patients as susceptible to develop UTIs, most importantly the length of catheterization, but also female sex, diabetes mellitus, bacterial colonization of the drainage bag, and errors in catheter care.[21] Other groups, such as the elderly[23] and patients with complex pelvic trauma,[24] pose as unique groups that make measuring CAUTIs for the Hospital VBP program difficult. Without clearly identifying all of the different groups that have a high propensity for developing CAUTIs, hospitals may face unfairly high or low reductions in their Medicare reimbursements simply because of their typical patient population. Another important concern is whether or not increased reporting of CAUTIs via the CMS's definition will reduce the incentive for getting urinary cultures and, thus, not diagnosing UTIs, even if antibiotics are given. This may result in the treatment of undocumented UTIs without a confirmed infection. Regardless, it will be important to highlight and study these issues before CAUTI becomes active as a measure in 2016, as the outcome measure may inspire a culture of premature or prolonged prophylaxis using antibiotics.

THIRTY-DAY MORTALITY FOR PNEUMONIA

MORT-30 PN is a 30-day mortality measure for pneumonia, an infection of the lung, that is calculated via claims data and data for public reporting that is mandated each fiscal year.[25] It was initially created as a general measure for public reporting that was first introduced by the CMS in 2007 as a part of its effort to publicize the quality of care that hospitals were providing. In 2013, since it was already a reported measure, it was introduced into the Hospital VBP program as well.[26] The CMS explains that pneumonia is studied as a mortality measure, rather than an incidence measure, because it is already reported in Medicare *Hospital Compare* as a part of core process and readmission measure. Furthermore, pneumonia has a high morbidity/mortality, and thus exerts a heavy burden on both patients and the healthcare system.[27]

Major forms of pneumonia include hospital-acquired pneumonia (HAP), ventilator-associated pneumonia (VAP), and health care–acquired pneumonia (HCAP). VAP, one of the most common types especially in the acute care setting, is pneumonia that develops within 48 hours of starting mechanical ventilation. HAP, on the other hand, is pneumonia that develops 48 hours after admission into the hospital. Furthermore, HCAP is pneumonia that nonhospitalized patients develop as a result of their interaction with the health care system; for example, this can occur through interaction as a result of therapy administration, wound care, chemotherapy administration, residency in a nursing home, acute care hospitalization, or a hemodialysis session at a clinic.[28] VAP, one of the most important types, is typically caused by colonization of the common aerodigestive tract and then subsequent aspiration of these bacteria into the distal airways.[29,30]

The diagnosis of pneumonia is difficult because the clinical findings are nonspecific. However, despite a lack of specific guidelines by the 2005 guidelines of the American Thoracic Society/IDSA, this group concluded that pneumonia, regardless of whether it is HAP, VAP, or HCAP, should be suspected if patients have any of the following: fever, purulent sputum, leukocytosis, or decline in oxygenation. The development of progressive radiographic infiltrates along with two or three of these signs should prompt the clinician to consider pneumonia as a diagnosis.[28]

The surgical patients at highest risk for pneumonia include those that undergo abdominal aortic aneurysm repair, thoracic surgery, or emergency surgery as well as patients that receive general anesthesia or will have received greater than 4 units of blood before surgery. Aside from this, patients that are aged 60 years or older, chronically use steroids as a treatment, have a recent history of alcohol use, have a recent history of cerebrovascular accident, or have a low (<8 mg/dL) or high (>22 mg/dL) blood urea nitrogen level are also at high risk.[31] Similar to CAUTI, the presence of high-risk patient groups that are not adjusted for has the potential to make MORT-30 PN a complex measure. Patients undergoing these high-risk surgeries may unfairly cost the hospital more money to treat, due to a lack of reimbursement. This may consequently affect prophylactic treatment behaviors. Currently risk adjustments include only age, past medical history, and comorbidities.[31] Lastly, it is unclear regarding who is following 30-day mortality. If hospitals are required to do this, it will require increased resources. Another concern with the 30-day mortality measure is that it is unclear on who is following the patients over a 30-day period. If hospitals are required to do this, it will require increased resources in order to assure proper documentation.

CENTRAL LINE–ASSOCIATED BLOOD STREAM INFECTION

CLABSIs are bloodstream infections that occur as a result of the presence of a central line that has been in place for greater than 2 days, including even those due to umbilical dialysis catheters- the Centers for Disease Control and Prevention (CDC) stresses that the central line must be present on the day of the event or have been removed the day before. The CDC outlines several ways to diagnose CLABSI:

1. There is the presence of a recognized pathogen in one or more blood cultures, when the pathogen is not the cause of infection elsewhere.
2. Patients have positive blood culture results, unrelated to other infections, containing the same common commensal, and in multiple cultures that are drawn at different times. The patient also has one of the following symptoms: fever (>38°), chills, or hypotension.
3. The patient is ≤ 1 year of age, has at least one of the following symptoms: fever (>38° core), hypothermia (<36° core), apnea, or bradycardia, and is found with positive blood culture results. These results are unrelated to other infections, are found in multiple cultures that are drawn at different times on the same day or on following days, and contain the same common commensal.[32]

The CDC stresses that the skill of the clinician performing the procedure, the use of appropriate antisepsis, the duration of central line use, insertion site, and the number of catheter lumens all play a significant role in determining the risk of CLABSI. Furthermore, it states that emergency central lines are at higher risk than elective central lines.[33] However, there may be other unidentified risk factors that classify specific groups or types of surgery as being more prone to CLABSI. As the authors highlighted for previous measures, these can have a significant impact on increasing or decreasing prophylactic treatments as well as impacting reimbursement payment via the Hospital VBP program. Accordingly, more attention is needed on risk factors and prophylactic prescribing behaviors regarding CLABSI.

SURGICAL SITE INFECTIONS

SSIs are postoperative infections that take place in the region of the body where the surgery was performed. Although these infections can be restricted to the skin and superficial tissues, they can also be more serious, involving tissues, organs, or implanted material in the region of the surgery.[34] The CDC further states that these infections must occur at or near the surgical incision within 30 days or within 1 year if prosthetic material was implanted during the surgery.[35,36] The CDC also highlights diagnostic criteria for SSIs and separates these into superficial incisional SSI, deep incisional SSI, and organ space SSI.[35] CMS will be evaluating SSI outcomes related to colorectal surgery and abdominal hysterectomy in 2016.[6]

Several risk factors have been identified as impacting the incidence of SSI: surgical technique, duration of surgery, hospital/operating room environment, instrument sterilization, preoperative preparation and management, and the underlying medical condition of the patients. In addition, specific to the surgical environment and operative practices, the following have been linked to SSI: a lack of preoperative hair removal, excessive personal traffic during operation, excessive use of electrosurgical cautery, presence of prosthesis/foreign body, amount of tissue trauma, and need for blood transfusion. With respect to patient characteristics, the risk factors include age, diabetes, obesity, cigarette smoking, immunosuppression, malnutrition, preoperative infection or the presence of infection at a nonsurgical site, recent surgery, length of preoperative hospitalization, and severity of preexisting illnesses.[36] It is unclear whether CMS has risk adjusted for all of these factors. This may bias patient selection by practitioners and hospital systems. Another potential issue is that concern for penalties for any superficial wound infections may lead to surgeons keeping wounds open more frequently.

SUMMARY

In FY 2013, the Hospital VBP program became active, introducing an incentive program into the already established IPPS. Although this program was created to replace volume-based medicine with value-based medicine through a *pay-for-value* system, the Hospital VBP program may be more accurately described as a *not-pay-for-value* or not-pay-for-services system. Because the stakes are high when hospitals risk losing Medicare funding, up to 2% by 2017, it is essential for health care teams to understand these complex rules. With respect to surgical infections, there are 8 measures that have affected or will affect payment in FY 2013 to 2017; these measures include SCIP-Inf measures 1 to 3 and 9, MORT-30 PN, CLABSI, CAUTI, and SSI. Although the SCIP guidelines have been assessed in great deal, the outcome measures have not been discussed or studied as thoroughly. There are still many key concerns and questions around VBP and reimbursement. First, it is unclear how these CMS' rules will be generalized or adopted by other insurance providers. A second key concern is whether hospitals will transfer high-risk patients to larger tertiary or "safety net" hospitals in order to keep their own infection rates low. Another issue is that it is unclear how these rules will affect surgeons relative to other health care providers. Finally, there is a concern that reimbursement may be withheld for complications that occur despite high-quality care. These are just some of the important issues that will need to be followed over the next several years as the newer models of reimbursement that were described in this article evolve.

REFERENCES

1. Millenson ML, Macri J. Will the Affordable Care Act move patient-centeredness to center stage? Urban quick strike series. 2012. Available at: http://www.rwjf.org/en/research-publications/find-rwjf-research/2012/03/will-the-affordable-care-act-move-patient-centeredness-to-center.html. Accessed October 15, 2014.

2. Azoulay E, Chevret S, Leleu G, et al. Half the families of intensive care unit patients experience inadequate communication with physicians. Crit Care Med 2000;28(8):3044–9.

3. Sayek I. Surgery, surgeon, and measurement of value and quality of surgeons' work. Scand J Surg 2013;102(3):141–4.

4. Patterson P. SCIP measures to weigh in Medicare pay starting in 2013. OR Manager 2011;27(3):1–5.

5. Acute Inpatient Prospective Payment System (IPPS) 2013; description of acute IPPS as defined by CMS. Available at: http://www.cms.gov/Medicare/Medicare-Fee-for-Service-Payment/AcuteInpatientPPS/index.html. Accessed October 15, 2014.

6. Services CfMM. Federal Register. In: Services DoHaH, editor. vol. 78. 2013. p. 50676–705.

7. Frequently asked questions hospital value-based purchasing program. Description of what it means for a measure, such as SCIP-Inf 1, to be "topped-out". 2012. Available at: http://www.cms.gov/Medicare/Quality-Initiatives-Patient-Assessment-Instruments/hospital-value-based-purchasing/Downloads/FY-2013-Program-Frequently-Asked-Questions-about-Hospital-VBP-3-9-12.pdf. Accessed October 15, 2014.

8. Hospital value-based purchasing program. Breakdown of hospital VBP domains and domain weights for FY 2013–2015. 2013. Available at: http://www.cms.gov/Outreach-and-Education/Medicare-Learning-Network-MLN/MLNProducts/downloads/Hospital_VBPurchasing_Fact_Sheet_ICN907664.pdf.

9. Berger A, Edelsberg J, Yu H, et al. Clinical and economic consequences of postoperative infections following major elective surgery in U.S. hospitals. Surg Infect (Larchmt) 2014;15(3):322–7.

10. Cataife G, Weinberg DA, Wong HH, et al. The effect of surgical care improvement project (SCIP) compliance on surgical site infections (SSI). Med Care 2014;52: S66–73. http://dx.doi.org/10.1097/MLR.0000000000000028.

11. Bratzler DW, Houck PM, Richards C, et al. Use of antimicrobial prophylaxis for major surgery: baseline results from the national surgical infection prevention project. Arch Surg 2005;140(2):174–82.

12. Miliani K, L'Heriteau F, Astagneau P. Non-compliance with recommendations for the practice of antibiotic prophylaxis and risk of surgical site infection: results of a multilevel analysis from the INCISO Surveillance Network. J Antimicrob Chemother 2009;64(6):1307–15. Accessed October 15, 2014.

13. Specifications manual for Joint Commission national quality core measures (2010B). Description of SCIP-Inf 3 and the rationale behind this measure. 2010. Available at: https://manual.jointcommission.org/releases/archive/TJC2010B1/MIF0112.html.

14. Kelly CP. Clostridium difficile in adults: treatment. In: Calderwood SB, editor. UpToDate. Waltham (MA): UpToDate; 2014. Available at: http://www.uptodate.com/contents/clostridium-difficile-in-adults-treatment?source=search_result&search=clostridium+difficile+in+adults%3A+treatment&selectedTitle=1~150. Accessed on July 16, 2014.

15. Owens RC Jr, Donskey CJ, Gaynes RP, et al. Antimicrobial-associated risk factors for clostridium difficile infection. Clin Infect Dis 2008;46(Suppl 1):S19–31. Accessed October 15, 2014.

16. Owen RM, Perez SD, Bornstein WA, et al. Impact of surgical care improvement project inf-9 on postoperative urinary tract infections: do exemptions interfere with quality patient care? Arch Surg 2012;147(10):946–53.

17. Palmer JA, Lee GM, Dutta-Linn MM, et al. Including catheter-associated urinary tract infections in the 2008 CMS payment policy: a qualitative analysis. Urol Nurs 2013;33(1):15–23.

18. Morgan DJ, Meddings J, Saint S, et al. Does nonpayment for hospital-acquired catheter-associated urinary tract infections lead to overtesting and increased antimicrobial prescribing? Clin Infect Dis 2012;55(7):923–9.

19. Prevention CfDCa. Catheter-associated urinary tract infections. Frequently asked questions about CAUTIs. 2010. Available at: http://www.cdc.gov/HAI/ca_uti/cauti_faqs.html. Accessed October 15, 2014.

20. NHSN CfDCaPa. Catheter-associated urinary tract infection (CAUTI) event PDF. A device associated infection: CAUTI manual put out by the CDC and NHSN. 2014. Available at: http://www.cdc.gov/nhsn/pdfs/pscmanual/7psccauticurrent.pdf. Accessed October 15, 2014.

21. Fekete T. Catheter-associated urinary tract infection in adults. In: Calderwood SB, editor. UpToDate. Waltham (MA): UpToDate; 2014. Available at: http://www.uptodate.com/contents/catheter-associated-urinary-tract-infection-in-adults?source=search_result&search=catheter+associated+urinary+trac+infection+in+adults&selectedTitle=4~150. Accessed July 16, 2014.

22. Trautner BW. Asymptomatic bacteriuria: when the treatment is worse than the disease. Nat Rev Urol 2012;9(2):85–93.

23. Holroyd-Leduc JM, Sen S, Bertenthal D, et al. The relationship of indwelling urinary catheters to death, length of hospital stay, functional decline, and nursing home admission in hospitalized older medical patients. J Am Geriatr Soc 2007; 55(2):227–33.

24. Wald H, Epstein A, Kramer A. Extended use of indwelling urinary catheters in postoperative hip fracture patients. Med Care 2005;43(10):1009–17.

25. Outcome measures. Description of 30-day mortality as a form of outcome measure. 2013. Available at: http://www.cms.gov/Medicare/Quality-Initiatives-Patient-Assessment-Instruments/HospitalQualityInits/OutcomeMeasures.html. Accessed October 15, 2014.

26. CMS. Medicare Hospital Quality Chartbook 2013; Available at: http://www.cms.gov/Medicare/Quality-Initiatives-Patient-Assessment-Instruments/HospitalQualityInits/Downloads/-Medicare-Hospital-Quality-Chartbook-2013.pdf. Accessed October 15, 2014.

27. Services CfMaM. Frequently asked questions: CMS publicly reported risk-standardized outcome measures. 2013. Available at: http://quality.knowledgebase.co/assets/riskstndoutcomemsrs_faqs_092013.pdf. Accessed October 15, 2014.

28. File TM Jr. Treatment of hospital-acquired, ventilator-associated, and healthcare-associated pneumonia in adults. In: Bartlett JG, editor. UpToDate. Waltham (MA): UpToDate; 2014. Available at: http://www.uptodate.com/contents/treatment-of-hospital-acquired-ventilator-associated-and-healthcare-associated-pneumonia-in-adults?source=search_result&search=treatment+of+hospital-acquired%2C+ventilator-associated%2C+and+healthcare-associated+pneumonia+in+adults&selectedTitle=1~150. Accessed July 16, 2014.

29. Hess D. The ventilator circuit and ventilator-associated pneumonia. In: Scott Manaker M, Finlay G, editors. UpToDate. Waltham (MA): UpToDate; 2014. Available at: http://www.uptodate.com/contents/the-ventilator-circuit-and-ventilator-associated-pneumonia?source=search_result&search=the+ventilator+circuit+an+dventilator-associated+pneumonia&selectedTitle=1~150. Accessed July 16, 2014.

30. Ofelia C, Tablan MD, Anderson LJ, et al. Guidelines for preventing health-care–associated pneumonia 2003. Available at: http://www.cdc.gov/mmwr/preview/mmwrhtml/rr5303a1.htm. Accessed October 15, 2014.

31. 30-Day death and readmission measures. Description of the 30-day mortality measure by CMS. Available at: http://www.medicare.gov/hospitalcompare/data/30-day-measures.html?AspxAutoDetectCookieSupport=1.

32. NHSN CfDCaPa. Central Line-Associated Blood Stream Infections(CLABSI) Event PDF. 2014; A device associated infection: CAUTI manual put out by the CDC and NHSN. Available at: http://www.cdc.gov/nhsn/pdfs/pscmanual/4psc_clabscurrent.pdf. Accessed October 15, 2014.

33. Alex Kallen M, Patel P. Central line-associated bloodstream infections (CLABSI) in non-intensive care unit (non-ICU) settings toolkit 2014; contains descriptions of various CLABSI risk factors. Available at: http://www.cdc.gov/hai/pdfs/toolkits/clabsitoolkit_white020910_final.pdf. Accessed October 15, 2014.

34. Surgical site infection (SSI). 2012. Available at: http://www.cdc.gov/hai/ssi/ssi.html. Accessed October 15, 2014.

35. Prevention CfDCa. Guideline for prevention of surgical site infection, 1999. Criteria for defining a surgical site infection (SSI). 1999. Available at: http://www.cdc.gov/hicpac/SSI/table1-SSI.html. Accessed October 15, 2014.

36. Deverick J, Anderson M, Sexton DJ. Epidemiology of surgical site infection in adults. In: Anthony Harris M, Baron EL, editors. *UpToDate*. Waltham, MA: UpToDate; 2014.

Bloodstream Infections and Central Line– Associated Bloodstream Infections

Christopher M. Watson, MD[a],*, Majdi N. Al-Hasan, MD[b]

KEYWORDS

- Bloodstream infection(s) • Catheter-related bloodstream infection(s) • Bacteremia
- Septicemia

KEY POINTS

- Bloodstream infections are costly to the patient and society.
- An understanding of the various definitions associated with bloodstream infections allows for better interpretation and use of the literature.
- A knowledge of regional and local epidemiology of bloodstream infections allows treatment to be tailored and more appropriate empirical antibiotics to be used.
- In addition to appropriate antibiotic selection, source control of secondary bloodstream infections is important.

INTRODUCTION

Bloodstream infections (BSI) are common, and the consequences of developing these infections are grave. It is estimated that more than 575,000 individuals develop BSI annually in North America, accounting for nearly 80,000 deaths. In addition, central line-associated BSI (CLABSI) is a major contributor to the cost of health care.

Although primary BSI may be seen by the surgeon, a secondary BSI is more likely to be encountered, especially CLABSI. Prompt identification of the source of infection in patients with secondary BSI is paramount. This practice allows early source control and initiation of appropriate antimicrobial therapy, with subsequent improvement in

Funding Sources: None.
Conflict of Interest: Consultant for Medtronic Advanced Energy (C.M. Watson); none (M.N. Al-Hasan).
[a] Division of Acute Care Surgery, Department of Surgery, Palmetto Health Richland, 9 Medical Park Drive, Suite 450, Columbia, SC 29203, USA; [b] Division of Infectious Diseases, Department of Medicine, University of South Carolina School of Medicine, 2 Medical Park, Suite 502, Columbia, SC 29203, USA
* Corresponding author.
E-mail address: christopher.watson@palmettohealth.org

outcomes. An understanding of evidence-based preventative measures and bundles is important to any surgeon's practice.

DEFINITIONS

BSI are defined by the presence of an organism within the bloodstream with or without signs or symptoms of an infection. The Centers for Disease Control and Prevention (CDC) categorize BSI for the purpose of surveillance into 3 types of laboratory-confirmed BSI (LCBSI).[1]

- LCBSI 1 requires that a recognized pathogen be cultured from 1 or more samples of blood.
- LCBSI 2 requires that a patient have fever, hypotension, or chills and the same common commensal be cultured from 2 or more blood cultures on separate occasions not more than 1 calendar day apart.
- LCBSI 3 adds different signs and symptoms for children younger than 1 year from LCBSI 2.

All 3 definitions of LCBSI require that the BSI cannot be attributable to an infection at another site, which defines the infection as a secondary BSI.

It is vital to know which organisms are considered recognized pathogens and which are considered common commensals; a list of these organisms can be found on the CDC Web site.[2] A common example in clinical practice is the scenario in which 1 of 2 sets of blood cultures is positive for *Staphylococcus aureus* versus coagulase-negative staphylococci (CoNS), including *Staphylococcus epidermidis*. The former is treated as a true BSI, whereas the latter is considered a skin contaminate if no signs or symptoms of infection are present or a third blood culture the following day does not grow the same organism. This situation emphasizes the importance of obtaining 2 sets of blood cultures from 2 different sites in patients with suspected infections, to allow differentiation of true BSI from positive blood cultures caused by skin contamination.

It is also important to understand the definitions of CLABSI and catheter-related BSI (CRBSI). The CDC defines CLABSI as a BSI in a patient with a central line that had been in place for at least 2 calendar days before the positive culture date in the absence of an identifiable source of BSI. The CDC goes further to define a central line as any catheter, temporary or permanent, with a tip that terminates in a central vein, the aorta, pulmonary artery, or the umbilical vein. These catheters may be long-term or short-term.

- A long-term catheter is defined as any catheter that is surgically implanted through a tunnel with a subcutaneous cuff used for prolonged home delivery of medications, chemotherapy, or hemodialysis. This term is used interchangeably with cuffed central line and tunneled central line.
- Short-term catheters are peripherally inserted central catheter (PICC) or an uncuffed, short-term central line, both of which are also tunneled through a subcutaneous track.

The definition of CRBSI is more complex, but more relevant clinically than epidemiologically. The Infectious Diseases Society of America (IDSA) defines CRBSI as the following:

- The same organism grows from at least 1 percutaneous culture and from the catheter tip in question or
- The same organism grows from at least 1 percutaneous blood culture and from blood cultures obtained through the catheter hub, which meets criteria for quantitative blood cultures (3-fold difference) or differential time to positivity ($\geq$2 hour

difference). An alternative definition is that the same organism grows from blood cultures obtained through 2 lumens of a central line, with one being 3-fold greater on quantitative culture.[3]

Until recently, BSIs were categorized as either community acquired or hospital acquired (nosocomial). The former infections were typically associated with a more benign pathogen and clinical course, whereas the latter were associated with pathogens that were likely resistant to antimicrobials and had a more malignant clinical course. As more data have been collected, it has become clear that there is a subgroup of patients with community-onset BSI that behave more like nosocomial infections. In an observational study, Friedman and colleagues[4] challenged the binary classification system by adding the definition of health care–associated (HCA) BSI. The investigators concluded that patients with HCA BSI suffered comparable clinical consequences to patients with nosocomial BSI. The investigators defined HCA acquisition as BSI occurring outside the hospital or within 48 hours of hospital admission with any of the following criteria:

- Receiving specialized home wound care or intravenous medication or chemotherapy administration within the previous 30 days or
- Attending a hospital or hemodialysis clinic within the previous 30 days or
- Having been hospitalized for 2 or more days within the previous 90 days or
- Residing in a nursing home or long-term care facility.

EPIDEMIOLOGY

Although the complete list of commensals and pathogens is too burdensome to commit to memory, it is important to know the relatively few pathogens and commensals that are common to one's clinical practice. There have been multiple studies addressing the epidemiology of BSI. There are differences in the results of epidemiologic studies of BSI, depending on the setting in which these studies were performed. The classic example is in regard to the most common organism causing BSI. Whereas almost all population-based studies show that *Escherichia coli* is the most common bloodstream isolate, large referral hospital-based surveillance studies report *S aureus* as the most common pathogen causing BSI.

Population-based studies, which include all the residents of a predefined geographic region, avoid referral bias that could occur in selected populations, such as tertiary-care hospitals or intensive care unit (ICU) settings.[5] Such population-based studies allow determination of the incidence rates within a population and comparison of these rates across different geographic areas. This strategy allows evaluation of risk factors for acquiring specific pathogens, detection of emerging pathogens, and establishment of effectiveness of preventative measures within that population.

Laupland[6] reviewed all population-based studies of BSI since the 1970s and reported an overall incidence of BSI in high-income populations of 80 to 189 episodes per 100,000 patient-years. Filice and colleagues[7] reported an overall incidence rate of BSI of 80 per 100,000 person-years in Charleston County, South Carolina between 1974 and 1976. The most commonly isolated pathogens were *E coli*, *S aureus*, *Klebsiella* species, and *Streptococcus pneumoniae*, because the study excluded common skin contaminants, including CoNS. Nearly 30 years later, a similar population-based study[8] in Olmstead County, Minnesota from 2003 to 2005 reported an overall incidence rate of BSI of 189 per 100,000 person-years. The most common bloodstream isolates were *E coli*, *S aureus*, CoNS, and *Klebsiella* species. Uslan and colleagues excluded CoNS only if it was clinically defined as a skin contaminant. The study also reported an increase in the incidence rate of BSI with age- and sex-specific differences in the incidence rates of E coli and S aureus BSI, with the former being more common in women and the latter more common in men.

It seems that the case-fatality rate (CFR) of BSI has declined over the past 3 decades. CFRs were reported as high as 30% in outcome studies from the 1970s and 1980s. However, more recent population-based studies have reported an overall CFR of 13% to 20%.[8,9]

On a broader scale, Goto and Al-Hasan estimated the overall burden of BSI in North America. Based on the reported age-adjusted and sex-adjusted incidence and mortality of BSI in population-based studies, it is estimated that nearly 600,000 individuals develop BSI annually in North America. In addition, BSI is the sixth and seventh leading cause of death in Canada and the United States, respectively, and the leading cause of death caused by infections in both countries, contributing to approximately 80,000 deaths each year.[10]

Regarding CLABSI, it is estimated that there have been 41,000 episodes of CLABSI in US hospitals in 2009, 18,000 of those occurring in ICUs.[11] An economic study of CLABSI in the United States estimated an average payment for a hospitalized patient with CLABSI of $64,894, an average expense of $91,733, with a gross negative margin of $26,839 per case in 2006. The investigators further estimated that CLABSI and its complications averaged 43% of the total health care cost.[12] Other sources have estimated that the cost of a case of CLABSI is between $3700 and $36,441, with CDC estimating a more moderate cost of $16,550 per CLABSI episode.[13] Aside from the economic impact, Klevens and colleagues,[14] after reviewing 3 different national databases, estimated a CFR of 12% for CLABSI.

DIAGNOSIS
History and Physical Examination

- In patients with suspected infections, the first order of business is a full history and physical examination.
- Symptoms and signs of systemic inflammatory response (eg, fever/hypothermia, hypotension, tachycardia) raise the clinical concern for BSI. However, elderly patients, immune-compromised hosts, and individuals with liver cirrhosis or end-stage renal disease may not mount a temperature response. Surgeons should have low threshold for suspicion of BSI in these patients when they present with hypotension and tachycardia.
- History should primarily focus on the likely source of infection and any potential complications from hematogenous seeding.
- Documentation of recent contact with the health care system is essential to determine the site of infection acquisition.
- Past medical history should include any recent infections, particularly those caused by resistant pathogens, such as methicillin-resistant S aureus (MRSA), vancomycin-resistant Enterococcus species, extended-spectrum β-lactamase (ESBL)-producing gram-negative bacilli, carbapenem-resistant Enterobacteriaceae (CRE), and multidrug-resistant Pseudomonas aeruginosa and Acinetobacter baumanii.
- Documentation of previous antibiotic exposure is important to determine risk factors for antimicrobial resistance.
- Physical examination is key to confirm a suspected source of infection.
- In patients with central lines, inspection of the catheter exit site for signs of infection (erythema or drainage) and palpation of catheter tunnel for tenderness are important clinical clues for central line infection.

- Careful cardiac and musculoskeletal examinations are of particular importance to detect new heart murmurs and hematogenous seeding of the joints, respectively.
- In patients with hemodynamic instability, a brief history and physical examination focusing on the source of infection followed by immediate resuscitation, collection of 2 sets of blood cultures, and initiation of empirical antimicrobial therapy is more appropriate, with completion of the rest of the history from the patient or family members afterward.

Laboratory and Imaging Data

- Only after the history and physical examination should specialized laboratory or imaging studies be obtained.
- Directed cultures can be obtained by this strategy rather than a shotgun approach of obtaining multiple unnecessary imaging studies and cultures of all known body fluids. It is uncommon that pan-cultures need to be obtained after a thorough history and physical examination are performed. Rather, cultures should be obtained from the blood and clinically suspected sites of infection.
- Initial imaging studies should also focus on the likely source of infection and potential complications.

It is important that blood cultures are properly acquired. The 2009 IDSA Guidelines contain specific recommendations on obtaining cultures, and all institutions should develop protocols using these guidelines.[3] However, multiple sterile samples of similar volume from all intravascular devices should be obtained, as well as 1 or more samples from peripheral new sticks. These samples should be obtained simultaneously and before initiation of any antimicrobials.

- If a CRBSI is suspected, and there is an indication for catheter removal, then, the distal 5 cm of the catheter should be sent for culture. A clinically important positive culture of the catheter tip depends on the particular method that a laboratory uses: either roll-plate or sonication (>15 CFU for the roll-plate method and >10^2 CFU for sonication). Both methods reliably detect colonization of the catheter; however, the roll-plate technique is recommended by the 2009 IDSA Guidelines, especially for catheters that have been in place for less than 14 days. These guidelines further recommend culturing the material inside a subcutaneous port rather than the catheter itself, should one of these devices be suspected as the source of a BSI.
- It is optimal that appropriate cultures be obtained before starting antimicrobial agents. This principle does not negate the urgency with which these patients should be treated. The recent update to the Surviving Sepsis Campaign Guidelines recommends starting antimicrobials within the first hour of recognizing septic shock or severe sepsis without shock, thus giving a limited window for obtaining blood cultures.[15] However, this strategy highlights the importance of blood cultures, in that it gives the clinician meaningful data for antimicrobial modification, surveillance, antibiogram composition, and de-escalation practices.
- New microbiology rapid diagnostic technology such as matrix-assisted laser desorption/ionization time-of-flight have allowed rapid identification of microorganisms in blood cultures and potential improvement of empirical antimicrobial therapy.[16]

TREATMENT
Empirical Antimicrobial Therapy

- Once blood cultures are obtained, appropriate selection of empirical antimicrobials is imperative, because inappropriate antimicrobial therapy has been associated with increased mortality (**Table 1**).[17,18]

Table 1
Suggested antimicrobial agents for empirical therapy for BSI based on suspected microbiological cause, site of infection acquisition, and acute severity of illness[a]

Suspected Microbiology (Source of Infection Examples)	Site of Infection Acquisition	
	Community Acquired	Hospital Acquired or Health Care Associated
Gram-positive cocci (skin, soft tissue, bone, and joint)	Vancomycin 15 mg/kg every 8–12 h	Vancomycin 15 mg/kg every 8–12 h
Aerobic gram-negative bacilli[b] (urinary tract)	Ceftriaxone 2 g every 24 h	Cefepime 2 g every 8–12 h or piperacillin-tazobactam 3.375–4.5 g every 6 h
Aerobic and anaerobic gram-negative bacilli[b] (intra-abdominal)	Cefoxitin 2 g every 8 h or ceftriaxone (as above) plus metronidazole 500 mg every 8 h	Piperacillin-tazobactam or cefepime plus metronidazole (as above)
Candida species (central line, intra-abdominal)	Fluconazole 400 mg every 24 h	Micafungin 100 mg every 24 h or caspofungin 70 mg x 1, then 50 mg every 24 h
Severe sepsis or septic shock[b] (undetermined source)	Piperacillin-tazobactam 4.5 g every 6 h plus vancomycin (as above) or cefepime 2 g every 8 h plus vancomycin (as above)	

[a] Provided dosing is for intravenous route in adults. Dose adjustment may be required for patients with renal or hepatic impairment. Local antimicrobial resistance rates, institutional antibiograms, and individual risk factors for antimicrobial resistance are important tools for optimization of empirical antimicrobial therapy.
[b] Critically ill patients with high acute severity of illness scores (ie, Pitt bacteremia score ≥4) may be treated with antipseudomonal agents regardless of the site of acquisition.

- Factors that influence the initial selection of antimicrobial therapy include likely source of BSI, site of infection acquisition, regional and local antimicrobial resistance rates, acute severity of illness, and risk factors for antimicrobial resistance.
- The primary source of infection may predict the likely microbiological cause of BSI. For example, skin, soft tissue, bone, and joint sources of infection suggest BSI caused by gram-positive cocci such as S aureus, streptococci, and enterococci. On the other hand, a urinary source of infection raises the suspicion for BSI caused by gram-negative bacilli such as E coli and Klebsiella species. BSI with a biliary or a gastrointestinal source is usually caused by gram-negative bacilli, including obligate anaerobes such as Bacteroides fragilis.
- The site of infection acquisition increases the risk of BSI caused by certain pathogens. This concept is particularly useful in patients with suspicion of BSI caused by gram-negative bacilli, such as those with a urinary or intra-abdominal source of infection. In these patients, hospital-acquired and HCA sites of acquisition are risk factors for BSI caused by gram-negative bacilli that harbor antimicrobial resistance genes such as P aeruginosa and Enterobacter cloacae.[19] This situation dictates the need for using antipseudomonal agents for the empirical therapy for patients with suspected or confirmed nosocomial or HCA gram-negative BSI. However, the site of infection acquisition has little clinical usefulness in patients with likely BSI caused by gram-positive cocci. Since the emergence of community-acquired methicillin-resistant S aureus (MRSA), the site of acquisition no longer predicts the risk of BSI caused by MRSA compared with methicillin-susceptible S aureus.

- Knowledge of regional antimicrobial resistance rates as reported from population-based or large surveillance studies is helpful when making empirical treatment decisions. Institutional antibiograms also provide useful tools for optimizing the initial selection of antibiotics based on local data.
- A high acute severity of illness such as severe sepsis or septic shock dictates the urgency of appropriate antimicrobial therapy and a relatively lower margin of error when choosing an antimicrobial agent. Several scores for the acute severity of illness are available. However, the Pitt bacteremia score and BSI mortality risk score contain variables that are pertinent only to patients with BSI.[20,21]

However, the nonstratified use of broad-spectrum antibiotics without taking into account individual risk factors for antimicrobial resistance, such as previous infections or colonization with resistant pathogens and recent use of broad-spectrum antimicrobial agents, should be discouraged. A comprehensive discussion of risk factors of BSI caused by gram-negative bacilli with specific mechanisms of resistance such as ESBLs and CRE is beyond the scope of this review.[22,23] Consultation with an infectious diseases specialist is useful for the optimal selection of empirical antimicrobial therapy in patients with risk factors for BSI caused by resistant pathogens.

Source Control

- If BSI is primary, then antimicrobials alone may suffice, but for the more likely scenario of a secondary BSI, the control of the source of sepsis is just as urgent as early delivery of appropriate antimicrobials.
- BSI secondary to abscesses require early drainage, whether by catheter-based or open surgical techniques. Infected tissues, such as skin and soft tissue, bowel and appendix, gallbladder, and infected pancreatic necrosis, likewise require prompt surgical intervention. Early aggressive resuscitation is required, but often it is difficult to return a patient to a normal physiologic state without source control. In patients with septic shock, it is not optimal to hold source control procedures until they are fully resuscitated. In this scenario, a discussion with the patient and family about realistic outcomes is necessary.

It is important to stratify patients with suspected CRBSI according to acute severity of illness into critically ill (septic shock or Pitt bacteremia score ≥ 4) and noncritically ill (without shock or Pitt bacteremia score <4). In critically ill patients, it is imperative that the catheter is removed as soon as possible. Antibiotics can be administered through a peripheral line or a newly placed central venous catheter at another location, given the likely need for vasopressors, inotropes, and invasive monitoring in such patients. Exchange of the potentially infected catheter over a guide wire may serve only to colonize the new line, because the subcutaneous track to the vein is the likely site of colonization, not the catheter lumen itself. Therefore, the option of catheter exchange over a guide wire should be considered only in critically ill patients with limited access sites, such as patients with end-stage renal disease on hemodialysis with extensive venous thrombosis caused by previous catheters.[24]

In noncritically ill patients with mild to moderate physiologic derangement from a suspected or documented CLABSI, treatment options are broader, and hence, the decision becomes more complicated. In general, all nontunneled catheters should be removed, if at all possible, with placement of a peripheral access for intravenous antibiotics. Placement of a new central line, if needed, should be delayed until repeat blood cultures show no growth for at least 48 hours. In patients with tunneled catheters, the decision to remove the central line depends on the microbiological cause of BSI and response to antimicrobial therapy. CLABSI caused by high-virulence organisms such as *S aureus*, *P aeruginosa*, and *Candida* species dictate removal of the tunneled catheter. This situation is mostly the result of the relatively high risk of mortality, recurrence, and distant complications, including infective endocarditis, secondary to BSI caused by these pathogens, if not treated properly. However, in patients with CLABSI caused by low-virulence organisms such as CoNS and favorable response to antimicrobial therapy, the option of retaining the tunneled catheter and use of antimicrobial catheter lock therapy is reasonable. In this situation, patients with long-term catheters may tolerate catheter lock techniques to preserve the central line. This option is particularly useful in patients with limited options for new venous access and those with severe thrombocytopenia, in whom removal of tunneled catheters may be complicated. The concept that a guide wire exchange increases the infection rate of the new catheter has been challenged in both retrospective and prospective comparisons of guide wire exchanged and new site catheters.[25–27] A systematic review by Cook and colleagues of 151 randomized, controlled trials comparing central line replacement at a new site versus over a guide wire showed trends toward higher catheter colonization rates, higher catheter exit site infections, and CRBSI in the catheters exchanged over a wire. However, none was statistically significant.[28] Routine exchange of noncolonized catheters at certain time intervals is not necessary.[29]

Identification of Bloodstream Infection Complications

In addition to establishing and controlling the primary source of infection, it is essential to identify potential complications from BSI such as suppurative thrombophlebitis, endocarditis, septic arthritis, osteomyelitis or epidural abscesses. The risk of such complications increases based on the microbiological cause of BSI, duration of bacteremia, and individual risk factors for such complications. In 1 study,[30] 43% of patients with *S aureus* BSI developed complicated bacteremia. Persistent bacteremia despite appropriate antimicrobial therapy also raises the suspicion for complications. In addition, patients with prosthetic heart valves or joints are at higher risk of prosthetic valve endocarditis and prosthetic joint infections, respectively. A history with full review of systems and complete physical examination are the key for identification of such complications. Repeat blood cultures are important for diagnosis of persistent bacteremia and for documentation of resolution of bacteremia before placement of new central venous catheters, if needed. Echocardiography is required in all patients with *S aureus* BSI, continuous bacteremia caused by viridans group streptococci, community-acquired *Enterococcus* species BSI of undetermined source, and other typical microorganisms for endocarditis.[31] Eye examination is of particular importance in patients with prolonged candidemia or *S aureus* BSI with visual symptoms to identify patients with endophthalmitis.

Definitive Antimicrobial Therapy

- Once the microorganism in blood cultures is identified and in vitro antimicrobial susceptibility results are available, antimicrobial regimen should be streamlined to the single narrowest spectrum, cheapest, most effective antimicrobial agent against the bloodstream pathogen, with the lowest risk of serious adverse events **(Table 2)**.
- The duration of antimicrobial therapy in patients with BSI depends on the pathogen, clinical course, and presence or absence of complications. In general, the optimal duration of antimicrobial therapy for BSI, in the absence of complications, is nearly 2 weeks of effective therapy, that is from the date of optimal source control or first negative blood culture, whichever comes last. A notable

Table 2
Suggested antimicrobial agents for definitive therapy for BSI caused by common microorganisms[a]

Microorganism	Preferred Agents[b]	Alternative Agents[b]
Methicillin-susceptible staphylococci	Nafcillin 2 g every 4 h or cefazolin 2 g every 8 h	Vancomycin[c] 15 mg/kg every 8–12 h
Methicillin-resistant staphylococci	Vancomycin (as above)	Daptomycin 6 mg/kg every 24 h
β-Hemolytic streptococci (eg, group A, B, C)	Penicillin G 18–24 million units daily divided every 4–6 h	Cefazolin (as above)
Viridans group streptococci	Penicillin G (as above)	Ceftriaxone 2 g every 24 h
Enterococcus species	Ampicillin 3 g every 6 h	Vancomycin (as above)
Escherichia coli, Klebsiella species, and Proteus mirabilis	Ampicillin-sulbactam 3 g every 6 h or ceftriaxone (as above) or ciprofloxacin 400 mg every 8 h	Levofloxacin 750 mg every 24 h
Enterobacter, Citrobacter, and Serratia species	Cefepime 2 g every 12 h or ciprofloxacin (as above)	Piperacillin-tazobactam 3.375–4.5 g every 6 h or levofloxacin 750 mg every 24 h
Pseudomonas aeruginosa	Piperacillin-tazobactam 4.5 g every 6 h or cefepime 2 g every 8 h	Ciprofloxacin (as above)
Bacteroides species	Metronidazole 500 mg every 8 h	Ampicillin-sulbactam or piperacillin-tazobactam (as above)

[a] For strains that are susceptible in vitro to the listed antimicrobial agents. Resistant strains should be treated based on in vitro antimicrobial susceptibility testing results.
[b] Provided dosing is for intravenous route in adults. Dose adjustment may be required for patients with renal or hepatic impairment.
[c] Alternative therapy for patients with severe penicillin allergy, such as anaphylaxis, angioedema, and hives.

exception is CRBSI caused by CoNS, in which 7 to 10 days of appropriate antibiotics after catheter removal may be adequate. Patients with complicated BSI, including infective endocarditis, deep abscesses, or hematogenous seeding of bones or joints require prolonged antimicrobial therapy for a minimum of 4 to 6 weeks, depending on the pathogen, adequacy of source control, and clinical response to therapy.

- Most patients with BSI require intravenous antibiotics for the course of treatment. However, patients with BSI caused by fluoroquinolone-susceptible gram-negative bacilli may be switched to high-dose oral fluoroquinolones, which have high bioavailability, after initial clinical improvement on intravenous antibiotics, given the ability to take and keep down oral medications.

Prevention of Bloodstream Infections

The role of infection control programs at local institutions is pivotal for prevention of BSI. Early removal of urinary catheters and emergently placed central venous catheters is an important measure for the prevention of hospital-acquired BSI, including CRBSI. A recent multicenter, cluster-randomized trial reported a reduction in the incidence rate of nosocomial BSI using daily bathing with chlorhexidine-impregnated washcloths.[32] Evidence-based preventative guidelines have been published in an effort to stem the tide of increasing health care costs and morbidity related to CRBSI.[29] Details of the recommendations are beyond the scope of this article, but specifically address:

- Education
- Insertion techniques and catheter selection, including hand hygiene, barrier precautions, and skin preparation
- Catheter maintenance techniques and dressing regimens
- Performance improvement strategies using bundles

SUMMARY

- High clinical suspicion for BSI in patients with symptoms and signs of infection and appropriate collection of 2 sets of blood cultures before starting antibiotics is key for diagnosis.
- Establishment and control of the source of infection is essential for successful treatment of BSI.
- In patients with CLABSI, the decision to remove the central line is complex and depends on:
  - Acute severity of illness at initial presentation
  - Type of catheter
  - Virulence of pathogen causing BSI
  - Difficulty of catheter removal, availability, and need of new venous access
- Early initiation of appropriate empirical antimicrobial therapy in patients with suspected or confirmed BSI improves survival and should be tailored to:
  - Likely microbiology based on suspected source of infection
  - Site of infection acquisition
  - Acute severity of illness and predicted prognosis at initial presentation
  - Local antimicrobial susceptibility rates
  - Individual risk factors for antimicrobial resistance
- Definitive antimicrobial therapy should be streamlined based on blood culture and in vitro antimicrobial susceptibility testing results
- Identification of potential complications of BSI is vital for both source control and determination of optimal duration of antimicrobial therapy.

REFERENCES

1. CDC. Central Line-Associated Bloodstream Infection (CLABSI) Event. 2014. Available at: http://www.cdc.gov/nhsn/PDFs/pscManual/17pscNosInfDef_current.pdf. Accessed on September 25, 2014.
2. CDC. Complete List of Common Commensals. 2013. Available at: http://www.cdc.gov/nhsn/XLS/master-organism-Com-Commensals-Lists.xlsx. Accessed on September 25, 2014.
3. Mermel LA, Allon M, Bouza E, et al. Clinical practice guidelines for the diagnosis and management of intravascular catheter-related infection: 2009 update by the Infectious Diseases Society of America. Clin Infect Dis 2009;49:1–45.
4. Friedman ND, Kaye KS, Stout JE, et al. Health care-associated bloodstream infections in adults: a reason to change the accepted definition of community-acquired infections. Ann Intern Med 2002;137:792–7.
5. Al-Hasan MN, Eckel-Passow JE, Baddour LM. Influence of referral bias on the clinical characteristics of patients with gram-negative bloodstream infection. Epidemiol Infect 2011;139:1750–6.

6. Laupland KB. Incidence of bloodstream infection: a review of population-based studies. Clin Microbiol Infect 2013;19(6):492–500.

7. Filice GA, Van Etta LL, Darby CP, et al. Bacteremia in Charleston County, South Carolina. Am J Epidemiol 1986;123:128–36.

8. Uslan DZ, Crane SJ, Steckelberg JM, et al. Age- and sex-associated trends in bloodstream infection: a population-based study in Olmstead County, Minnesota. Arch Intern Med 2007;167:834–9.

9. Sogaard M, Norgaard M, Dethlefsen C. Temporal changes in the incidence and 30-day mortality associated with bacteremia in hospitalized patients from 1992 through 2006: a population-based cohort study. Clin Infect Dis 2011;52:61–9.

10. Goto M, Al-Hasan MN. Overall burden of bloodstream infection and nosocomial bloodstream infection in North America and Europe. Clin Microbiol Infect 2013;19(6):501–9.

11. US Centers for Disease Control and Prevention. Vital signs: central line–associated blood stream infections–United States, 2001, 2008, and 2009. MMWR Morb Mortal Wkly Rep 2011;60(8):243–8.

12. Shannon RP, Patel B, Cummins D, et al. Economics of central line-associated bloodstream infections. Am J Med Qual 2006;21(6 Suppl):7S–16S.

13. The Joint Commission. Preventing central line-associated bloodstream infections: a global challenge, a global perspective. 2012. Available at: http://www.jointcommission.org/assets/1/18/CLABSI_Monograph.pdfhttp://www.jointcommission.org/assets/1/18/CLABSI_Monograph.pdf. Accessed on February 25, 2014.

14. Klevens RM, Edwards JR, Richards CL Jr, et al. Estimating health care–associated infections and deaths in U.S. hospitals, 2002. Public Health Rep 2007;122(2):160–6.

15. Dellinger RP, Levy MM, Rhodes A, et al. Surviving sepsis campaign: international guidelines for management of severe sepsis and septic shock, 2012. Intensive Care Med 2013;39:165–228.

16. Huang AM, Newton D, Kunapuli A, et al. Impact of rapid organism identification via matrix-assisted laser desorption/ionization time-of-flight combined with antimicrobial stewardship team intervention in adult patients with bacteremia and candidemia. Clin Infect Dis 2013;57:1237–45.

17. Retamar P, Portillo MM, López-Prieto MD, et al. Impact of inadequate empirical therapy on the mortality of patients with bloodstream infections: a propensity score-based analysis. Antimicrob Agents Chemother 2012;56:472–8.

18. Paul M, Shani V, Muchtar E, et al. Systematic review and meta-analysis of the efficacy of appropriate empiric antibiotic therapy for sepsis. Antimicrob Agents Chemother 2010;54:4851–63.

19. Al-Hasan MN, Eckel-Passow JE, Baddour LM. Impact of healthcare-associated acquisition on community-onset gram-negative bloodstream infection: a population-based study. Eur J Clin Microbiol Infect Dis 2012;31:1163–71.

20. Paterson DL, Ko WC, Von Gottberg A, et al. International prospective study of *Klebsiella pneumoniae* bacteremia: implications of extended-spectrum beta-lactamase production in nosocomial infections. Ann Intern Med 2004;140:26–32.

21. Al-Hasan MN, Lahr BD, Eckel-Passow JE, et al. Predictive scoring model of mortality in gram-negative bloodstream infection. Clin Microbiol Infect 2013;19:948–54.

22. Tumbarello M, Trecarichi EM, Bassetti M, et al. Identifying patients harboring extended-spectrum-beta-lactamase-producing Enterobacteriaceae on hospital admission: derivation and validation of a scoring system. Antimicrob Agents Chemother 2011;55:3485–90.

23. Orsi GB, Bencardino A, Vena A, et al. Patient risk factors for outer membrane permeability and KPC-producing carbapenem-resistant *Klebsiella pneumoniae* isolation: results of a double case-control study. Infection 2013;41:61–7.

24. Casey J, Davies J, Balshaw-Greer A, et al. Inserting tunneled hemodialysis catheters using elective guidewire exchange from nontunnelled catheters: is there a greater risk of infection when compared with new-site replacement? Hemodial Int 2008;12(1):52–4.

25. Mokrzycki MH, Singhal A. Cost-effectiveness of three strategies of managing tunneled, cuffed haemodialysis catheters in clinically mild or asymptomatic bacteraemias. Nephrol Dial Transplant 2002;17(12):2196–203.

26. Erbay A, Ergonul O, Stoddard GJ, et al. Recurrent catheter-related bloodstream infections: risk factors and outcome. Int J Infect Dis 2006;10(5):396–400.

27. Badley AD, Steckelberg JM, Wollan PC, et al. Infectious rates of central venous pressure catheters: comparison between newly placed catheters and those that have been changed. Mayo Clin Proc 1996;71(9):838–46.

28. Cook D, Randolph A, Kernerman P, et al. Central venous catheter replacement strategies: a systematic review of the literature. Crit Care Med 1997;25(8): 1417–24.

29. O'Grady NP, Alexander M, Burns LA, et al. Guidelines for the prevention of intravascular catheter-related infections, 2011. Clin Infect Dis 2011;52(9):e162–93.

30. Fowler VG, Olsen MK, Corey GR, et al. Clinical identifiers of complicated *Staphylococcus aureus* bacteremia. Arch Intern Med 2003;163:2066–72.

31. Baddour LM, Wilson WR, Bayer AS, et al. Infective endocarditis: diagnosis, antimicrobial therapy, and management of complication: a statement for healthcare professionals from the committee on rheumatic fever, endocarditis, and Kawasaki disease, Council on Cardiovascular Disease in the Young, and the Councils on Cardiology, Stroke, and Cardiovascular Surgery and Anesthesia, American Heart Association: endorsed by the Infectious Diseases Society of America. Circulation 2005;111:394–434.

32. Climo MW, Yokoe DS, Warren DK, et al. Effect of daily chlorhexidine bathing on hospital-acquired infections. N Engl J Med 2013;368:533–42.

Surgical Site Infections

Pang Y. Young, MD[a], Rachel G. Khadaroo, MD, PhD, FRCSC[a,b],*

KEYWORDS

- Surgical site infection • Surgical wound infections • Antibiotic prophylaxis
- Infection control • Postoperative complication

KEY POINTS

- Surgical site infections (SSIs) are major contributors to patient morbidity and mortality in hospital settings.
- Risk for SSI is multifactorial and includes modifiable and nonmodifiable factors.
- Basic and clinical research has expanded evidence-based guidelines for SSI prevention.
- SSIs are increasingly used as outcome and surrogate measures for examining the quality of surgical care.
- A culture of safety and quality is an important element to reducing SSI.

INTRODUCTION

Surgical site infections (SSIs) have played a major role in the evolution of medical care throughout history. Wound complications contributed significantly to the historical surgical mortality rates before the development of Lister's aseptic approach in the nineteenth century.[1] The impact of the antiseptic/aseptic techniques was readily apparent in its adaptation to battlefield medicine. During the Civil War in America, surgeons routinely operated bare-handed, with wound suppuration considered to be a beneficial aspect of wound healing.[2] With the gradual acceptance of the principles of antisepsis, and the usage of sterile dressings and aseptic surgical technique, there was a dramatic reduction in mortality from wounds to 7.4% in the Spanish-American War.[3]

Despite nearly 2 centuries of medical progress, the management of surgical infection remains a pressing concern, and SSIs continue to be a leading component of nosocomial morbidity and mortality. In this article, the epidemiology, pathogenesis,

Disclosures: No conflicts of interest to disclose.
[a] Division of General Surgery, Department of Surgery, Faculty of Medicine and Dentistry, University of Alberta, 8440–112 Street Northwest, Edmonton, Alberta T6G 2B7, Canada; [b] Division of Critical Care Medicine, Faculty of Medicine and Dentistry, University of Alberta, 8440–112 Street Northwest, Edmonton, Alberta T6G 2B7, Canada
* Corresponding author. 2D Walter C. Mackenzie Health Sciences Centre, 8440–112 Street Northwest, Edmonton, Alberta T6G 2R7, Canada.
E-mail address: khadaroo@ualberta.ca

Surg Clin N Am 94 (2014) 1245–1264
http://dx.doi.org/10.1016/j.suc.2014.08.008
0039-6109/14/$ – see front matter © 2014 Elsevier Inc. All rights reserved.

surgical.theclinics.com

risk factors, and approach to prevention of SSIs are reviewed. This review highlights the multifaceted and multidisciplinary approach to management of SSIs, which are a critical aspect of infection control outcomes.

DEFINITIONS

To assist with appropriate surveillance of SSIs, establishing clear definitions for cases of SSIs was critical. The Centers for Disease Control and Prevention (CDC) established the National Healthcare Safety Network (NHSN) to monitor quality control measures, including SSIs, and has defined widely used definitions for SSI (**Box 1**).[4] SSI are classified based on the depth of involvement of the infection, which may be confined to the skin and subcutaneous tissues (superficial incisional SSI), involve the deep soft tissue, such as the fascial and muscular layers (deep incisional SSI), or extend further beyond these anatomic boundaries (organ/space SSI) (**Fig. 1**).[5] Incisional SSIs are further subdivided into primary and secondary for cases with more than one incision. For instance, a primary incisional SSI involves the primary incision (eg, chest incision for coronary artery bypass grafting), and a secondary incisional SSI involves secondary incisions (eg, leg incision for donor site in coronary artery bypass grafting).

EPIDEMIOLOGY

Recognizing the historical context of surgical infection can highlight the gains that have been made over the past few centuries. Before the antisepsis era, the risk of surgery was exceedingly high due to the enormous rates of surgical infection. Compounded by the absence of the effective anesthesia, early surgical procedures had limited success compared with the modern era. Acknowledgment of the aseptic approach made a significant impact on outcomes. The simple introduction of hand washing by Semmelweis resulted in a decrease in mortality due to puerperal sepsis from 12% to 2%.[6]

The development of multiple aspects of modern surgical care has led to significant improvements in the historical context described. Nevertheless, SSIs remain a frequent postoperative complication, developing in 3% to 20% of surgical procedures.[7] The rate of SSI is highly variable depending on the specific operative procedure, with rates that can be even higher depending on the number of risk factors present.

There is a substantial impact of SSI on both morbidity and mortality. However, establishing the exact impact of SSI is difficult because of the dependence on accuracy of reporting and the variability of patient follow-up. In the 1980s, it was observed that SSI led to a 10-day increase in hospital length of stay.[8] Even a decade later, another study reported persistent delayed discharge from hospital and increased requirement for post-discharge care.[9] In a study of 288,906 patients, in-hospital mortality for the patients with SSIs was 14.5% versus 1.8% of patients with no SSI. SSIs are estimated to be responsible for more than 8000 deaths annually in the United States.[7] SSIs may be of even greater consequence in developing countries, because surveillance rates of SSI in a study conducted by the International Nosocomial Infection Control Consortium were higher for most surgical procedures compared with CDC-NHSN rates.[10]

RISK FACTORS FOR SURGICAL SITE INFECTION

From a general perspective, the microbes responsible for infection of surgical wounds originate from either the surrounding skin or associated structures that are contiguous

Box 1
Centers for Disease Control and Prevention–National Healthcare Safety Network definitions for surgical site infections

Superficial incisional surgical site infection

Infection occurs within 30 days after the operative procedure *and*

Involves only skin and subcutaneous tissue of the incision *and*

Patient has at least 1 of the following:

a. Purulent drainage from the superficial incision

b. Organisms isolated from an aseptically obtained culture of fluid or tissue from the superficial incision

c. At least 1 of the following signs or symptoms of infection: pain or tenderness, localized swelling, redness, or heat, and superficial incision is deliberately opened by surgeon and is culture positive or not cultured. A culture-negative finding does not meet this criterion

d. Diagnosis of superficial incisional SSI by the surgeon or attending physician

Deep incisional surgical site infection

Infection occurs within 30 days after the operative procedure if no implant is left in place or within 1 year if implant is in place and the infection appears to be related to the operative procedure *and*

Involves deep soft tissues (eg, fascial and muscle layers) of the incision *and*

Patient has at least 1 of the following:

a. Purulent drainage from the deep incision but not from the organ/space component of the surgical site

b. A deep incision spontaneously dehisces or is deliberately opened by a surgeon and is culture-positive or not cultured when the patient has at least 1 of the following signs or symptoms: fever (>38°C) or localized pain or tenderness. A culture-negative finding does not meet this criterion

c. An abscess or other evidence of infection involving the deep incision is found on direct examination, during reoperation, or by histopathologic or radiologic examination

d. Diagnosis of a deep incisional SSI by a surgeon or attending physician

Organ/space surgical site infection

Infection occurs within 30 days after the operative procedure if no implant is left in place or within 1 year if implant is in place and the infection appears to be related to the operative procedure and infection involves any part of the body, excluding the skin incision, fascia, or muscle layers, that is opened or manipulated during the operative procedure *and*

Patient has at least 1 of the following:

a. Purulent drainage from a drain that is placed through a stab wound into the organ/space

b. Organisms isolated from an aseptically obtained culture of fluid or tissue in the organ/space

c. An abscess or other evidence of infection involving the organ/space that is found on direct examination, during reoperation, or by histopathologic or radiologic examination

d. Diagnosis of an organ/space SSI by a surgeon or attending physician.

From Horan TC, Andrus M, Dudeck MA. CDC/NHSN surveillance definition of health care-associated infection and criteria for specific types of infections in the acute care setting. Am J Infect Control 2008;36:313–4; with permission.

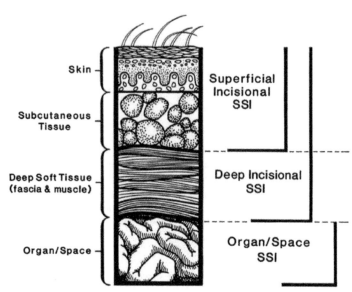

Fig. 1. Schematic for CDC classification of surgical site infection. (*From* Horan TC, Gaynes RP, Martone WJ, et al. CDC definitions of nosocomial surgical site infections, 1992: a modification of CDC definitions of surgical wound infections. Infect Control Hosp Epidemiol 1992; 13(10):606–8.)

with the regions of the surgical procedure. The logical extension of this principle is that the risk of wound contamination and subsequent SSI depends on location, the nature of the surgical wound/incision, and the procedure performed. The CDC wound classification system defines wound class based on risk and is divided into 4 categories: clean, clean-contaminated, contaminated, and dirty (**Table 1**).[5] With clean wounds, the expected risk is from microbes located directly on the surface of the skin, or introduced from the external environment. With increasing wound class, there is increased exposure to microorganisms that are present on internal structures of the body, such as epithelial surfaces of the gastrointestinal tract and genitourinary tract. In the early epidemiologic studies, the SSI rate increased with wound class (I, 2.1%; II, 3.3%; III, 6.4%; IV, 7.1%).[11]

Appropriate risk stratification for SSI cannot be limited to the wound alone. There are a variety of patient-related factors and perioperative factors that can significantly affect the risk of SSI in a surgical patient (**Box 2**). One system of risk stratification is the National Nosocomial Infection Surveillance (NNIS) System risk score, based on 3 factors. These factors are (1) an American Society of Anesthesiology preoperative assessment score of greater than or equal to 3; (2) an operation with a wound classification as contaminated or dirty; and (3) an operation longer than the 75th percentile in duration for the specific procedure.[11] In the original development of the NNIS risk score, each additional risk factor resulted in increasing rates of SSI, even within the same traditional wound class. In the most recent publication of aggregate data from the NHSN SSI surveillance system, the effects of risk factors remain apparent (**Table 2**), with escalating SSI rates with the number of risk factors. The NNIS score has been further modified to account for some specific instances of laparoscopic cases, as the risk for SSI can be lower.

The risk factors identified in the NNIS risk scoring system are useful from surveillance and monitoring perspectives. However, prevention requires identification of

Table 1 Surgical wound classification		
Class	Type	Description
I	Clean	An uninfected operative wound in which no inflammation is encountered and the respiratory, alimentary, genital, or uninfected urinary tract is not entered. In addition, clean wounds are primarily closed and, if necessary, drained with closed drainage. Operative incisional wounds that follow nonpenetrating (blunt) trauma should be included in this category if they meet the criteria.
II	Clean—contaminated	An operative wound in which the respiratory, alimentary, genital, or urinary tracts are entered under controlled conditions and without unusual contamination. Specifically, operations involving the biliary tract, appendix, vagina, and oropharynx are included in this category, provided no evidence of infection or major break in technique is encountered.
III	Contaminated	Open, fresh, accidental wounds. In addition, operations with major breaks in sterile technique (eg, open cardiac massage) or gross spillage from the gastrointestinal tract, and incisions in which acute, nonpurulent inflammation is encountered are included in this category.
IV	Dirty—infected	Old traumatic wounds with retained devitalized tissue and those that involve existing clinical infection or perforated viscera. This definition suggests that the organisms causing postoperative infection were present in the operative field before the operation.

From Mangram AJ, Horan TC, Pearson ML, et al. Guideline for prevention of surgical site infection, 1999. Am J Infect Control 1999;27:109; with permission.

risk factors that are more readily modifiable than those listed in the NNIS scoring system. An approach to the risk factors of SSIs can be categorized into a schematic of microbial factors, patient factors, and perioperative factors.

MICROBIAL FACTORS

The predominant source of microbes involved in SSIs originate from either the skin or the surrounding tissues of the incision, or from deeper structures involved in the operative procedure (eg, enteric organisms in bowel-related surgeries). In the most recent NHSN surveillance report on 21,100 isolates from 2009 to 2010, the most frequently identified pathogens were, in order, *Staphylococcus aureus*, Coagulase-negative *Staphylococci*, *Escherichia coli*, *Enterococcus faecalis*, and *Pseudomonas aeruginosa*.[12] The overall distribution of pathogens associated with SSI has changed to some extent over the past couple decades (**Table 3**).[12–14] The proportion of gram-negative bacilli has decreased coinciding with a relative increase in the proportion of *S aureus*–related infection. In the most recently published 2010 NHSN data, *S aureus* accounted for 30.4% of SSI, up from 20% in the early 1990s. Individual institutions may have variations in the proportions of specific species, due to differences in the volumes of various surgical specialties.

The temporal trend of significance is the substantial growth in multidrug resistance (MDR). The most apparent example is the increase in methicillin-resistant *Staphylococcus aureus* (MRSA).[15] In a study of community hospitals in southeastern United States, the incidence of MRSA-associated SSI increased from 12% in 2000 to 23% in 2005.[16] In the 2010 NHSN update, the proportion of SSI due to MRSA was 43.7%.[12] Increases in MRSA prevalence internationally show similar temporal trends.

Box 2
Risk factors for surgical site infection

Patient factors

  Age

  Nutritional status

  Diabetes

  Smoking

  Obesity

  Coexistent infections at a remote body site

  Colonization with microorganisms

  Altered immune response

  Length of preoperative stay

Operative factors

  Duration of surgical scrub

  Skin antisepsis

  Preoperative shaving

  Preoperative skin preparation

  Duration of operation

  Antimicrobial prophylaxis

  Operating room ventilation

  Inadequate sterilization of instruments

  Foreign material in the surgical site

  Surgical drains

  Surgical technique

    Poor hemostasis

    Failure to obliterate dead space

    Tissue trauma

From Mangram AJ, Horan TC, Pearson ML, et al. Guideline for prevention of surgical site infection, 1999. Am J Infect Control 1999;27:105; with permission.

In a Japanese study of 702 isolates, methicillin resistance in S aureus isolates was 72.0%.[17] Community-acquired MRSA is increasing in prevalence, with the prevalence of nasal colonization with MRSA in the general population increasing from 0.8% to 1.5% from 2001–2002 to 2003–2004.[18] Studies have attempted to clarify the relationship between colonization and risk for MRSA SSI. In a study of 9006 patients in a Pennsylvania tertiary care hospital by Kalra and colleagues,[19] 4.3% of patients were positive for nasal MRSA screening; the MRSA SSI rate was 1.86% in MRSA-screen-positive patients compared with 0.20% in MRSA-screen-negative patients.

An important aspect of the temporal changes in MDR pathogens is the significant alteration in the pharmacodynamics of the antibiotics used to manage these infections. Several studies have shown an upward shift in minimal inhibitory concentration (MIC) of vancomycin in clinically isolated strains of MRSA, described as "MIC creep."

Table 2
Surgical site infection rates, based on risk index for various surgical procedures

Procedure	Risk Index (%)			
	0	1	2	3
CABG with chest and donor incision	0.35	2.55	4.26	8.49
Breast surgery	0.95	2.95	6.46	
Colon surgery	3.99	5.59	7.06	9.47
Gallbladder surgery (inpatient)	0.23	0.61	1.72	
Herniorrhaphy (inpatient)	0.74	2.42	5.25	
Rectal surgery	3.47	7.99		26.67
Small bowel surgery	3.44	6.75		
Thoracic surgery	0.76		2.04	

Abbreviation: CABG, coronary artery bypass grafting.
Data from Edwards JR, Peterson KD, Mu Y, et al. National Healthcare Safety Network (NHSN) report: data summary for 2006 through 2008, issued December 2009. Am J Infect Control 2009;37:783–805.

During a period between 2000 and 2004, Wang and colleagues[20] reported on 6003 clinical isolates, showing a large significant increase in the proportion of isolates with vancomycin MIC of 1 mg/L from 19.9% to 70.4%. In a 5-year period between 2001 and 2005, Steinkraus and colleagues[21] reported a significant increase in the MIC of vancomycin, oxacillin, and linezolid in 662 isolates collected over the 5-year period. For vancomycin, in particular, there was a significant shift in proportion of isolates with MIC $\leq$0.5 mg/L, from 46% in 2001 to 5% in 2006.

There have been conflicting data with respect to "MIC creep." Several surveillance studies from Canadian, United Kingdom, and American centers have not demonstrated the same degree of MIC creep.[22–24] Additional controversy lies in the methodologies to represent changes in MIC. In general, these trends remain cause for concern as higher MIC is predictive of vancomycin treatment failure in MRSA.[25] In some series, MRSA infection has been independently associated with mortality.[26] Narrowing of the therapeutic window will increase the risk for adverse effects as dosing targets are adjusted.[27] Management of MRSA as a single example of antibiotic resistance carries a significant burden of cost.

Table 3
Distribution of causative pathogenic organisms in surgical site infection, reported by the National Healthcare Safety Network at various reporting dates

Pathogen	Year		
	1990–1996	2007	2010
S aureus	20%	30.0%	30.4%
Coagulase-negative *Staphylococcus*	14%	13.7%	11.7%
Enterococcus sp.	12%	11.2%	11.6%
E coli	8%	9.6%	9.4%
P aeruginosa	8%	5.6%	5.5%
Enterobacter sp	7%	4.2%	4.0%
K pneumoniae	3%	3.0%	4.0%

Data from Refs.[12–14]

The concerns of antibiotic resistance are increasing as new mechanisms for multidrug resistance are continuing to develop. For instance, New Delhi metallo-β-lactamase 1 (NDM-1) was first reported in Sweden in 2008.[28] It has been increasingly identified in isolates from India, Pakistan, and the United Kingdom.[29] The global spread of NDM-1 is now broad, with identification in Canada, United States, Australia, China, and Russia.[30–34] The resistance mechanism was first identified in *Klebsiella pneumoniae* and *E coli*.[28] Other species of *Enterobacteriaceae* have now also been identified to harbor NDM-1, including *Acinetobacter, Enterobacter, Providencia*, and *Raoultella*. It has been primarily identified in patients with community-acquired pneumonia, urinary tract infections, and bacteremia.[29] Nevertheless, like the spread geographically and in speciation, there is significant potential impact with SSI. In one case report, *Acinetobacter baumanii* expressing NDM-1 was isolated from a Dacron graft infection.[35] NDM-1 is just one example of an MDR mechanism that has spread globally in a few short years.[36]

A discussion on microbial factors in surgical infection can extend far beyond a discussion on cause alone. There is a growing body of research literature that suggests that there is an important role of the host microbiome in response to disease.[37] The most well-studied interactions are within inflammatory bowel disease, which demonstrates a clear relationship with altered microbiome composition.[38,39] Understanding of the interaction of the host microbiome with wound healing is evolving. As an example, in an animal model of anastomotic leak, there is an association of anastomotic leak with specific virulence factors in *P aeruginosa*.[40] Further research may significantly alter the understanding of surgical infection and the interaction with microbial etiologies.

PATIENT FACTORS

Patient comorbidities can contribute significantly to the potential risk of SSIs. These factors include age, obesity, smoking, diabetes mellitus, malnutrition, dyslipidemia, and immunosuppression (see **Box 2**).[41] These factors are not directly accounted for in the NNIS classification scheme but can contribute significantly to the risk of SSI. Identification of these risk factors with appropriate preoperative history and physical examination is critical. The core principle for management of these patient-related risk factors is preoperative optimization.

Because many of the patient comorbidities are nonmodifiable, there can be a substantial increase in SSI risk. Particularly in urgent or emergent situations, there may not be an opportunity to optimize a patient's comorbid status fully. The rate of SSI is expected to be much higher in emergency surgery, as opposed to elective cases, which has been demonstrated in many studies.[41–43] The higher SSI rate in emergency cases also signifies patients that are more critically ill, with greater physiologic compromise, and expectedly, worse outcome.

Other patient-related risk factors are also often nonmodifiable in the timeline of preoperative planning. Although age is clearly a nonmodifiable risk factor, other comorbidities, such as diabetes, obesity, and immunosuppression, are not easily reversible in a short-term time frame. Optimization of these risk factors is critical. For diabetes, optimization of glucose control has been clearly demonstrated to have efficacy in reduction of SSI rates.[41,44,45] In the cardiac surgery literature, rates of sternal wound infection have been shown to improve with the quality of glycemic control.[46–48] Glycemic control optimization recommendations include a reduction in serum glucose levels and a reduction in HgbA1c to less than 7.0%.[45,49]

Smoking results in significantly increased risk of SSI because of its effects on local tissue perfusion. Large numbers of studies have consistently shown that smoking results in at least a 2-fold increased risk of SSI.[44] In one trial by Møller and colleagues[50] of 120 patients, smoking cessation therapy resulted in a reduction of wound-related complications from 31% to 5%. This finding has been confirmed by additional studies, and in meta-analyses of trial data.[51,52] Recommendations are for smoking cessation at least 30 days before operation.[41,44,45]

For patients that have significantly elevated risk because of risk factors that cannot be modified, additional preventative measures need to be considered and can include the use of altered protocols for antimicrobial prophylaxis (as discussed later), or consideration of additional risk reduction measures.

PERIOPERATIVE FACTORS

Preventative measures in the preoperative period have changed rapidly over the past few decades. A large volume of research has established the importance of a host of preventative measures in the operative period. Examples include skin decontamination, perioperative warming, and antimicrobial prophylaxis.[41,44,45] As additional studies have been conducted with increasing methodological rigor, from observational studies to randomized controlled trials, refinements of existing preventative measures have further improved the efficacy of these measures. This review focuses on areas of prevention that are the focus of significant active research or have seen recent changes in key guidelines or recommendations.

Skin Decontamination

The use of antiseptic agents topically has long been recommended for use in skin decontamination.[5] The 2 broad classes of topical agents include chlorhexidine-based preparations and iodophor-based agents. In addition, these agents can be combined with isopropyl alcohol (IPA) in solution. Several studies have sought to address potential differences in efficacy between the various available agents, although there has been significant inconsistency of results, which have been also been confounded by methodological differences between the studies.

In the systematic review and meta-analysis conducted by Lee and colleagues,[53] chlorhexidine-based agents were found to reduce the risk of SSIs significantly, with an adjusted risk ratio of 0.64, and result in a net cost-savings over the use of iodophor-based agents. This analysis included 9 randomized controlled trials, but in several of the included trials, chlorhexidine-based solutions containing IPA were compared with povidone-iodine solutions not containing IPA, which confounded the results of the analysis.[54–56] In a nonrandomized study by Swenson and colleagues,[57] there was no significant difference between chlorhexidine/IPA and 1 of 2 forms of iodophor-based agents (povidone-iodine or iodine povacrylex in IPA).

In the most recently published cohort study by Hakkarainen and colleagues,[58] there were no significant differences between 4 different preparations of skin antisepsis agents (chlorhexidine/IPA, chlorhexidine, povidone-iodine, and iodine-povacrylex/IPA) in a cohort of primarily clean-contaminated general surgical cases. In their conclusion, there was minimal incremental benefit for chlorhexidine-based agent in their specific subset of clean-contaminated cases. As one prospective European study highlighted, there was no direct correlation between the residual bacterial flora following disinfection and subsequent SSI in a variety of surgical cases,[59] suggesting that in certain surgical disciplines, the choice of skin antisepsis has less effect, particularly when the microbial cause lies in noncutaneous sources, such as enteric sources for general surgical procedures.

Antibiotic Prophylaxis

From a historical perspective, routine antibiotic prophylaxis was questioned for its usefulness. With demonstrated clinical benefit in the clinical trials conducted separately by Polk and Lopez-Mayor and Stone and colleagues,[60,61] there has been tremendous improvement in SSI as an outcome. From the outset, the development of antibiotic prophylaxis has undoubtedly led to a clear reduction in rates of SSI. The complexity and nuance of clinical practice guidelines has continued to become more complex and refined.

Although there have been continual updates to the clinical practice guidelines, the general principles of antimicrobial prophylaxis are consistent.[41,62–64] First, the antimicrobial agent should be safe. Second, an appropriate antimicrobial agent should be selected that has a narrow spectrum of coverage for the expected relevant pathogens. Third, antimicrobial prophylaxis should be administered in the preoperative period to allow serum and tissue concentrations to reach appropriate levels at the time of incision. Last, the antimicrobial agent should be administered for the shortest effect period, with appropriate discontinuation of the agent.

Clinical practice guidelines for antimicrobial prophylaxis were recently updated in 2013 in a joint publication by the American Society of Health-System Pharmacists, the Infectious Diseases Society of America, the Surgical Infection Society, and the Society for Healthcare Epidemiology of America.[63] The revised guidelines replaced the previously published 1999 guidelines[65] and highlighted several focuses including timing of preoperative dosing, weight-based dosing, and duration of postoperative prophylaxis.

Selection of antibiotics for prophylaxis should be made with the primary consideration of the spectrum of coverage required. This consideration should be made because of the wound classification and the overall risk of infection. For example, in clean surgical procedures, the risk of SSI is relatively low and, in several cases, antimicrobial prophylaxis is not indicated.[41] Prophylaxis is considered in specific clean procedures where the consequence of infection is critical (eg, prosthetic implants, cardiac pacemakers). Consideration of intrinsic patient-related factors associated with increased risk of SSI (eg, age, malnutrition, immunosuppression) is relevant and appropriate justification for the use of antimicrobial prophylaxis.[63,65] A meta-analysis conducted by Bowater and colleagues[66] demonstrated that the relative risk reduction was the same across wound classes.

In clean procedures, the primary coverage is for the likely *Staphylococcus* sp. that will be the predominant cause. For clean-contaminated procedures, similar spectrum of coverage for *Staphylococus* sp. is required, with additional coverage as needed depending on the site of surgery. As such, first-generation and second-generation cephalosporins remain the recommended prophylactic antibiotics for a large number of surgical procedures.[41,63,65] For contaminated and dirty wound classes, prophylaxis is typically not indicated, because therapeutic antibiotic management is required.

Preoperative dosing of antibiotic prophylaxis is optimized to allow serum and tissue concentrations to reach sufficient levels at the time of incision. Several studies have studied the precise timeline for preoperative administration of prophylaxis to achieve maximal benefit. In 1992, Classen and colleagues[67] showed a decreased SSI rate to 0.59% with administration within 2 hours of incision, compared with 3.8% for early (2–24 hours before incision) and 3.3% for postoperative administration. In a cardiac surgery study of 2048 patients, the rate of SSI was lowest in the group receiving vancomycin prophylaxis in the window of 16 to 60 minutes before incision.[68]

Trends have been seen in several studies that may suggest that the window for preoperative antibiotics could be narrowed to 30 minutes of incision. In the Trial to

Reduce Antimicrobial Prophylaxis Errors (TRAPE) study of 4722 patients undergoing cardiac, arthroplasty, or hysterectomy procedures, the effect of specific windows of antibiotic prophylaxis (in 30-minute intervals, preceding and following incision) was examined.[69] The lowest rate of SSI was in the 30-minute window immediately before incision. In an orthopedic study by van Kasteren and colleagues,[70] 1922 patients undergoing hip arthroplasty were examined. The rates of SSI in the groups receiving antibiotics in the 1- to 30-minute and 31- to 60-minute windows were 2.19% and 2.60%, respectively, which was not statistically significant. Both studies reinforced that the highest rate of SSI occurred in groups receiving antibiotics following incision. The potential incremental benefit of an earlier antibiotic window is likely small and would be difficult to detect without significantly larger sample sizes. Current guidelines emphasize prophylaxis administration within 60 minutes of incision, or within 120 minutes for antibiotics requiring longer infusion times.[63]

In the updated clinical practice guidelines, weight-based dosing is an additional focus.[63] Particularly in obese patients, studies have shown the pharmacokinetics of antibiotic administration are significantly altered. In a 1989 study on obese patients undergoing gastroplasty and normal-weight adults undergoing abdominal surgery, 1 g dosing of cefazolin resulted in significantly lower blood and tissue concentrations in obese patients.[71] However, 2 g dosing of cefazolin resulted in blood and tissue levels equivalent to normal-weight patients. Guidelines recommend increased dosing and fewer adjustments in renal impairment.[63,64]

Adequate redosing of antibiotics for longer operative procedures is necessary for risk reduction. With longer procedures, serum and tissue concentrations can drop below adequate levels, particularly in antibiotics with shorter half-lives (eg, cefazolin, cefoxitin, gentamicin).[63,72] The effect was seen even in smaller case series. In the study by Morita and colleagues[73] of 131 patients undergoing colorectal procedures, the SSI rates in procedures longer than 4 hours were 8.5% and 26.5%, in groups with or without redosing, respectively. In the TRAPE trial, the rate of SSI was increased with an absence of redosing, 5.5% versus 1.8%.[69] Guidelines emphasize repeated dosing at intervals of 2 half-lives of the antibiotic used.[63]

Additional routes of antibiotic administration have been investigated in the past and have been historically ruled out. Topical routes of antibiotic prophylaxis have been considered for some time. Recent reinvestigation into topical antibiotic prophylaxis has been most thorough in the cardiac surgery literature. Gentamicin-impregnated sponges have been studied in several randomized controlled trials for the prevention of sternal wounds.[74–77] A recent meta-analysis by Mavros and colleagues[78] demonstrated that gentamicin collagen sponges reduced the risk of deep sternal wound infections, although there was significant heterogeneity among the included randomized controlled trials. However, in a trial by Bennett-Guerrero and colleagues,[79] no benefit was seen in a group of 602 colorectal surgery patients, with significantly higher SSI rates in the gentamicin sponge group. Further interest is still present in examining topical antibiotics in general surgical populations,[80] but more rigorous evidence will need to be presented before any adoption. With the recent guidelines, there are no recommendations describing a role for topical routes of antibiotic administration.[63]

Additional Measures

Several additional measures have been investigated for implementation in the prevention of SSI. In many circumstances, recommendations have been equivocal due to the lack of evidence or the presence of often contradictory evidence. In these cases, guidelines are directed by expert opinion and experience. Further research is continuing to clarify controversial issues in SSI prevention, and in some cases, causing further controversy.

As a prime example, perioperative oxygenation was shown in 2 early trials to lead to a reduction in SSI rates with the use of 80% oxygen intraoperatively and immediately post-operatively.[81,82] Further investigations have been mixed, with 2 prominent studies showing negative findings for efficacy.[83,84] In the PROXI trial, a large Danish randomized controlled trial studied 1400 patients undergoing abdominal surgery, who received either 80% oxygen or 30% oxygen during and for 2 hours after surgery.[83] There was no significant difference in SSI rates with increased perioperative oxygen fraction. In addition, subsequent subgroup analysis of the PROXI study showed there was increased long-term mortality in the high inspired oxygen group, with patients undergoing cancer surgery,[85] although this secondary finding of mortality difference is controversial because of potential confounding, sample size, and lack of a convincing biological mechanism.

Several conducted meta-analyses of these trials do suggest an overall reduction of SSI rates.[86–88] There is significant heterogeneity of the trials performed, with variability of the type of surgical procedures, perioperative care, and delivery protocol for hyperoxia. Perioperative hyperoxia has been included in some recommendations for the prevention of SSIs.[44]

Perioperative measures with considerably less controversy include perioperative warming, hair removal, and optimization of the operating room environment. Perioperative hypothermia is associated with significantly increased risk of SSI.[41,89,90] With regards to hair removal, the lowest risk of SSI has always been associated with not removing hair. If hair needs to be removed because of interference with the procedure, then hair removal should be done immediately before the surgery with a clipper rather a razor.[41,44,91,92]

The development of further preventative measures will require additional research, combining both basic and clinical research. Even with the existing measures, there continue to be areas that are controversial due to the conflicting data available. As baseline SSI rates decline with improving standard of care, identification of additional methods of prevention will continue to become more challenging.

MAJOR LIMITATIONS IN PREVENTION

In an ideal scenario, primary prevention is completely effective and the burden of SSI-related morbidity is reduced to 0%. As described in later discussion, the relationship between compliance with evidence-based guidelines and SSI outcomes is imperfect. With the risk inherent with nonmodifiable risk factors, there will likely be a minimum prevalence that cannot be entirely eliminated. In addition, with the development of numerous evidence-based guidelines, there continue to be hurdles with implementation and translation of these guidelines to practice.

In several jurisdictions, there is incomplete compliance with guidelines, even when associated with checklists, pathways, and packages. Compliance itself is a multifactorial issue that can be limited by a host of factors. Compliance can be limited by lack of awareness of guidelines by members of the multidisciplinary health care team. Lack of awareness of specific guidelines can occur even though SSI outcomes are considered to be important and major determinants of health care outcomes.[93] Local regional campaigns to improve compliance with these measures are also resource-intensive and can be associated with marginal improvement in both compliance and outcomes.[94]

THERAPY

The general principle of SSI therapy remains control of the source of infection. For superficial SSI, the standard management remains the use of incision and drainage.[62,95] The wound should be sufficiently sized to promote adequate drainage. A variety of local wound care options are available, with the simplest being saline-soaked cotton gauze dressings.[62] For uncomplicated superficial SSIs, simple incision and drainage, with local wound care, are appropriate, with no antibiotic therapy required.[96,97]

Identification of deep SSI or complicated skin and soft tissue infection requires adequate clinical suspicion. The presence of systemic features (eg, fever or leukocytosis) with an absence of local signs of wound infection should raise suspicion for organ/space SSI, or for an infection arising from an alternate site. In addition, consideration should be made for antibiotic therapy in SSIs in patients with systemic features, or widening erythema (>5 cm in diameter).[97] Direct clinical examination should follow to ensure an appropriate clinical response, with consideration of alternative diagnoses, if atypical features were to appear.

For more complicated skin and soft tissue infections, antibiotic therapy is appropriate, particularly in patients demonstrating signs of systemic shock. The principle of source control remains important, with the appropriate selection of antibiotics based on the type of surgical procedure performed, and the expected microbial causes for the infection.[62,95] As highlighted earlier, the growing impact of MDR organisms will greatly increase the difficulty of treatment of SSIs. Effective prevention will help to limit the potential impact of increasing resistance.

THE ECONOMIC AND QUALITY OF CARE IMPACT OF SURGICAL SITE INFECTIONS

The economic costs of SSIs are significant because of the volumes of cases that are seen, with an annual 2.7 million operative procedures performed in the United States.[5] Even with a conservative estimate of more than 290,000 cases of SSI,[7] there is a substantial economic cost to the management of SSI. There is a wide variance in estimates of the attributable costs of SSI infection that depends heavily on the type of surgical procedure and the geographic region studied.[98] There is additional confounding of the economic cost estimates due the lack of risk stratification of patient populations studied, and methods of cost summation. The estimates vary from $3937 per infection (Canadian tertiary care hospital)[99] to about $20,000 per infection (American orthopedic surgery population).[100] These analyses may underestimate the economic impact, through a combination of underestimation of surgical infection rates, and the costs of the worst manifestations of SSI, such as organ/space SSI with accompanying sepsis and septic shock, which can exceed $22,100 per case.[101]

The rates of SSI are increasingly being used as outcome and surrogate measures for examining the quality of surgical care. The National Surgical Infection Prevention Project was developed in 2003 with the goal to standardize quality improvement measure to decrease the incidence of SSI in major surgical procedures nationally.[64] This project has now transitioned to the Surgical Care Improvement Project (SCIP) in 2005, which included the SSI measures (**Table 4**) and additional performance measures of cardiac, respiratory, and thromboembolic complications.

In some countries these quality indicators have become pay-performance measures. For example, in the United States, the Centers for Medicare and Medicaid Services linked Medicare payments to hospitals on their compliance to performance indicators.[102] The 2014 hospital payment rule finalized the general framework for the Hospital-Acquired Condition Reduction Program to be implemented in 2015.[103] The rule updated measures and financial incentives with the following areas related to SSI: postoperative sepsis rate, wound dehiscence rate, central line–associated bloodstream infection, and catheter-associated urinary tract infection. The 2 new

Table 4
Surgical care improvement project surgical site infection performance measures

SCIP INF-1	Prophylactic antibiotic received within 1 h before surgical incision
SCIP INF-2	Proper prophylactic antibiotic selected
SCIP INF-3	Prophylactic antibiotics discontinued within 24 h after surgery end time
SCIP INF-4	Cardiac surgery patients with controlled 6 AM postoperative blood glucose measurement
SCIP INF-6	Appropriate hair removal
SCIP INF-9	Urinary catheter removed on postoperative day 1 or 2
SCIP INF-10	Appropriate perioperative temperature management

measures added of health care–associated infections were hospital-onset MRSA bacteremia and *Clostridium difficile*.[103]

There have been conflicting results with studies examining the compliance of the SCIP and the effect on SSI rates. Some studies have shown significantly lower SSI rates in hospital groups with higher compliance rates with 2 specific SCIP measures (appropriate antibiotic timing and antibiotic selection).[104] Another study showed if at least 2 of the 7 (see **Table 3**) measures were done there was a significant decrease in the SSI rate; however, compliance of just one of the SCIP did not result in benefit.[105] Although other studies have shown that adherence to multiple SCIP measures did not correlate with a decrease of SSI,[106,107] these studies demonstrate it is more than just compliance to specific metric that influences outcome in SSI. The emphasis cannot be only on adherence reporting but instead focused on a culture of safety and quality within the team.

SUMMARY

SSIs remain a very important component of patient outcome, contributing to substantial patient morbidity. From a historical perspective, there has been a significant improvement in postsurgical outcomes, but these incremental gains have slowed in the recent decades. The translation of basic and clinical research has expanded the complexity of evidence-based guidelines for SSI prevention. The importance of SSI prevention has been heightened because of its association with institutional and regulatory quality control measures. Sustained research in multiple aspects of SSI prevention needs to continue to realize further gains in SSI prevention. A multidisciplinary and multifaceted approach to SSI is absolutely necessary to continue to improve these critical outcomes of surgery.

REFERENCES

1. Newsom S. Pioneers in infection control—Joseph Lister. J Hosp Infect 2003; 55(4):246–53.
2. Blaisdell FW. Medical advances during the Civil War. Arch Surg 1988;123(9):1045.
3. Manring MM, Hawk A, Calhoun JH, et al. Treatment of war wounds: a historical review. Clin Orthop 2009;467(8):2168–91.
4. Horan TC, Gaynes RP, Martone WJ, et al. CDC definitions of nosocomial surgical site infections, 1992: a modification of CDC definitions of surgical wound infections. Am J Infect Control 1992;20(5):271–4.
5. Mangram AJ, Horan TC, Pearson ML, et al. Guideline for prevention of surgical site infection, 1999. Am J Infect Control 1999;27(2):97–134.

6. Nespoli A, Geroulanos S, Nardone A, et al. The history of surgical infections. Surg Infect (Larchmt) 2011;12(1):3–13.

7. Klevens RM, Edwards JR, Richards CL Jr, et al. Estimating health care-associated infections and deaths in U.S. hospitals, 2002. Public Health Rep 2007;122(2):160–6.

8. Cruse PJ, Foord R. The epidemiology of wound infection. A 10-year prospective study of 62,939 wounds. Surg Clin North Am 1980;60(1):27–40.

9. DiPiro JT, Martindale RG, Bakst A, et al. Infection in surgical patients: effects on mortality, hospitalization, and postdischarge care. Am J Health Syst Pharm 1998;55(8):777–81.

10. Rosenthal VD, Richtmann R, Singh S, et al. Surgical site infections, International Nosocomial Infection Control Consortium (INICC) report, data summary of 30 countries, 2005-2010. Infect Control Hosp Epidemiol 2013;34(6):597–604.

11. Culver DH, Horan TC, Gaynes RP, et al. Surgical wound infection rates by wound class, operative procedure, and patient risk index. National Nosocomial Infections Surveillance System. Am J Med 1991;91(3B):152S–7S.

12. Sievert DM, Ricks P, Edwards JR, et al. Antimicrobial-resistant pathogens associated with healthcare-associated infections: summary of data reported to the National Healthcare Safety Network at the Centers for Disease Control and Prevention, 2009-2010. Infect Control Hosp Epidemiol 2013;34(1):1–14.

13. Hidron AI, Edwards JR, Patel J, et al. NHSN annual update: antimicrobial-resistant pathogens associated with healthcare-associated infections: annual summary of data reported to the National Healthcare Safety Network at the Centers for Disease Control and Prevention, 2006-2007. Infect Control Hosp Epidemiol 2008;29(11):996–1011.

14. National Nosocomial Infections Surveillance (NNIS) report, data summary from October 1986–April 1996, issued May 1996: A report from the National Nosocomial Infections Surveillance (NNIS) System. Am J Infect Control 1996;24(5):380–8.

15. Jernigan JA. Is the burden of Staphylococcus aureus among patients with surgical-site infections growing? Infect Control Hosp Epidemiol 2004;25(6):457–60.

16. Anderson DJ, Sexton DJ, Kanafani ZA, et al. Severe surgical site infection in community hospitals: epidemiology, key procedures, and the changing prevalence of methicillin-resistant Staphylococcus aureus. Infect Control Hosp Epidemiol 2007;28(9):1047–53.

17. Takesue Y, Watanabe A, Hanaki H, et al. Nationwide surveillance of antimicrobial susceptibility patterns of pathogens isolated from surgical site infections (SSI) in Japan. J Infect Chemother 2012;18(6):816–26.

18. Gorwitz RJ, Kruszon-Moran D, McAllister SK, et al. Changes in the prevalence of nasal colonization with Staphylococcus aureus in the United States, 2001-2004. J Infect Dis 2008;197(9):1226–34.

19. Kalra L, Camacho F, Whitener CJ, et al. Risk of methicillin-resistant Staphylococcus aureus surgical site infection in patients with nasal MRSA colonization. Am J Infect Control 2013;41(12):1253–7.

20. Wang G, Hindler JF, Ward KW, et al. Increased vancomycin MICs for Staphylococcus aureus clinical isolates from a university hospital during a 5-year period. J Clin Microbiol 2006;44(11):3883–6.

21. Steinkraus G, White R, Friedrich L. Vancomycin MIC creep in non-vancomycin-intermediate Staphylococcus aureus (VISA), vancomycin-susceptible clinical methicillin-resistant S. aureus (MRSA) blood isolates from 2001-05. J Antimicrob Chemother 2007;60(4):788–94.

22. Adam HJ, Louie L, Watt C, et al. Detection and characterization of heterogeneous vancomycin-intermediate Staphylococcus aureus isolates in Canada: results from the Canadian Nosocomial Infection Surveillance Program, 1995-2006. Antimicrob Agents Chemother 2010;54(2):945–9.

23. Reynolds R, Hope R, Warner M, et al. Lack of upward creep of glycopeptide MICs for methicillin-resistant Staphylococcus aureus (MRSA) isolated in the UK and Ireland 2001-07. J Antimicrob Chemother 2012;67(12):2912–8.

24. Sader HS, Fey PD, Limaye AP, et al. Evaluation of vancomycin and daptomycin potency trends (MIC creep) against methicillin-resistant Staphylococcus aureus isolates collected in nine U.S. medical centers from 2002 to 2006. Antimicrob Agents Chemother 2009;53(10):4127–32.

25. van Hal SJ, Paterson DL. Systematic review and meta-analysis of the significance of heterogeneous vancomycin-intermediate Staphylococcus aureus isolates. Antimicrob Agents Chemother 2011;55(1):405–10.

26. Engemann JJ, Carmeli Y, Cosgrove SE, et al. Adverse clinical and economic outcomes attributable to methicillin resistance among patients with Staphylococcus aureus surgical site infection. Clin Infect Dis 2003;36(5):592–8.

27. van Hal SJ, Fowler VG Jr. Is it time to replace vancomycin in the treatment of methicillin-resistant Staphylococcus aureus infections? Clin Infect Dis 2013;56(12):1779–88.

28. Yong D, Toleman MA, Giske CG, et al. Characterization of a new metallo-beta-lactamase gene, bla(NDM-1), and a novel erythromycin esterase gene carried on a unique genetic structure in Klebsiella pneumoniae sequence type 14 from India. Antimicrob Agents Chemother 2009;53(12):5046–54.

29. Kumarasamy KK, Toleman MA, Walsh TR, et al. Emergence of a new antibiotic resistance mechanism in India, Pakistan, and the UK: a molecular, biological, and epidemiological study. Lancet Infect Dis 2010;10(9):597–602.

30. Hardy EJ, Mermel LA, Chapin KC, et al. Carbapenem-resistant Enterobacteriaceae containing New Delhi metallo-beta-lactamase in two patients - Rhode Island, March 2012. MMWR Morb Mortal Wkly Rep 2012;61(24):446–8.

31. Mulvey MR, Grant JM, Plewes K, et al. New Delhi metallo-beta-lactamase in Klebsiella pneumoniae and Escherichia coli, Canada. Emerg Infect Dis 2011;17(1):103–6.

32. Poirel L, Lagrutta E, Taylor P, et al. Emergence of metallo-beta-lactamase NDM-1-producing multidrug-resistant Escherichia coli in Australia. Antimicrob Agents Chemother 2010;54(11):4914–6.

33. Zhou G, Guo S, Luo Y, et al. NDM-1-producing strains, family Enterobacteriaceae, in hospital, Beijing, China. Emerg Infect Dis 2014;20(2):340–2.

34. Barantsevich EP, Churkina IV, Barantsevich NE, et al. Emergence of Klebsiella pneumoniae producing NDM-1 carbapenemase in Saint Petersburg, Russia. J Antimicrob Chemother 2013;68(5):1204–6.

35. Göttig S, Pfeifer Y, Wichelhaus TA, et al. Global spread of New Delhi metallo-β-lactamase 1. Lancet Infect Dis 2010;10(12):828–9.

36. Nordmann P, Naas T, Poirel L. Global spread of Carbapenemase-producing Enterobacteriaceae. Emerg Infect Dis 2011;17(10):1791–8.

37. Morowitz MJ, Babrowski T, Carlisle EM, et al. The human microbiome and surgical disease. Ann Surg 2011;253(6):1094–101.

38. Frank DN, St Amand AL, Feldman RA, et al. Molecular-phylogenetic characterization of microbial community imbalances in human inflammatory bowel diseases. Proc Natl Acad Sci U S A 2007;104(34):13780–5.

39. Seksik P, Rigottier-Gois L, Gramet G, et al. Alterations of the dominant faecal bacterial groups in patients with Crohn's disease of the colon. Gut 2003;52(2): 237–42.
40. Olivas AD, Shogan BD, Valuckaite V, et al. Intestinal tissues induce an SNP mutation in Pseudomonas aeruginosa that enhances its virulence: possible role in anastomotic leak. PLoS One 2012;7(8):e44326.
41. Mangram AJ, Horan TC, Pearson ML, et al. Guideline for prevention of surgical site infection, 1999. Hospital Infection Control Practices Advisory Committee. Infect Control Hosp Epidemiol 1999;20(4):250–78 [quiz: 279–80].
42. Neumayer L, Hosokawa P, Itani K, et al. Multivariable predictors of postoperative surgical site infection after general and vascular surgery: results from the patient safety in surgery study. J Am Coll Surg 2007;204(6):1178–87.
43. Watanabe A, Kohnoe S, Shimabukuro R, et al. Risk factors associated with surgical site infection in upper and lower gastrointestinal surgery. Surg Today 2008;38(5):404–12.
44. Alexander JW, Solomkin JS, Edwards MJ. Updated recommendations for control of surgical site infections. Ann Surg 2011;253(6):1082–93.
45. Anderson DJ, Kaye KS, Classen D, et al. Strategies to prevent surgical site infections in acute care hospitals. Infect Control Hosp Epidemiol 2008; 29(Suppl 1):S51–61.
46. Furnary AP, Zerr KJ, Grunkemeier GL, et al. Continuous intravenous insulin infusion reduces the incidence of deep sternal wound infection in diabetic patients after cardiac surgical procedures. Ann Thorac Surg 1999;67(2):352–60 [discussion: 360–2].
47. Latham R, Lancaster AD, Covington JF, et al. The association of diabetes and glucose control with surgical-site infections among cardiothoracic surgery patients. Infect Control Hosp Epidemiol 2001;22(10):607–12.
48. Zerr KJ, Furnary AP, Grunkemeier GL, et al. Glucose control lowers the risk of wound infection in diabetics after open heart operations. Ann Thorac Surg 1997;63(2):356–61.
49. Dronge AS, Perkal MF, Kancir S, et al. Long-term glycemic control and postoperative infectious complications. Arch Surg 2006;141(4):375–80 [discussion: 380].
50. Møller AM, Villebro N, Pedersen T, et al. Effect of preoperative smoking intervention on postoperative complications: a randomised clinical trial. Lancet 2002; 359(9301):114–7.
51. Lindstrom D, Sadr Azodi O, Wladis A, et al. Effects of a perioperative smoking cessation intervention on postoperative complications: a randomized trial. Ann Surg 2008;248(5):739–45.
52. Thomsen T, Tonnesen H, Moller AM. Effect of preoperative smoking cessation interventions on postoperative complications and smoking cessation. Br J Surg 2009;96(5):451–61.
53. Lee I, Agarwal RK, Lee BY, et al. Systematic review and cost analysis comparing use of chlorhexidine with use of iodine for preoperative skin antisepsis to prevent surgical site infection. Infect Control Hosp Epidemiol 2010;31(12):1219–29.
54. Darouiche RO, Wall MJ Jr, Itani KM, et al. Chlorhexidine-alcohol versus povidone-iodine for surgical-site antisepsis. N Engl J Med 2010;362(1):18–26.
55. Paocharoen V, Mingmalairak C, Apisarnthanarak A. Comparison of surgical wound infection after preoperative skin preparation with 4% chlorhexidine [correction of chlohexidine] and povidone iodine: a prospective randomized trial. J Med Assoc Thai 2009;92(7):898–902.

56. Brown TR, Ehrlich CE, Stehman FB, et al. A clinical evaluation of chlorhexidine gluconate spray as compared with iodophor scrub for preoperative skin preparation. Surg Gynecol Obstet 1984;158(4):363–6.

57. Swenson BR, Hedrick TL, Metzger R, et al. Effects of preoperative skin preparation on postoperative wound infection rates: a prospective study of 3 skin preparation protocols. Infect Control Hosp Epidemiol 2009;30(10):964–71.

58. Hakkarainen TW, Dellinger EP, Evans HL, et al. Comparative effectiveness of skin antiseptic agents in reducing surgical site infections: a report from the Washington State Surgical Care and Outcomes Assessment Program. J Am Coll Surg 2014;218(3):336–44.

59. Tschudin-Sutter S, Frei R, Egli-Gany D, et al. No risk of surgical site infections from residual bacteria after disinfection with povidone-iodine-alcohol in 1014 cases: a prospective observational study. Ann Surg 2012;255(3):565–9.

60. Polk HC Jr, Lopez-Mayor JF. Postoperative wound infection: a prospective study of determinant factors and prevention. Surgery 1969;66(1):97–103.

61. Stone HH, Hooper CA, Kolb LD, et al. Antibiotic prophylaxis in gastric, biliary and colonic surgery. Ann Surg 1976;184(4):443–52.

62. Barie PS, Eachempati SR. Surgical site infections. Surg Clin North Am 2005; 85(6):1115–35, viii–ix.

63. Bratzler DW, Dellinger EP, Olsen KM, et al. Clinical practice guidelines for antimicrobial prophylaxis in surgery. Am J Health Syst Pharm 2013;70(3): 195–283.

64. Bratzler DW, Houck PM, Surgical Infection Prevention Guideline Writers Workgroup. Antimicrobial prophylaxis for surgery: an advisory statement from the National Surgical Infection Prevention Project. Am J Surg 2005;189(4):395–404.

65. ASHP Therapeutic Guidelines on Antimicrobial Prophylaxis in Surgery. American Society of Health-System Pharmacists. Am J Health Syst Pharm 1999;56(18): 1839–88.

66. Bowater RJ, Stirling SA, Lilford RJ. Is antibiotic prophylaxis in surgery a generally effective intervention? Testing a generic hypothesis over a set of meta-analyses. Ann Surg 2009;249(4):551–6.

67. Classen DC, Evans RS, Pestotnik SL, et al. The timing of prophylactic administration of antibiotics and the risk of surgical-wound infection. N Engl J Med 1992; 326(5):281–6.

68. Garey KW, Dao T, Chen H, et al. Timing of vancomycin prophylaxis for cardiac surgery patients and the risk of surgical site infections. J Antimicrob Chemother 2006;58(3):645–50.

69. Steinberg JP, Braun BI, Hellinger WC, et al. Timing of antimicrobial prophylaxis and the risk of surgical site infections: results from the Trial to Reduce Antimicrobial Prophylaxis Errors. Ann Surg 2009;250(1):10–6.

70. van Kasteren ME, Mannien J, Ott A, et al. Antibiotic prophylaxis and the risk of surgical site infections following total hip arthroplasty: timely administration is the most important factor. Clin Infect Dis 2007;44(7):921–7.

71. Forse RA, Karam B, MacLean LD, et al. Antibiotic prophylaxis for surgery in morbidly obese patients. Surgery 1989;106(4):750–6 [discussion: 756–7].

72. Zelenitsky SA, Ariano RE, Harding GK, et al. Antibiotic pharmacodynamics in surgical prophylaxis: an association between intraoperative antibiotic concentrations and efficacy. Antimicrob Agents Chemother 2002;46(9):3026–30.

73. Morita S, Nishisho I, Nomura T, et al. The significance of the intraoperative repeated dosing of antimicrobials for preventing surgical wound infection in colorectal surgery. Surg Today 2005;35(9):732–8.

74. Bennett-Guerrero E, Ferguson TB Jr, Lin M, et al. Effect of an implantable gentamicin-collagen sponge on sternal wound infections following cardiac surgery: a randomized trial. JAMA 2010;304(7):755–62.

75. Eklund AM, Valtonen M, Werkkala KA. Prophylaxis of sternal wound infections with gentamicin-collagen implant: randomized controlled study in cardiac surgery. J Hosp Infect 2005;59(2):108–12.

76. Friberg O, Svedjeholm R, Soderquist B, et al. Local gentamicin reduces sternal wound infections after cardiac surgery: a randomized controlled trial. Ann Thorac Surg 2005;79(1):153–61 [discussion: 161–2].

77. Schimmer C, Ozkur M, Sinha B, et al. Gentamicin-collagen sponge reduces sternal wound complications after heart surgery: a controlled, prospectively randomized, double-blind study. J Thorac Cardiovasc Surg 2012;143(1):194–200.

78. Mavros MN, Mitsikostas PK, Alexiou VG, et al. Gentamicin collagen sponges for the prevention of sternal wound infection: a meta-analysis of randomized controlled trials. J Thorac Cardiovasc Surg 2012;144(5):1235–40.

79. Bennett-Guerrero E, Pappas TN, Koltun WA, et al. Gentamicin-collagen sponge for infection prophylaxis in colorectal surgery. N Engl J Med 2010;363(11):1038–49.

80. Alexander JW, Rahn R, Goodman HR. Prevention of surgical site infections by an infusion of topical antibiotics in morbidly obese patients. Surg Infect (Larchmt) 2009;10(1):53–7.

81. Greif R, Akca O, Horn EP, et al. Supplemental perioperative oxygen to reduce the incidence of surgical-wound infection. N Engl J Med 2000;342(3):161–7.

82. Belda FJ, Aguilera L, Garcia de la Asuncion J, et al. Supplemental perioperative oxygen and the risk of surgical wound infection: a randomized controlled trial. JAMA 2005;294(16):2035–42.

83. Meyhoff CS, Wetterslev J, Jorgensen LN, et al. Effect of high perioperative oxygen fraction on surgical site infection and pulmonary complications after abdominal surgery: the PROXI randomized clinical trial. JAMA 2009;302(14): 1543–50.

84. Pryor KO, Fahey TJ 3rd, Lien CA, et al. Surgical site infection and the routine use of perioperative hyperoxia in a general surgical population: a randomized controlled trial. JAMA 2004;291(1):79–87.

85. Meyhoff CS, Jorgensen LN, Wetterslev J, et al. Increased long-term mortality after a high perioperative inspiratory oxygen fraction during abdominal surgery: follow-up of a randomized clinical trial. Anesth Analg 2012;115(4):849–54.

86. Hovaguimian F, Lysakowski C, Elia N, et al. Effect of intraoperative high inspired oxygen fraction on surgical site infection, postoperative nausea and vomiting, and pulmonary function: systematic review and meta-analysis of randomized controlled trials. Anesthesiology 2013;119(2):303–16.

87. Qadan M, Akca O, Mahid SS, et al. Perioperative supplemental oxygen therapy and surgical site infection: a meta-analysis of randomized controlled trials. Arch Surg 2009;144(4):359–66 [discussion: 366–7].

88. Chura JC, Boyd A, Argenta PA. Surgical site infections and supplemental perioperative oxygen in colorectal surgery patients: a systematic review. Surg Infect (Larchmt) 2007;8(4):455–61.

89. Kurz A, Sessler DI, Lenhardt R. Perioperative normothermia to reduce the incidence of surgical-wound infection and shorten hospitalization. Study of Wound Infection and Temperature Group. N Engl J Med 1996;334(19):1209–15.

90. Walz JM, Paterson CA, Seligowski JM, et al. Surgical site infection following bowel surgery: a retrospective analysis of 1446 patients. Arch Surg 2006; 141(10):1014–8 [discussion: 1018].

91. Bratzler DW, Hunt DR. The surgical infection prevention and surgical care improvement projects: national initiatives to improve outcomes for patients having surgery. Clin Infect Dis 2006;43(3):322–30.

92. Tanner J, Woodings D, Moncaster K. Preoperative hair removal to reduce surgical site infection. Cochrane Database Syst Rev 2006;(3):CD004122.

93. Eskicioglu C, Gagliardi AR, Fenech DS, et al. Surgical site infection prevention: a survey to identify the gap between evidence and practice in University of Toronto teaching hospitals. Can J Surg 2012;55(4):233–8.

94. Larochelle M, Hyman N, Gruppi L, et al. Diminishing surgical site infections after colorectal surgery with surgical care improvement project: is it time to move on? Dis Colon Rectum 2011;54(4):394–400.

95. Kirby JP, Mazuski JE. Prevention of surgical site infection. Surg Clin North Am 2009;89(2):365–89, viii.

96. Nichols RL, Florman S. Clinical presentations of soft-tissue infections and surgical site infections. Clin Infect Dis 2001;33(Suppl 2):S84–93.

97. Stevens DL, Bisno AL, Chambers HF, et al. Practice guidelines for the diagnosis and management of skin and soft-tissue infections. Clin Infect Dis 2005;41(10): 1373–406.

98. Fry DE. The economic costs of surgical site infection. Surg Infect (Larchmt) 2002;3(s1):s37–43.

99. Zoutman D, McDonald S, Vethanayagan D. Total and attributable costs of surgical-wound infections at a Canadian tertiary-care center. Infect Control Hosp Epidemiol 1998;19(4):254–9.

100. Whitehouse JD, Friedman ND, Kirkland KB, et al. The impact of surgical-site infections following orthopedic surgery at a community hospital and a university hospital: adverse quality of life, excess length of stay, and extra cost. Infect Control Hosp Epidemiol 2002;23(4):183–9.

101. Angus DC, Linde-Zwirble WT, Lidicker J, et al. Epidemiology of severe sepsis in the United States: analysis of incidence, outcome, and associated costs of care. Crit Care Med 2001;29(7):1303–10.

102. Awad SS. Adherence to surgical care improvement project measures and postoperative surgical site infections. Surg Infect (Larchmt) 2012;13(4):234–7.

103. Fact sheet: CMS final rule to improve quality of care during hospital inpatient stays. 2013. Available at: http://www.cms.gov/newsroom/mediareleasedatabase/fact-sheets/2013-fact-sheets-items/2013-08-02-3.html. Accessed March 9, 2014.

104. Cataife G, Weinberg DA, Wong HH, et al. The effect of Surgical Care Improvement Project (SCIP) compliance on surgical site infections (SSI). Med Care 2014;52(2 Suppl 1):S66–73.

105. Stulberg JJ, Delaney CP, Neuhauser DV, et al. Adherence to surgical care improvement project measures and the association with postoperative infections. JAMA 2010;303(24):2479–85.

106. Hawn MT, Vick CC, Richman J, et al. Surgical site infection prevention: time to move beyond the surgical care improvement program. Ann Surg 2011;254(3): 494–9 [discussion: 499–501].

107. Tillman M, Wehbe-Janek H, Hodges B, et al. Surgical care improvement project and surgical site infections: can integration in the surgical safety checklist improve quality performance and clinical outcomes? J Surg Res 2013;184(1): 150–6.

Prosthetic Joint Infections

Antonia F. Chen, MD, MBA, Snir Heller, MD, Javad Parvizi, MD, FRCS*

KEYWORDS

- Prosthetic joint infection • Diagnosis • Suppressive antibiotics
- Irrigation and debridement • One-stage exchange arthroplasty
- Two-stage exchange arthroplasty

KEY POINTS

- The diagnosis of prosthetic joint infection is multifactorial, and is based on history, physical examination, serum laboratory tests, synovial fluid analysis, microbiology results, and biomarkers from the serum and synovial fluid.
- Patients with prosthetic joint infections who have high medical comorbidities that make them poor candidates for surgical intervention may be treated with suppressive, oral antibiotics.
- Acute prosthetic joint infections that occur less than 4 weeks after the initial surgery or 4 weeks within an acute hematogenous event may be treated with irrigation and debridement, although the success rate may not be as high as other treatment options.
- Chronic prosthetic joint infections that occur greater than 4 weeks after the initial surgery may be treated by 1-stage or 2-stage exchange arthroplasty.
- One-stage exchange arthroplasty is beneficial, because only 1 surgery is required, but the success rate may be lower than 2-stage exchange arthroplasty, which requires 2 procedures and a period with an antibiotic cement spacer and intravenous antibiotics.

INTRODUCTION

Periprosthetic joint infections (PJIs) are devastating complications after total joint arthroplasty, which lead to increased morbidity and mortality.[1] Treatment options for PJIs include medical management with chronic suppressive antibiotics, as well as surgical treatment with irrigation and debridement (I&D) for acute infections, and 1-stage or 2-stage exchange arthroplasty for chronic infections. The pros and cons of each surgical approach, along with the complications, postoperative care, and comparison of outcomes, are discussed in this article.

Disclosures: A.F. Chen and S. Heller have no disclosures that are relevant for the topic discussed within this article. J. Parvizi is a consultant and receives royalties from Zimmer.
Department of Orthopaedic Surgery at the Sidney Kimmel School of Medicine, Rothman Institute, 925 Chestnut Street, Philadelphia, PA 19107, USA
* Corresponding author.
E-mail address: parvj@aol.com

DIAGNOSIS OF INFECTION

The diagnosis of infection requires a multifactorial approach. The patient must first be assessed by performing a complete history and physical examination. Signs of inflammation at an operative site include rubor (redness), tumor (swelling), calor (increased heat), dolor (pain), and functio laesa (loss of function), which may be manifest with decreased range of motion, pain with ambulation, and difficulty walking up and down stairs, when a previous problem did not exist. Patients may also present with evidence of a sinus tract, which is pathognomonic for diagnosis of a PJI. Radiographic analysis may show evidence of prosthetic loosening and bone loss if an indolent infection has been present for some time.

Diagnosing PJI is also performed by laboratory tests, looking at acute phase reactants like erythrocyte sedimentation rate (ESR) and C-reactive protein (CRP). However, these laboratory test results can be increased in any inflammatory condition and are not specific to PJI. Thus, a joint aspiration and analyzing the synovial fluid for white blood cell (WBC) count and neutrophil percentage (% PMN) and microbiology culture results can provide a more concrete diagnosis of PJI. It is recommended that a minimum of 3 cultures be taken for analysis and that the cultures be taken of tissue and not swabs.[2,3]

Using these factors, the Musculoskeletal Infection Society developed a definition of PJI based on major and minor criteria, of which the 2 major criteria are the presence of a sinus tract communicating to the implant and positive culture taken from separate samples. Patients may also meet 4 of 6 minor criteria to be diagnosed with a PJI: (1) increased ESR or CRP level, (2) increased synovial WBC count, (3) increased synovial % PMN, (4) purulence in the joint, (5) positive culture taken from 1 sample, and (6) greater than 5 neutrophils per high power field under a 400× magnified microscope.[4,5] These factors should be combined to determine the diagnosis of PJI, as shown in **Fig. 1**.

Newer biomarkers for determining infection are being investigated. Synovial fluid cytokines, such as interleukin 1β (IL-1β), IL-6, IL-8, tumor necrosis factor α (TNF-α), interferon δ, and vascular endothelial growth factor, are increased in inflammatory conditions such as PJI.[6] Also, synovial fluid biomarkers with antimicrobial function such as CRP, leukocyte esterase, α-defensin, human β-defensin-2 (HBD-2) and HBD-3, and LL-37 may be increased.[7–9] Serum biomarkers such as procalcitonin, IL-6, TNF-α, and soluble intercellular adhesion molecule-1 (sICAM-1) may also be elevated in PJI.[10]

MEDICAL TREATMENT OF INFECTION

The gold standard for treatment of infection is surgical management, as described later, but some patients have high medical comorbidities that make them poor candidates to undergo surgical intervention. These patients, or patients who refuse surgical treatment, can be managed with chronic suppressive antibiotics, which may not fully eradicate the infection but may reduce the bioburden enough so that the patient's innate immune system can continue to fight the infection. Rao and colleagues[11] reported that a combination of surgical debridement and short course (4–6 weeks) of intravenous antibiotics followed by chronic oral antibiotic suppression eradicated infection in 86% of patients at 5 years and in 69% of staphylococcal infections at 5 years, when using their organism-specific treatments.

SURGICAL TREATMENT OF INFECTION

The mainstay of PJI treatment is surgery. Depending on the chronicity of an infection, an acute PJI that presents less than 4 weeks since the index surgery or within 4 weeks

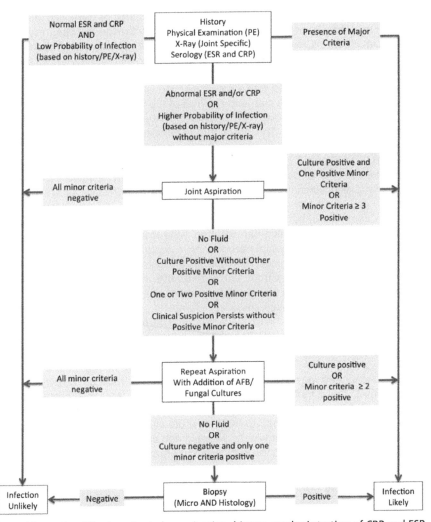

Major Criteria:
- Sinus tract communicating with the joint

Minor Criteria:
- Culture
- Leukocyte Esterase
- Synovial White Blood Cell Count
- Synovial Neutrophil Percentage

Fig. 1. Diagnosing PJI using physical examination, history, serologic testing of CRP and ESR, and analyzing synovial fluid. (*From* Parvizi J, Gehrke T. Proceedings of the International Consensus Meeting on Periprosthetic Joint Infection. Towson (MD): Data Trace Publishing Company; 2013. p. 160; with permission.)

after an acute event such as bacterial seeding from a dental cleaning may be treated with I&D. Infections of greater duration than 4 weeks after the index procedure or greater than 4 weeks after an inciting event should be treated with a removal of implants, because bacteria preferentially adhere to metal and create biofilms. The following sections describe the risks and benefits of performing these various surgical procedures, as well as other surgical options for treating PJI.

Irrigation and Debridement

I&D of a joint entails performing an arthrotomy, performing a thorough debridement of infected soft tissues, washing all the soft tissue and implant thoroughly with irrigation, changing out modular components, and placing patients on a postoperative short course of intravenous antibiotics tailored to the organisms isolated during surgery. To gain adequate exposure to the joint, the modular parts of the joint should be removed. For a total knee arthroplasty (TKA), the polyethylene between the femur and the tibia should be removed, and for a total hip arthroplasty (THA), the femoral head and acetabular liner should be removed. In the knee, this strategy allows the surgeon to gain better access to the posterior capsule of the knee so that a thorough debridement can be performed with a complete synovectomy. Removing the acetabular liner allows access to the cup, and removal of the femoral head permits evaluation of the trunnion. A thorough debridement of the synovium and periarticular muscles must be performed. This procedure is followed by a mechanical irrigation, preferentially with pulse lavage, with antibiotics such as bacitracin (50,000 U) and polymixin B (500,000 U). A minimum of 9 L of irrigation should be washed throughout the joint. The use of other bactericidal solutions, such as dilute betadine[12] and sodium hypochlorite (Dakin solution),[13] have been shown to be effective as antimicrobial solutions.

I&D is an attractive option for treating acute PJI, because the existing implants do not need to be removed, which can result in bone loss, increased blood loss, and increased pain. However, multiple studies have reported that a low success rate may be achieved by this surgical technique, as measured by the recurrence of infection. The success rate ranges from 15.8% to 90.0%, with an average success rate of 51.3% (**Table 1**).[14–41] The studies that reported a higher rate of success treated patients with oral antimicrobials, including rifampicin and fusidic acid,[14] or 2-stage debridement with antibiotic bead placement.[22] The addition of rifampin for 3 to 6 months as an oral antibiotic showed a 100% infection eradication when compared with 58% eradication when using ciprofloxacin alone, in a randomized prospective study.[42]

Higher failure rates were seen in infections by methicillin-resistant *Staphylococcus aureus* (MRSA),[16] I&Ds that were performed greater than 2 weeks after presentation,[20] and in patients who were infected with gram-negative organisms.[35] Thus, it is recommended that I&Ds are performed to treat an acute infection as soon as the infected patient presents and that multiple debridements and antibiotic choice be considered, especially when treating infections with resistant organisms.

One-Stage Exchange Arthroplasty

Although I&D may be an appropriate treatment of a PJI that presents within 4 weeks of surgery or when symptoms appear, exchange arthroplasty is the gold standard of treatment of chronic infections where all the components are removed. This treatment allows for removal of bacteria that may adhere to the implant surfaces, where biofilm is formed that may not be easily removed by mechanical or chemical debridement.

There are 2 methods to perform exchange arthroplasty. The first is 1-stage exchange arthroplasty, in which 1 operative procedure is performed to exchange out the infected component. During this procedure, the previous incision is incorporated into the surgical approach, if possible, and the implant is exposed. A radical debridement of infected soft tissue and scar tissue is performed.[43] It is recommended for knees that the tourniquet not be applied until after the debridement has occurred, to allow for better delineation of devascularized infected soft tissue and scar tissue

Table 1
Success rate of PJI treatment using I&D, as determined by the percentage of eradicated infections

Authors, Year	Site	Number of Eradicated Infections	Number of Total Implants	Success Rate (%)
Aboltins et al,[14] 2007	Hip, knee	18	20	90.0
Azzam et al,[15] 2010	Hip, knee	40	104	38.4
Bradbury et al,[16] 2009	Knee	3	19	15.8
Brandt et al,[17] 1997	Hip, knee	12	33	36.3
Chiu Chen,[18] 2007	Knee	12	20	60.0
Choi et al,[19] 2011	Knee	10	32	31.3
Crockarell et al,[20] 1998	Hip	4	19	21.1
Deirmengian et al,[21] 2003	Knee	11	31	35.4
Estes et al,[22] 2010	Hip, knee	18	20	90.0
Fehring et al,[23] 2013	Hip, knee	32	86	37.2
Gardner et al,[24] 2011	Knee	5	10	50.0
Hartman et al,[25] 1991	Knee	8	11	72.7
Ivey et al,[26] 1990	Knee	3	10	30.0
Klouche et al,[27] 2011	Hip	9	12	75.0
Koyonos et al,[28] 2011	Hip, knee	64	102	62.7
Krasin et al,[29] 2001	Hip	5	7	71.4
Marculescu et al,[30] 2006	Hip, knee	56	91	56.5
Mont et al,[31] 1997	Knee	10	24	41.7
Odum et al,[32] 2011	Hip, knee	46	150	30.7
Peel et al,[33] 2013	Hip, knee	94	112	83.9
Rasul et al,[34] 1991	Knee	2	6	33.3
Schoifet Morrey,[35] 1990	Knee	7	31	22.6
Segawa et al,[36] 1999	Knee	5	10	50.0
Tsukayama et al,[37] 1996	Hip	25	35	71.4
Tsumura et al,[38] 2005	Knee	6	10	60.0
Van Kleunen et al,[39] 2010	Hip, knee	10	18	55.6
Vilchez et al,[40] 2011	Hip, knee	40	65	69.2
Wasielewski et al,[41] 1996	Knee	8	10	80.0

from healthy, viable tissue. Once the implant is exposed, all hardware, cement, and devitalized bone should be removed. Intramedullary canals should be curetted, and the surgical site should be thoroughly irrigated with pulse lavage. Before performing the next stage of the operation, the femur and tibia for knees and the femur and acetabulum for hips should be packed with polyhexanid swabs. The operative team rescrubs, new instruments are used, and a new prosthesis is implanted. Often, revision components including the use of stems, augments, cones, and sleeves can be used to create a stable construct. Bone allograft impregnated with antibiotics can be used to provide prolonged release of local antibiotics and provide a scaffold for new bone growth, because there is often bone loss in the light of infected revisions.[44] Antibiotic-loaded cement is often used in the reimplantation, with vancomycin and tobramycin as the most common antibiotics.[45,46] Postoperatively, the administration of antibiotics can vary according to geographic and institutional preferences, ranging from 2 to 6 weeks postoperatively.[47–49]

Although a 1-stage exchange arthroplasty has been shown to be effective for treating PJI, especially in Europe, it is imperative that patients have a known organism before surgery (by joint aspiration or soft tissue identification), so the correct antibiotic can be administered as antibiotic prophylaxis and within the antibiotic cement. Contraindications to a 1-stage exchange arthroplasty are if there have been 2 previous failures of 1-stage exchange arthroplasty, if a patient is actively septic, if the infection affects the neurovascular bundle, if the organism is unknown because the samples are culture negative, if the organism shows high antibiotic resistance, and the specific antibiotic needed to eradicate the known organism is not available.[50] In addition, if a draining sinus is present, performing a 1-stage exchange arthroplasty may not be feasible, because obtaining primary closure over the implant may not be possible.[51]

The benefit of performing a 1-stage exchange arthroplasty is that there is only 1 operative procedure and that it is a cost-effective approach for treating PJI.[33] Performing this treatment within 1 stage may also decrease hospital length of stay and allow for quicker mobilization, instead of waiting for delayed implantation in 2-stage exchange arthroplasty. However, studies have shown that there is no difference in function when comparing 1-stage with 2-stage exchange arthroplasty knee patients.[52,53] The success rate of 1-stage exchange arthroplasty ranges from 55.6% to 100.0%, with an average success rate of 85.0% (**Table 2**).[46,48,49,51,52,54–60] The average success rate was higher than the success for an incision and drainage.

Two-Stage Exchange Arthroplasty

Two-stage exchange arthroplasty is similar to 1-stage exchange arthroplasty, in that all the components are removed at the time of surgery. However, in contrast, 2-stage exchange arthroplasty places a temporary antibiotic delivery device to eradicate the infection locally, and systemic antibiotics are given intravenously for 4 to 6 weeks.[61] Two-stage exchange arthroplasty should be considered the treatment of choice for

Table 2
Success rate of PJI treatment using 1-stage exchange arthroplasty, as determined by the percentage of eradicated infections

Authors, Year	Site	Number of Eradicated Infections	Number of Total Implants	Success Rate (%)
Buechel et al,[49] 2004	Knee	20	22	90.9
Callaghan et al,[51] 1999	Hip	22	24	91.7
Göksan Freeman,[54] 1992	Knee	16	18	88.9
Hansen et al,[48] 2013	Hip	15	27	55.6
Jenny et al,[52] 2013	Knee	41	47	87.2
Klouche et al,[55] 2012	Hip	38	38	100.0
Lu et al,[56] 1997	Knee	8	8	100.0
Raut et al,[46] 1996	Hip	14	15	93.3
Romanò et al,[57] 2012	Knee	167	204	81.9
Scott et al,[58] 1993	Knee	7	10	70.0
Von Foerster et al,[59] 1991	Knee	76	104	73.1
Zeller et al,[60] 2014	Hip	149	157	94.9

PJI if a patient is septic, when a diagnosis of PJI has been made but no organism has been isolated so the antibiotic cannot be tailored for the patient, the culture shows an antibiotic-resistant organism, there is a sinus tract present, and the soft tissue cover is not adequate.

The approach to a 2-stage exchange arthroplasty is similar to the 1-stage, because the skin incision can be made in the same location as the previous incision, an arthrotomy is performed, the components are removed, a thorough debridement of the infected soft tissue is performed, and a mechanical and antibiotic irrigation is completed. All infected instruments should be removed, and clean instruments should be used to finish the procedure. In the 2-stage approach, instead of reimplanting a prosthesis, an antibiotic delivery device is implanted, which is often polymethylmethacrylate (PMMA) cement mixed with antibiotics. They can be molded into static spacers, in which the joint is immobilized by the cement, articulating spacers (**Fig. 2**), in which the joint can flex because the cement pieces articulate with one another and can move, antibiotic beads that go within the intramedullary canal, and intramedullary rods with antibiotic cement for infected knees that provide joint stability (**Fig. 3**).[62,63] Studies have reported that the use of an articulating spacer improves range of motion between stages in total knees[64–67] and total hips[68–70] and is as efficacious if not more at eradicating infections when compared with static spacers.[57,71]

Once an antibiotic delivery device is in place, patients also receive intravenous antibiotics to allow for infection eradication, repeat surgical debridement if necessary, and soft tissue healing if soft tissue coverage was compromised from the first stage. Often, the duration of treatment ranges from 2 to 6 weeks, with an antibiotic holiday of

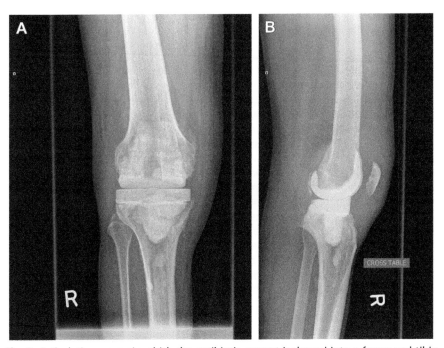

Fig. 2. Articulating spacer in which the antibiotic cement is shaped into a femur and tibia for a knee that allows for improved motion in the immediate postoperative period between stages. (*A*) Anteroposterior radiograph, (*B*) lateral radiograph.

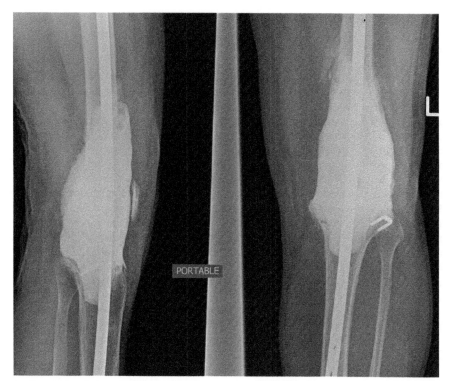

Fig. 3. Intramedullary rods with antibiotic cement for treating infected knees that provide joint stability in the light of PJI.

2 to 8 weeks before reimplantation to ensure that the infection is eradicated.[72] To monitor the treatment of infection, inflammatory laboratory values of CRP and ESR can be regularly drawn between stages to ensure that the antibiotics used are effective.[73] These laboratory values should slowly trend downwards as the infection is clearing, and implantation may occur once these values are low and the joint aspirate is negative. However, there is no clear biomarker of infection that can be used to signal when reimplantation should occur, and studies are being conducted to define an ideal serum biomarker. A time interval greater than 6 months between stages may result in poor patient function and may not eradicate the infection any greater than those who underwent reimplantation within 6 months.[74]

Reimplantation should be performed only once the infection is believed to be eradicated. The antibiotic delivery device should be removed, and a minimum of 3 tissue cultures should be taken at the time of surgery. Further debridement of devitalized tissue should be conducted, as well as preparation of the intramedullary canals using curettes and reverse curettes. Reimplantation is often performed with revision, stemmed components, with or without the use of structural and metal augments. For total knee reimplantations, it is recommended that antibiotic-loaded cement be used to prevent infection recurrence.

The success rate for 2-stage exchange arthroplasty ranges from 74.5% to 100.0% with an average success rate of 90.1% (**Table 3**), which is comparable with rates reported in literature.[55,58,64,67,70,75–103] This success rate is comparable with the success rate for 1-stage exchange arthroplasty, and studies support the fact that

Table 3
Success rate of PJI treatment using 2-stage exchange arthroplasty, as determined by the percentage of eradicated infections

Authors, Year	Site	Number of Eradicated Infections	Number of Total Implants	Success Rate (%)
Anderson et al,[80] 2009	Knee	24	25	96.0
Borden Gearen,[87] 1987	Knee	10	11	90.9
Emerson et al,[88] 2002	Knee	44	48	91.7
Fehring et al,[64] 2000	Knee	51	55	92.7
Freeman et al,[89] 2007	Knee	69	76	90.8
Gacon et al,[90] 1997	Knee	24	29	82.8
Goldman et al,[81] 1996	Knee	58	64	90.6
Gooding et al,[77] 2011	Knee	101	115	87.8
Haddad et al,[76] 2000	Knee	41	45	91.1
Haleem et al,[78] 2004	Knee	81	96	84.4
Hanssen et al,[91] 1994	Knee	79	89	88.8
Hirakawa et al,[92] 1998	Knee	41	55	74.5
Hoad-Reddick et al,[75] 2005	Knee	34	38	89.5
Hofmann et al,[67] 2005	Knee	44	50	88.0
Hofmann et al,[70] 2005	Hip	26	27	96.3
Hsieh et al,[86] 2004	Hip	122	128	95.3
Hsu et al,[79] 2007	Knee	25	28	89.3
Huang et al,[93] 2006	Knee	20	21	95.2
Insall et al,[83] 1983	Knee	10	11	90.9
Karpas Sponer,[82] 2003	Hip	18	18	100.0
Klouche et al,[55] 2012	Hip	45	46	97.8
Lonner et al,[94] 2001	Knee	44	53	83.0
Masri et al,[84] 1994	Knee	22	24	91.7
McPherson et al,[95] 1997	Knee	20	21	95.2
Meek et al,[96] 2004	Knee	52	54	96.3
Ocguder et al,[97] 2010	Knee	15	17	88.2
Pietsch et al,[98] 2003	Knee	22	24	91.7
Pitto et al,[99] 2005	Knee	19	19	100.0
Rosenberg et al,[100] 1988	Knee	12	15	80.0
Scott et al,[58] 1993	Knee	7	7	100
Van Thiel et al,[101] 2011	Knee	53	60	88.3
Whiteside,[102] 1994	Knee	28	33	84.8
Windsor et al,[103] 1990	Knee	34	38	89.5
Younger et al,[85] 1997	Hip	45	48	93.8

explanting components to provide adequate access to perform radical debridement of infected soft tissue aids with the eradication of the infection.

Other Surgical Situations

Most patients are able to undergo prosthetic reconstruction of their limb after a PJI; however, there are subsets of patients who have failed multiple attempts at reconstruction, have massive bone loss, or prefer to undergo a single operation for definitive treatment of their PJI. These patients may undergo resection arthroplasty, in which the prosthetic joint is removed and no additional prosthesis is reimplanted.[104] In the hip, this is called a Girdlestone procedure, and patients may ambulate on this construct. However, for knees, performing a resection arthroplasty may result in a less functional limb, so performing a fusion of the femur to the tibia does not allow range of motion but may provide stability when ambulating. In other patients who may have wound healing problems, removal of the limb or amputation may be the best option to prevent further complications. For a TKA, an above-knee amputation needs to be performed, and for a THA, a hindquarter amputation needs to be performed.

POSTOPERATIVE CARE

Patient postoperative care depends on the procedure performed (**Table 4**). For all surgical treatment modalities, using antibiotics to help eradicate the infection is paramount. In the early surgical postoperative period, I&D and 2-stage exchange patients should receive 4 to 6 weeks intravenous antibiotics. It is recommended that 1-stage exchange patients receive antibiotics for only 10 to 14 days.[47,105] For 2-stage exchange patients, antibiotics need to be administered only between the 2 stages, and patients may or may not receive oral suppressive antibiotics after the second stage. In between the 2 stages, a knee immobilizer may be applied when a spacer is in place, but this strategy should not be necessary in other patients who have prostheses in place. Patients between stages are permitted often touchdown weight bearing to reduce the likelihood of fracturing an antibiotic cement spacer. Patients are often permitted full weight bearing if a prosthesis is present, either after an I&D and 1-stage exchange arthroplasty, or after the second stage is complete.

COMPLICATIONS

After treatment of PJI, there are multiple surgical and medical complications that may occur after surgery. One common complication after treating PJI is that a patient can have a recurrent infection.[106,107] Increased risk for recurrent infection includes multiple

Table 4 Postoperative care after prosthetic joint infections			
	I&D	**One-Stage Exchange**	**Two-Stage Exchange**
Weight bearing status	Weight bearing as tolerated	Weight bearing as tolerated	Spacer: touchdown or non–weight bearing Second stage reimplantation: weight bearing as tolerated
Bracing	None	None	Consider knee immobilizer during spacer stage
Postoperative antibiotics duration	4–6 wk intravenous antibiotics after surgical intervention	10–14 d intravenous antibiotics after surgical intervention	4–6 wk intravenous antibiotics between stages
Laboratory monitoring	None	None	ESR/CRP

previous surgical procedures, compromised patient immune status, bone loss, necrosis, and the presence of a resistant organism, such as MRSA, which is associated with older patient age, thyroid disease, and higher body mass index.[36,108,109] There may be reduced mechanical stability, and hip dislocations and femoral fractures may occur after treatment of PJI.[110,111] In addition, the use of intravenous antibiotics may lead to acute renal failure, ototoxicity, or allergic reactions.[111] Patients who undergo multiple operative procedures for PJI also have an increased risk of mortality, because 90-day mortality was found to be 4%, and 5-year mortality was found to be 26%, which was significantly higher than patients who underwent revision for aseptic reasons.[1,112]

OUTCOMES

The outcomes of surgical treatment of PJI vary, with success being determined as prevention of recurrence of infection. An I&D and polyethylene exchange has the lowest success rate, and 2-stage exchange arthroplasty has the highest success rate for preventing subsequent PJI (see **Tables 1–3**). This finding is especially true in situations in which resistant organisms are found, such as MRSA, in which the success rate of I&D for preventing a subsequent infection in MRSA PJIs was as low as 18%.[16] A subsequent retrospective, multicenter study later reported that the success rate was low regardless if sensitive *Staphylococcus* was present (28% success) compared with resistant *Staphylococcus* (24% success).[32] There has been no prospective, randomized clinical trial conducted comparing 1-stage and 2-stage exchange arthroplasty, and there has only been a Markov model that has shown that 1-stage exchange predicted better life expectancy at 10 years and better quality of life for patients when compared with 2-stage exchange.[113] Thus, selecting the type of exchange arthroplasty depends on the surgeon's comfort with the procedure, the complete debridement of the soft tissue, and the knowledge of which organism is present so that appropriate antibiotics can be administered.

SUMMARY

PJIs are complications that are often managed by surgical treatment of I&D in acute infections, and 1-stage or 2-stage exchange arthroplasty in chronic infections. Patients who undergo I&D have had lower success rates compared with patients who undergo exchange arthroplasty, especially if resistant organisms are encountered. In patients who cannot undergo surgical reconstruction, resection arthroplasty, fusion, or amputation may be performed. Patients who are poor surgical candidates may be treated with chronic antibiotic suppression. Despite these treatments, PJIs may not be fully eradicated, and future research should be performed to prevent the development of PJIs.

REFERENCES

1. Zmistowski B, Karam JA, Durinka JB, et al. Periprosthetic joint infection increases the risk of one-year mortality. J Bone Joint Surg Am 2013;95(24):2177.
2. DeHaan A, Huff T, Schabel K, et al. Multiple cultures and extended incubation for hip and knee arthroplasty revision: impact on clinical care. J Arthroplasty 2013;28(8 Suppl):59.
3. Aggarwal VK, Higuera C, Deirmengian G, et al. Swab cultures are not as effective as tissue cultures for diagnosis of periprosthetic joint infection. Clin Orthop Relat Res 2013;471(10):3196.

4. Workgroup Convened by the Musculoskeletal Infection Society. New definition for periprosthetic joint infection. J Arthroplasty 2011;26(8):1136.

5. Parvizi J, Zmistowski B, Berbari EF, et al. New definition for periprosthetic joint infection: from the Workgroup of the Musculoskeletal Infection Society. Clin Orthop Relat Res 2011;469(11):2992.

6. Gollwitzer H, Dombrowski Y, Prodinger PM, et al. Antimicrobial peptides and proinflammatory cytokines in periprosthetic joint infection. J Bone Joint Surg Am 2013;95(7):644.

7. Parvizi J, Jacovides C, Adeli B, et al. Coventry Award: synovial C-reactive protein: a prospective evaluation of a molecular marker for periprosthetic knee joint infection. Clin Orthop Relat Res 2012;470(1):54.

8. Parvizi J, Jacovides C, Antoci V, et al. Diagnosis of periprosthetic joint infection: the utility of a simple yet unappreciated enzyme. J Bone Joint Surg Am 2011; 93(24):2242.

9. Deirmengian C. Diagnosing PJI: the era of the biomarker has arrived. Philadelphia: Musculoskeletal Infection Society; 2013.

10. Drago L, Vassena C, Dozio E, et al. Procalcitonin, C-reactive protein, interleukin-6, and soluble intercellular adhesion molecule-1 as markers of postoperative orthopaedic joint prosthesis infections. Int J Immunopathol Pharmacol 2011; 24(2):433.

11. Rao N, Crossett LS, Sinha RK, et al. Long-term suppression of infection in total joint arthroplasty. Clin Orthop Relat Res 2003;(414):55.

12. Brown NM, Cipriano CA, Moric M, et al. Dilute betadine lavage before closure for the prevention of acute postoperative deep periprosthetic joint infection. J Arthroplasty 2012;27(1):27.

13. Levine JM. Dakin's solution: past, present, and future. Adv Skin Wound Care 2013;26(9):410.

14. Aboltins CA, Page MA, Buising KL, et al. Treatment of staphylococcal prosthetic joint infections with debridement, prosthesis retention and oral rifampicin and fusidic acid. Clin Microbiol Infect 2007;13(6):586.

15. Azzam KA, Seeley M, Ghanem E, et al. Irrigation and debridement in the management of prosthetic joint infection: traditional indications revisited. J Arthroplasty 2010;25(7):1022.

16. Bradbury T, Fehring TK, Taunton M, et al. The fate of acute methicillin-resistant *Staphylococcus aureus* periprosthetic knee infections treated by open debridement and retention of components. J Arthroplasty 2009;24(6 Suppl): 101.

17. Brandt CM, Sistrunk WW, Duffy MC, et al. *Staphylococcus aureus* prosthetic joint infection treated with debridement and prosthesis retention. Clin Infect Dis 1997;24(5):914.

18. Chiu FY, Chen CM. Surgical debridement and parenteral antibiotics in infected revision total knee arthroplasty. Clin Orthop Relat Res 2007;461:130.

19. Choi HR, von Knoch F, Zurakowski D, et al. Can implant retention be recommended for treatment of infected TKA? Clin Orthop Relat Res 2011;469(4):961.

20. Crockarell JR, Hanssen AD, Osmon DR, et al. Treatment of infection with debridement and retention of the components following hip arthroplasty. J Bone Joint Surg Am 1998;80(9):1306.

21. Deirmengian C, Greenbaum J, Lotke PA, et al. Limited success with open debridement and retention of components in the treatment of acute *Staphylococcus aureus* infections after total knee arthroplasty. J Arthroplasty 2003; 18(7 Suppl 1):22.

22. Estes CS, Beauchamp CP, Clarke HD, et al. A two-stage retention debridement protocol for acute periprosthetic joint infections. Clin Orthop Relat Res 2010; 468(8):2029.

23. Fehring TK, Odum SM, Berend KR, et al. Failure of irrigation and debridement for early postoperative periprosthetic infection. Clin Orthop Relat Res 2013; 471(1):250.

24. Gardner J, Gioe TJ, Tatman P. Can this prosthesis be saved?: implant salvage attempts in infected primary TKA. Clin Orthop Relat Res 2011;469(4):970.

25. Hartman MB, Fehring TK, Jordan L, et al. Periprosthetic knee sepsis. The role of irrigation and debridement. Clin Orthop Relat Res 1991;(273):113.

26. Ivey FM, Hicks CA, Calhoun JH, et al. Treatment options for infected knee arthroplasties. Rev Infect Dis 1990;12(3):468.

27. Klouche S, Lhotellier L, Mamoudy P. Infected total hip arthroplasty treated by an irrigation-debridement/component retention protocol. A prospective study in a 12-case series with minimum 2 years' follow-up. Orthop Traumatol Surg Res 2011;97(2):134.

28. Koyonos L, Zmistowski B, Della Valle CJ, et al. Infection control rate of irrigation and debridement for periprosthetic joint infection. Clin Orthop Relat Res 2011; 469(11):3043.

29. Krasin E, Goldwirth M, Hemo Y, et al. Could irrigation, debridement and antibiotic therapy cure an infection of a total hip arthroplasty? J Hosp Infect 2001; 47(3):235.

30. Marculescu CE, Berbari EF, Hanssen AD, et al. Outcome of prosthetic joint infections treated with debridement and retention of components. Clin Infect Dis 2006;42(4):471.

31. Mont MA, Waldman B, Banerjee C, et al. Multiple irrigation, debridement, and retention of components in infected total knee arthroplasty. J Arthroplasty 1997;12(4):426.

32. Odum SM, Fehring TK, Lombardi AV, et al. Irrigation and debridement for periprosthetic infections: does the organism matter? J Arthroplasty 2011;26(6 Suppl):114.

33. Peel TN, Cheng AC, Lorenzo YP, et al. Factors influencing the cost of prosthetic joint infection treatment. J Hosp Infect 2013;85(3):213.

34. Rasul AT Jr, Tsukayama D, Gustilo RB. Effect of time of onset and depth of infection on the outcome of total knee arthroplasty infections. Clin Orthop Relat Res 1991;(273):98.

35. Schoifet SD, Morrey BF. Treatment of infection after total knee arthroplasty by debridement with retention of the components. J Bone Joint Surg Am 1990; 72(9):1383.

36. Segawa H, Tsukayama DT, Kyle RF, et al. Infection after total knee arthroplasty. A retrospective study of the treatment of eighty-one infections. J Bone Joint Surg Am 1999;81(10):1434.

37. Tsukayama DT, Estrada R, Gustilo RB. Infection after total hip arthroplasty. A study of the treatment of one hundred and six infections. J Bone Joint Surg Am 1996;78(4):512.

38. Tsumura H, Ikeda S, Ono T, et al. Synovectomy, debridement, and continuous irrigation for infected total knee arthroplasty. Int Orthop 2005;29(2):113.

39. Van Kleunen JP, Knox D, Garino JP, et al. Irrigation and debridement and prosthesis retention for treating acute periprosthetic infections. Clin Orthop Relat Res 2010;468(8):2024.

40. Vilchez F, Martinez-Pastor JC, Garcia-Ramiro S, et al. Outcome and predictors of treatment failure in early post-surgical prosthetic joint infections due to

Staphylococcus aureus treated with debridement. Clin Microbiol Infect 2011; 17(3):439.

41. Wasielewski RC, Barden RM, Rosenberg AG. Results of different surgical procedures on total knee arthroplasty infections. J Arthroplasty 1996;11(8):931.

42. Zimmerli W, Widmer AF, Blatter M, et al. Role of rifampin for treatment of orthopedic implant-related staphylococcal infections: a randomized controlled trial. Foreign-Body Infection (FBI) Study Group. JAMA 1998;279(19):1537.

43. Winkler H. Rationale for one stage exchange of infected hip replacement using uncemented implants and antibiotic impregnated bone graft. Int J Med Sci 2009;6(5):247.

44. Winkler H. Bone grafting and one-stage revision of THR–biological reconstruction and effective antimicrobial treatment using antibiotic impregnated allograft bone. Hip Int 2012;22(Suppl 8):S62.

45. Elson R. One-stage exchange in the treatment of the infected total hip arthroplasty. Semin Arthroplasty 1994;5(3):137.

46. Raut VV, Orth MS, Orth MC, et al. One stage revision arthroplasty of the hip for deep gram negative infection. Int Orthop 1996;20(1):12.

47. Kordelle J, Frommelt L, Kluber D, et al. Results of one-stage endoprosthesis revision in periprosthetic infection cause by methicillin-resistant *Staphylococcus aureus*. Z Orthop Ihre Grenzgeb 2000;138(3):240 [in German].

48. Hansen E, Tetreault M, Zmistowski B, et al. Outcome of one-stage cementless exchange for acute postoperative periprosthetic hip infection. Clin Orthop Relat Res 2013;471(10):3214.

49. Buechel FF, Femino FP, D'Alessio J. Primary exchange revision arthroplasty for infected total knee replacement: a long-term study. Am J Orthop (Belle Mead NJ) 2004;33(4):190.

50. Lichstein P, Gehrke T, Lombardi A, et al. One-stage vs two-stage exchange. J Arthroplasty 2013;29(2 Suppl):108–11.

51. Callaghan JJ, Katz RP, Johnston RC. One-stage revision surgery of the infected hip. A minimum 10-year followup study. Clin Orthop Relat Res 1999;(369):139.

52. Jenny JY, Barbe B, Gaudias J, et al. High infection control rate and function after routine one-stage exchange for chronically infected TKA. Clin Orthop Relat Res 2013;471(1):238.

53. Jamsen E, Stogiannidis I, Malmivaara A, et al. Outcome of prosthesis exchange for infected knee arthroplasty: the effect of treatment approach. Acta Orthop 2009;80(1):67.

54. Göksan SB, Freeman MA. One-stage reimplantation for infected total knee arthroplasty. J Bone Joint Surg Br 1992;74(1):78.

55. Klouche S, Leonard P, Zeller V, et al. Infected total hip arthroplasty revision: one- or two-stage procedure? Orthop Traumatol Surg Res 2012;98(2):144.

56. Lu H, Kou B, Lin J. One-stage reimplantation for the salvage of total knee arthroplasty complicated by infection. Zhonghua wai ke za zhi 1997;35(8):456 [in Chinese].

57. Romanò CL, Gala L, Logoluso N, et al. Two-stage revision of septic knee prosthesis with articulating knee spacers yields better infection eradication rate than one-stage or two-stage revision with static spacers. Knee Surg Sports Traumatol Arthrosc 2012;20(12):2445.

58. Scott IR, Stockley I, Getty CJ. Exchange arthroplasty for infected knee replacements. A new two-stage method. J Bone Joint Surg Br 1993;75(1):28.

59. von Foerster G, Kluber D, Kabler U. Mid- to long-term results after treatment of 118 cases of periprosthetic infections after knee joint replacement using one-stage exchange surgery. Orthopade 1991;20(3):244 [in German].

60. Zeller V, Ghorbani A, Strady C, et al. *Propionibacterium acnes*: an agent of prosthetic joint infection and colonization. J Infect 2007;55(2):119.

61. Bernard L, Legout L, Zurcher-Pfund L, et al. Six weeks of antibiotic treatment is sufficient following surgery for septic arthroplasty. J Infect 2010; 61(2):125.

62. Kotwal SY, Farid YR, Patil SS, et al. Intramedullary rod and cement static spacer construct in chronically infected total knee arthroplasty. J Arthroplasty 2012; 27(2):253.

63. Antoci V, Phillips MJ, Antoci V Jr, et al. The treatment of recurrent chronic infected knee arthroplasty with a 2-stage procedure. J Arthroplasty 2009;24(1): 159.e13.

64. Fehring TK, Odum S, Calton TF, et al. Articulating versus static spacers in revision total knee arthroplasty for sepsis. The Ranawat Award. Clin Orthop Relat Res 2000;(380):9.

65. Chiang ER, Su YP, Chen TH, et al. Comparison of articulating and static spacers regarding infection with resistant organisms in total knee arthroplasty. Acta Orthop 2011;82(4):460.

66. Evans RP. Successful treatment of total hip and knee infection with articulating antibiotic components: a modified treatment method. Clin Orthop Relat Res 2004;(427):37.

67. Hofmann AA, Goldberg T, Tanner AM, et al. Treatment of infected total knee arthroplasty using an articulating spacer: 2- to 12-year experience. Clin Orthop Relat Res 2005;(430):125.

68. Fleck EE, Spangehl MJ, Rapuri VR, et al. An articulating antibiotic spacer controls infection and improves pain and function in a degenerative septic hip. Clin Orthop Relat Res 2011;469(11):3055.

69. Romano CL, Romano D, Meani E, et al. Two-stage revision surgery with preformed spacers and cementless implants for septic hip arthritis: a prospective, non-randomized cohort study. BMC Infect Dis 2011;11:129.

70. Hofmann AA, Goldberg TD, Tanner AM, et al. Ten-year experience using an articulating antibiotic cement hip spacer for the treatment of chronically infected total hip. J Arthroplasty 2005;20(7):874.

71. Guild GN 3rd, Wu B, Scuderi GR. Articulating vs. static antibiotic impregnated spacers in revision total knee arthroplasty for sepsis. A systematic review. J Arthroplasty 2014;29(3):558–63.

72. Osmon DR, Berbari EF, Berendt AR, et al, Infectious Diseases Society of America. Executive summary: diagnosis and management of prosthetic joint infection: clinical practice guidelines by the Infectious Diseases Society of America. Clin Infect Dis 2013;56(1):1.

73. Ghanem E, Azzam K, Seeley M, et al. Staged revision for knee arthroplasty infection: what is the role of serologic tests before reimplantation? Clin Orthop Relat Res 2009;467(7):1699.

74. Joseph J, Raman R, Macdonald D. Time interval between first and second stage revision hip arthroplasty for infection, the effect on outcome. J Bone Joint Surg Br 2003;85-B(Suppl):58.

75. Hoad-Reddick DA, Evans CR, Norman P, et al. Is there a role for extended antibiotic therapy in a two-stage revision of the infected knee arthroplasty? J Bone Joint Surg Br 2005;87(2):171.

76. Haddad FS, Masri BA, Campbell D, et al. The PROSTALAC functional spacer in two-stage revision for infected knee replacements. Prosthesis of antibiotic-loaded acrylic cement. J Bone Joint Surg Br 2000;82(6):807.

77. Gooding CR, Masri BA, Duncan CP, et al. Durable infection control and function with the PROSTALAC spacer in two-stage revision for infected knee arthroplasty. Clin Orthop Relat Res 2011;469(4):985.

78. Haleem AA, Berry DJ, Hanssen AD. Mid-term to long-term followup of two-stage reimplantation for infected total knee arthroplasty. Clin Orthop Relat Res 2004;(428):35.

79. Hsu YC, Cheng HC, Ng TP, et al. Antibiotic-loaded cement articulating spacer for 2-stage reimplantation in infected total knee arthroplasty: a simple and economic method. J Arthroplasty 2007;22(7):1060.

80. Anderson JA, Sculco PK, Heitkemper S, et al. An articulating spacer to treat and mobilize patients with infected total knee arthroplasty. J Arthroplasty 2009;24(4):631.

81. Goldman RT, Scuderi GR, Insall JN. 2-Stage reimplantation for infected total knee replacement. Clin Orthop Relat Res 1996;(331):118.

82. Karpas K, Sponer P. Management of the infected hip arthroplasty by two-stage reimplantation. Acta Medica (Hradec Kralove) 2003;46(3):113.

83. Insall JN, Thompson FM, Brause BD. Two-stage reimplantation for the salvage of infected total knee arthroplasty. J Bone Joint Surg Am 1983; 65(8):1087.

84. Masri BA, Kendall RW, Duncan CP, et al. Two-stage exchange arthroplasty using a functional antibiotic-loaded spacer in the treatment of the infected knee replacement: the Vancouver experience. Semin Arthroplasty 1994; 5(3):122.

85. Younger AS, Duncan CP, Masri BA, et al. The outcome of two-stage arthroplasty using a custom-made interval spacer to treat the infected hip. J Arthroplasty 1997;12(6):615.

86. Hsieh PH, Shih CH, Chang YH, et al. Two-stage revision hip arthroplasty for infection: comparison between the interim use of antibiotic-loaded cement beads and a spacer prosthesis. J Bone Joint Surg Am 2004;86-A(9):1989.

87. Borden LS, Gearen PF. Infected total knee arthroplasty. A protocol for management. J Arthroplasty 1987;2(1):27.

88. Emerson RH Jr, Muncie M, Tarbox TR, et al. Comparison of a static with a mobile spacer in total knee infection. Clin Orthop Relat Res 2002;(404):132.

89. Freeman MG, Fehring TK, Odum SM, et al. Functional advantage of articulating versus static spacers in 2-stage revision for total knee arthroplasty infection. J Arthroplasty 2007;22(8):1116.

90. Gacon G, Laurencon M, Van de Velde D, et al. Two stages reimplantation for infection after knee arthroplasty. Apropos of a series of 29 cases. Rev Chir Orthop Reparatrice Appar Mot 1997;83(4):313 [in French].

91. Hanssen AD, Rand JA, Osmon DR. Treatment of the infected total knee arthroplasty with insertion of another prosthesis. The effect of antibiotic-impregnated bone cement. Clin Orthop Relat Res 1994;(309):44.

92. Hirakawa K, Stulberg BN, Wilde AH, et al. Results of 2-stage reimplantation for infected total knee arthroplasty. J Arthroplasty 1998;13(1):22.

93. Huang HT, Su JY, Chen SK. The results of articulating spacer technique for infected total knee arthroplasty. J Arthroplasty 2006;21(8):1163.

94. Lonner JH, Beck TD Jr, Rees H, et al. Results of two-stage revision of the infected total knee arthroplasty. Am J Knee Surg 2001;14(1):65.

95. McPherson EJ, Patzakis MJ, Gross JE, et al. Infected total knee arthroplasty. Two-stage reimplantation with a gastrocnemius rotational flap. Clin Orthop Relat Res 1997;(341):73.

96. Meek RM, Dunlop D, Garbuz DS, et al. Patient satisfaction and functional status after aseptic versus septic revision total knee arthroplasty using the PROSTALAC articulating spacer. J Arthroplasty 2004;19(7):874.

97. Ocguder A, Firat A, Tecimel O, et al. Two-stage total infected knee arthroplasty treatment with articulating cement spacer. Arch Orthop Trauma Surg 2010; 130(6):719.

98. Pietsch M, Wenisch C, Traussnig S, et al. Temporary articulating spacer with antibiotic-impregnated cement for an infected knee endoprosthesis. Orthopade 2003;32(6):490 [in German].

99. Pitto RP, Castelli CC, Ferrari R, et al. Pre-formed articulating knee spacer in two-stage revision for the infected total knee arthroplasty. Int Orthop 2005; 29(5):305.

100. Rosenberg AG, Haas B, Barden R, et al. Salvage of infected total knee arthroplasty. Clin Orthop Relat Res 1988;(226):29.

101. Van Thiel GS, Berend KR, Klein GR, et al. Intraoperative molds to create an articulating spacer for the infected knee arthroplasty. Clin Orthop Relat Res 2011;469(4):994.

102. Whiteside LA. Treatment of infected total knee arthroplasty. Clin Orthop Relat Res 1994;(299):169.

103. Windsor RE, Insall JN, Urs WK, et al. Two-stage reimplantation for the salvage of total knee arthroplasty complicated by infection. Further follow-up and refinement of indications. J Bone Joint Surg Am 1990;72(2):272.

104. Falahee MH, Matthews LS, Kaufer H. Resection arthroplasty as a salvage procedure for a knee with infection after a total arthroplasty. J Bone Joint Surg Am 1987;69(7):1013.

105. Frommelt L. Principles of systemic antimicrobial therapy in foreign material associated infection in bone tissue, with special focus on periprosthetic infection. Injury 2006;37(Suppl 2):S87.

106. Borowski M, Kusz D, Wojciechowski P, et al. Treatment for periprosthetic infection with two-stage revision arthroplasty with a gentamicin loaded spacer. The clinical outcomes. Ortop Traumatol Rehabil 2012;14(1):41.

107. Macheras GA, Koutsostathis SD, Kateros K, et al. A two stage re-implantation protocol for the treatment of deep periprosthetic hip infection. Mid to long-term results. Hip Int 2012;22(Suppl 8):S54.

108. Schwarzkopf R, Oh D, Wright E, et al. Treatment failure among infected periprosthetic patients at a highly specialized revision TKA referral practice. Open Orthop J 2013;7:264.

109. Kurd MF, Ghanem E, Steinbrecher J, et al. Two-stage exchange knee arthroplasty: does resistance of the infecting organism influence the outcome? Clin Orthop Relat Res 2010;468(8):2060.

110. Erhart J, Jaklitsch K, Schurz M, et al. Cementless two-staged total hip arthroplasty with a short term interval period for chronic deep periprosthetic infection. Technique and long-term results. Wien Klin Wochenschr 2010;122(9–10):303.

111. Jung J, Schmid NV, Kelm J, et al. Complications after spacer implantation in the treatment of hip joint infections. Int J Med Sci 2009;6(5):265.

112. Berend KR, Lombardi AV Jr, Morris MJ, et al. Two-stage treatment of hip periprosthetic joint infection is associated with a high rate of infection control but high mortality. Clin Orthop Relat Res 2013;471(2):510.

113. Wolf CF, Gu NY, Doctor JN, et al. Comparison of one and two-stage revision of total hip arthroplasty complicated by infection: a Markov expected-utility decision analysis. J Bone Joint Surg Am 2011;93(7):631.

Surgical Intervention for Thoracic Infections

Daniel Raymond, MD

KEYWORDS

- Infection • Parapneumonic effusion • Empyema • Pulmonary abscess
- Tuberculosis • Aspergilloma • Sternoclavicular joint infection

KEY POINTS

- Multidisciplinary management of thoracic infection, including experts in thoracic surgery, pulmonology, infectious disease, and radiology, is ideal for optimal outcomes.
- Initial assessment of parapneumonic effusion and empyema requires computed tomographic evaluation and consideration for fluid sampling or drainage.
- Goals for the treatment of parapneumonic effusion and empyema include drainage of the pleural space and complete lung reexpansion.
- Pulmonary abscess is often successfully treated with antibiotics and observation.
- Surgical intervention for the treatment of fungal or tuberculous lung disease should be undertaken by experienced surgeons following multidisciplinary assessment.
- Sternoclavicular joint infection often requires joint resection.

PARAPNEUMONIC EFFUSION AND EMPYEMA

Historically, open surgical drainage of the pleural space was the only available treatment for pleural infection from the time of Hippocrates until the early twentieth century.[1] In response to a rash of streptococcal respiratory infections, likely related to the influenza epidemic, the US Army established an empyema commission with mortality rates reaching 70%.[2] Evarts Graham subsequently published the results of this effort, outlining several key principles (**Box 1**), which remain the cornerstone of contemporary management of pleural space infection. The application of these principles led to a remarkable reduction in mortality, to 3.4%[2] in the military population. Despite many subsequent advances, including the introduction of antibiotics, ventilator technology, minimally invasive surgical techniques, and the many advances in critical care, mortality remains as high as 20% in modern series.[3]

Pathophysiology

Pleural fluid normally measures less than 15 mL (in a standard 70-kg individual) and serves to lubricate the pleural space. Lacunas in the pleural surface connect it with

Thoracic & Cardiovascular Surgery, Cleveland Clinic Foundation, 9500 Euclid Avenue, J4-1, Cleveland, OH 44195, USA
E-mail address: raymond3@ccf.org

Surg Clin N Am 94 (2014) 1283–1303
http://dx.doi.org/10.1016/j.suc.2014.08.004
0039-6109/14/$ – see front matter
surgical.theclinics.com

> **Box 1**
> **Essential principles of empyema management reported by Evarts Graham in 1925**
>
> 1. Careful avoidance of pneumothorax in the acute stage including the utilization of closed drainage systems
> 2. Prevention of chronic empyema by the rapid sterilization and obliteration of the infected cavity
> 3. Careful attention to the nutrition of the patient

lymphatics that ultimately drain into the thoracic duct.[4] Pleural effusions are due to either an increase in the production of pleural fluid or a decrease in drainage, and are a precursor to empyema. Parapneumonic effusions occur in response to a suppurative pulmonary process; up to 60% of pneumonias are associated with pleural effusion,[1] although less than 5% progress to empyema (**Table 1**).[4] Parapneumonic effusions begin as simple, free-flowing collections as the increased interstitial fluid from the pulmonary parenchyma traverses the pleura and enters the pleural space. Early on this is known as the exudative stage, in which the fluid analysis is characterized by glucose greater than 60 mg/dL, pH greater than 7.2, and negative Gram stain/cultures. Without intervention, this can progress to the fibrinopurulent stage, in which loculations caused by fibrinous septations occur. Fluid analysis at this point reveals glucose less than 60, pH less than 7.2, and positive bacterial studies. Subsequently fibroblasts may migrate into the pleural fluid, resulting the in the third stage, the organizing stage. At this point a fibrinous peel entraps the lung and prevents expansion (**Table 2**). Infection may progress at any point from the early fibrinopurulent stage, resulting in frank pus in the pleural space or empyema.

Diagnosis

The diagnosis of a parapneumonic effusion or empyema begins with a careful history and physical examination. Clinical features of pneumonia include productive cough, fever, dyspnea, and pleuritic chest pain. In general, history alone is not useful for differentiating patients with pneumonia from those with pneumonia and a parapneumonic process. The same is also true for physical examination, whereby diminished breath sounds, dullness to percussion, fremitus, and egophony can all be explained by consolidated lung parenchyma or a pleural fluid collection. Generally speaking, imaging is essential to making the correct diagnosis.

Imaging

Imaging generally begins with a simple chest radiograph. **Fig. 1**A and B display the typical radiographic appearance of a parapneumonic effusion/empyema including basilar consolidation, lateral meniscus sign, and opacification of the costophrenic sulcus on lateral images. Separate densities at the base suggest a loculated process. Decubitus views are helpful for identifying layering fluid collections implying a

Table 1 Etiology of empyema	
Pneumonia	60%
Postoperative	20%
Trauma	5%
Other	15%

Table 2
Stages of pleural effusion

Stage	Appearance	WBC (mm³)	pH	Glucose (mg/dL)	Gram Stain	LDH (IU)
I. Exudative	Clear	<1000	>7.2	>40	–	<500
II. Fibrinopurulent	Turbid	>5000	<7.2	<40	+	>1000
III. Organizing	Turbid or gelatinous	Variable	<7.2	<40	Variable	Variable

Abbreviations: LDH, lactate dehydrogenase; WBC, white blood cells.
Data from de Hoyos A, Sundaresan S. Thoracic empyema. Surg Clin North Am 2002;82(3):643–71, viii; and Light RW. Parapneumonic effusions and empyema. Proc Am Thorac Soc 2006;3(1):75–80.

free-flowing pleural process. Measurement of the thickness of a layering collection can help to estimate the volume of the collection and identify patients who may be treated conservatively. Unfortunately, with plain radiographs alone the differentiation between a loculated basilar fluid collection and dense parenchymal consolidation can be challenging (**Fig. 2**). In this circumstance ultrasonography can be a useful tool for differentiating fluid collections from solid tissue, identifying loculations, and choosing a location for thoracentesis. Ultrasonography is gaining in popularity because of its increasing accessibility and portability of the equipment; however, the results and interpretation are highly operator dependent. Ultrasound-guided thoracentesis has notably been shown to decrease hospital stay, cost, and complications such as hemorrhage and pneumothorax when compared with traditional thoracentesis.[5]

Computed tomography (CT) scanning remains the gold standard for radiographic evaluation of pleural abnormality. CT is useful for differentiating pleural fluid from consolidated parenchyma and for identification of loculations, central airway abnormality, and density changes implying mass or clot in pleural collections. Findings on the CT scan such as a dense peel and multiloculated collections (**Fig. 3**) are essential for diagnostic and therapeutic decisions. CT may also be useful for image-guided placement of percutaneous catheters for drainage of collections, in addition to obtaining specimens for pathologic and microbiologic analysis.

Pleural Fluid Sampling

Once a patient with a parapneumonic effusion is identified, pleural fluid sampling is essential for further diagnostic and therapeutic considerations. The exception is the

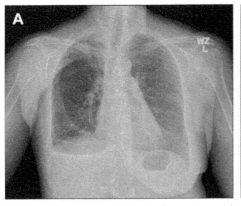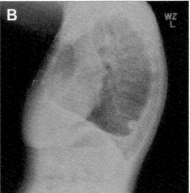

Fig. 1. (*A, B*) Chest radiographs of a patient with a parapneumonic effusion.

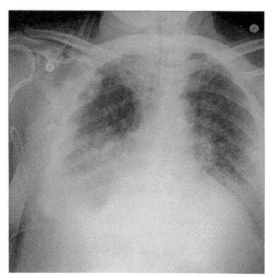

Fig. 2. Right lower lobe pneumonia without effusion on plain radiography.

patient with a small (<10 mm) free-flowing effusion on decubitus imaging, whose condition will usually resolve under appropriate antibiotic therapy for the pneumonic process and careful follow-up.[1,6] Pleural fluid sampling may be performed by the traditional, blind technique or with the aid of radiologic guidance. As mentioned previously, ultrasound guidance has been demonstrated to reduce complications and cost associated with thoracentesis,[7] and should be used when the technology is available. CT-guided drainage is an additional means of fluid sampling in challenging clinical scenarios.

Pleural fluid should be sent for the battery of tests listed in **Table 3**. Light's criteria (**Box 2**) may be used to differentiate transudative from exudative effusions.[8,9] The presence of any 1 of the criteria indicates that the fluid is an exudate, which would be consistent with a parapneumonic effusion. In the appropriate clinical scenarios additional testing may be useful, such as pleural fluid amylase for identifying

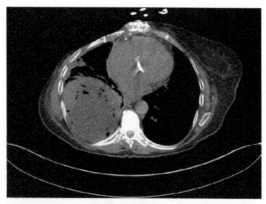

Fig. 3. Pleural thickening and microbubbles seen on computed tomography can identify patients who will require surgical drainage.

Table 3 Laboratory assessment of pleural effusion	
White blood cell count with differential	Bacterial culture
Total protein	Glucose
Lactate dehydrogenase	pH
Cytology	

esophageal perforation or pancreaticopleural fistulas. When tuberculosis infection is suspected, a pleural fluid adenosine deaminase (>40 IU/L indicates infection)[10] and pleural fluid cultures for acid-fast bacilli should be performed. Care should be taken with interpretation of these cultures, which are positive in only 20% to 30% of cases.[4] This caution should be extended to the interpretation of all pleural fluid cultures, as sensitivity is estimated at 40% to 60%[11] owing to various issues including sampling volume and presampling antibiotic therapy.[12,13] Pleural fluid pH is a valuable tool for differentiating simple from complicated parapneumonic effusion, and should be sent in a heparinized tube for analysis on a blood gas analyzer.[1]

To Drain or Not to Drain

Once the diagnosis of parapneumonic effusion or empyema has been made, treatment options should be considered, which center around antibiotic therapy and pleural drainage. Pleural drainage can include therapeutic thoracentesis, image-guided catheter placement, tube thoracostomy, and surgical drainage procedures. The American College of Chest Physicians has created useful consensus guidelines to aid the clinician with decisions regarding pleural drainage (**Table 4**). In essence, free-flowing effusions less than 10 cm on lateral decubitus can be managed with antibiotics and close observation. If the patient fails to clinically improve, fluid sampling is recommended. For small to moderate effusions the fluid should be sampled, but further drainage procedures are not necessary in the absence of symptoms. Close follow-up with chest imaging is vital. Often in this scenario the diagnostic thoracentesis can completely drain the pleural space, and thus also serve a therapeutic role. Once there is evidence of bacterial infection in the pleural space, either by bacteriology studies or chemistry studies, formal pleural drainage is indicated. Clinical judgment is required to determine which pleural drainage method has the best chance of success; paramount in this assessment is the CT scan and evidence of chronicity of infection.

For parapneumonic effusions in the early fibrinopurulent stage, chest tube drainage is generally sufficient, owing to the relative low viscosity of the fluid. There is some ambiguity, however, regarding the aforementioned nomenclature specifically regarding the definition of "chest tube". The broadest definition would include any drainage catheter placed into the chest for pleural drainage ranging from less than 10F catheters to 32F thoracostomy tubes. In surgical vernacular, chest tube is often interpreted as the surgical placement of a large-bore catheter, whereas smaller-bore,

Box 2 Light's criteria
Pleural fluid-to-serum protein ratio greater than 0.5
Pleural fluid lactate dehydrogenase (LDH) greater than 200 IU
Pleural fluid-to-serum LDH ratio greater than 0.6

Table 4
Outcome and drainage decisions for patients with parapneumonic effusion and empyema

Pleural Space Anatomy		Pleural Fluid Bacteriology		Pleural Fluid Chemistry[a]	Category	Risk of Poor Outcome	Drainage
Minimal, free-flowing effusion[b]					1	Very low	No
Small to moderate effusion[c]	AND	Negative	AND	pH$\geq$7.20	2	Low	No
Large, free-flowing, or loculated; effusion with pleural thickening[d]	OR	Positive	OR	pH<7.20	3	Moderate	Yes
		Pus			4	High	Yes

[a] pH should be obtained using a blood gas analyzer.
[b] <10 cm on lateral decubitus film.
[c] >10 mm to <$\frac{1}{2}$ hemithorax.
[d] On contrast-enhanced computed tomography.
Data from Colice GL, Curtis A, Deslauriers J, et al. Medical and surgical treatment of parapneumonic effusions: an evidence-based guideline. Chest 2000;118(4):1158–71.

radiographically placed catheters are often referred to as pigtails or pleural drains. This terminology generally lends to some confusion with respect to intraspecialty communication regarding management. Theoretically, smaller-bore catheters would become obstructed more easily, simply because of the relationship between resistance and lumen size (Poiseuille's law). However, a secondary analysis of the MIST1 randomized trial of intrapleural streptokinase did not reveal a difference in outcome when comparing patients managed with large (15–20F), medium (10–14F), or small (<10F) tubes.[14] On the other hand, the choice of catheter size was not part of the randomization, so there is certain to be a component of bias. In addition, this protocol included instillation of 30 mL of saline or streptokinase twice daily, which would mitigate some of the concerns regarding maintaining catheter patency. In general, a larger-bore catheter is preferable. However, this must be balanced against the increased pain associated with larger-bore tube insertion, which could compromise a patient with a tenuous respiratory status. When using smaller-bore tubes, the author urges all practitioners to develop protocols to assure catheter patency. This approach would include routine checks to identify catheter kinking including careful anchoring at the entry site, routine catheter flushes, and connection to a closed pleural drainage system with continuous, regulated suction.

Evidence of loculations, pleural thickening, and progressive organization in the chest (see **Fig. 3**) would suggest that less invasive drainage procedures may be unsuccessful. In this circumstance, options include attempts at intrapleural fibrinolysis or surgical intervention. Several large studies have identified intrapleural fibrinolytic therapy as a means of decreasing the need for surgical intervention,[15,16] although this is not a consistent finding.[12] The author generally reserves intrapleural fibrinolytic therapy for high-risk surgical candidates who have an early, small collection not drained successfully by chest drain placement. In these circumstances, pleural space clearance and complete lung expansion must be achieved for the treatment to be considered a success.

Once evidence of organization is documented on CT or ultrasonography, surgical intervention is often required to debride the pleural collection. Such intervention may only take place after attempts at less invasive means of drainage have failed, based on radiographic evidence revealing failure to achieve lung reexpansion or clearance of the pleura collection, or clinical deterioration of the patient. Patients must be assessed carefully before surgery and medically optimized. The patient must be able to tolerate single-lung ventilation, and any airway abnormalities should prompt a preoperative assessment by the anesthesia team. Blood loss can be significant during surgical decortication, so evaluation of coagulation profiles, treatment of anemia, and blood product preparation should be considered. Appropriate antibiotic selection is necessary, and assistance can be obtained from the Infectious Disease team. Hemodynamic instability can be encountered during decortication procedures; appropriate vascular access, arterial blood pressure monitoring, preoperative cardiac assessment, and blood product preparation should be considered.

Surgical Intervention

For patients whose disease has progressed to the organizing stage, surgical intervention is often required for optimal recovery.[17] The goals of surgical intervention include source control of the infection by thorough debridement of the pleural space and complete lung reexpansion. The decision for surgery can be made based on either clinical information, such as the demonstration of a multiloculated process with pleural thickening, or following failure of a less invasive attempt at pleural drainage. Failure of less invasive attempts at drainage can include a lack of clinical improvement implying inadequate source control, or radiographic evidence of persistent lung entrapment.

Fortunately patients with empyema are rarely in a toxic state, thus there is time for thorough preoperative evaluation, including an assessment of pulmonary function with a careful history and pulmonary function testing. One must be careful when interpreting these results, as indwelling drains or the presence of a bronchopleural fistula may affect the results. Cardiac testing may also be undertaken in appropriate patients, with consideration for tolerance to single-lung ventilation. Appropriate antibiosis should be assured, coagulation parameters optimized, and preparation for blood transfusion made.

Video-Assisted Thoracic Surgery and Thoracotomy

Management of pleural infection using video-assisted thoracic surgery (VATS) is gaining in popularity because of its perceived benefits, including improved postoperative pain, hastened recovery, and patient acceptance.[18] The procedure, often referred to as a VATS decortication, involves the use of small access incisions in the chest wall, under general anesthesia and single-lung ventilation, to thoroughly debride the pleural space and reexpand the lung (**Fig. 4**). If a more advanced process is encountered, the surgeon can easily convert the procedure to an open thoracotomy to accomplish the same goals.

In a prospective, randomized trial comparing immediate VATS drainage with tube thoracostomy with streptokinase for the management of multiloculated parapneumonic effusions and empyema, Wait and colleagues[19] demonstrated VATS to have a superior treatment success rate (91% vs 44%; $P<.05$), decreased duration of chest tube drainage (5.8 vs 9.8 days; $P = .03$), and decreased length of stay in hospital (8.7 vs 12.8 d; $P = .009$). These findings translated into a decreased cost for the VATS group, which did not reach statistical significance. The results of this study and similar retrospective studies[18,20–22] have resulted in the early application of VATS for patients with complex, multiloculated collections.

The decision regarding application of VATS or open thoracotomy for the treatment of empyema depends on clinical factors such as the duration of the infectious

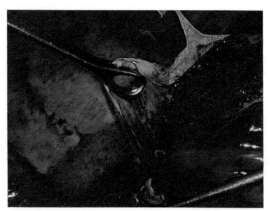

Fig. 4. Video-assisted thoracic surgery (VATS) decortication procedure. A restrictive peel is being removed from the lung surface.

process, radiographic evidence of pleural thickening, prior history of chest surgery or infection, and patient comorbidities, in addition to surgeon experience. VATS and thoracotomy are truly complementary techniques, thoracotomy being reserved for more complex cases. This situation is reflected in many retrospective studies that demonstrate superior outcomes in the VATS cases, which are often confounded by more favorable preoperative patient characteristics. Lardinois and colleagues[23] presented a series of 328 consecutive cases of empyema treated with surgical debridement including 178 patients who underwent a VATS approach, 44% of whom required conversion to open thoracotomy. Multivariate analysis identified prolonged time from symptoms to surgery and gram-negative organisms as predictors of conversion to thoracotomy. The patients in the VATS group had an average of 9.8 days from onset of symptoms to surgery, compared with 17.3 days in the group that required conversion to thoracotomy. Tong and colleagues[22] presented their experience with the use of VATS versus open decortication (OD) for the treatment of benign pleural disease including empyema, complex effusion, and hemothorax. The groups were surprisingly well balanced, although there were more patients with prior surgery and empyema in the OD group. In comparison with the OD group, the VATS group had fewer postoperative respiratory complications including ventilator dependency (13% vs 25.8%; $P = .006$), reintubation (2.5% vs 11.0%; $P = .002$), and tracheostomy (8.9% vs 17.0%; $P = .04$). The VATS group, furthermore, had a lower incidence of blood transfusion (33.8% vs 47.3%; $P = .02$), sepsis (1.2% vs 5.5%; $P = .03$), median postoperative length of stay (7 vs 10 d; $P<.001$), and 30-day mortality (7.5% vs 16.1%; $P = .02$). The conversion rate was 11.4% during the study, which demonstrated an increased utilization of VATS for primary therapy over the 10 years of the study. The investigators concluded that VATS is "an effective and reasonable first option for most patients with complex pleural effusions and empyema."[22]

Overall conversion rates from VATS to open thoracotomy seem to be declining as experience evolves and technology improves. Conversion, however, should not be considered a failure but good clinical judgment dictated by the patient's disease. The author suggests the following steps for practitioners building their VATS experience:

1. Use preoperative imaging carefully to assure appropriate access to the chest. Lung volume loss can contribute to diaphragm elevation to the infrascapular level, which

can lead to inadvertent diaphragmatic injury if the trocar sites are not selected appropriately.

2. After placing in the lateral decubitus position, mark the skin for a thoracotomy. Use a 2- to 3-cm portion of this incision for the initial VATS access port. Incise to the level of the pleura under direct visualization. If thickened rigid pleura is encountered, incise under direct visualization with a scalpel to avoid underlying lung injury.

3. Once access is gained to the pleural space, use CO_2 insufflation to aid in developing appropriate space for visualization. Observe the patient carefully for hemodynamic changes.

4. Place a second trocar incision at the site of the ultimate chest tube placement. A third trocar site can be triangulated from the prior 2 incisions.

5. If a thickened pleural peel is encountered on the lung, incise with a #15 blade on a long handle, choosing a location on the lung that is easily accessible. Visualize the knife at all times with the thoracoscope. Use techniques similar to OD to develop the peel. Specialty VATS instruments are very helpful in this regard.

6. Incise the pleural reflection at the hilum of the lung and divide the inferior pulmonary ligament. Often this will add significantly to lung mobilization and obliteration of the residual space.

7. At the end of the procedure, address major air leaks with sutures or surgical staplers, and drain the space widely with 2 to 3 chest tubes.

Open Thoracostomy

In some circumstances, decortication by either VATS or thoracotomy may not be feasible. The patient may be too ill for an extensive decortication or have comorbidities that preclude a safe operation (**Fig. 5**). There may be chronic contamination of the pleural space resulting from a fistula (eg, bronchopleural or esophagopleural) or chronic volume loss (eg, prior pneumonectomy, chronic lung entrapment). In these circumstances, source control of the infection may be achieved with an open thoracostomy, also known as a Clagett window or an Eloesser flap. In this procedure a portion of the chest wall is removed (generally 6–8 cm segments of 2–3 ribs) with marsupialization of the pleura to the skin (see **Fig. 5**B, C). The goal is to create a dependent defect in the chest wall of adequate size to permit drainage of fluid and debris. Pleural symphysis is necessary to avoid complete pneumothorax, which typically is due to chronic infection. The infected space is debrided and the wound is packed with dressings, which are changed daily. Patients may live indefinitely with the window, often with a family member becoming the primary wound care technician. Individuals with bronchopleural fistulas must avoid submerging the wound, and should be educated regarding the future difficulties of positive pressure ventilation that would require complex airway and ventilator management. Ultimately these windows may be closed after resolution of any fistula. Procedures include the transposition of a pedicled muscle flap (eg, serratus or latissimus muscle) to obliterate the space, or instillation of an antibiotic solution into the space followed by closure of the window (completion stage of the Clagett procedure). Alternatively, residual space may be obliterated by thoracoplasty, which entails removal of ribs and collapse of the chest wall soft tissue onto the lung and mediastinal structures. This procedure was initially used for the treatment of tuberculous lung disease in the early twentieth century, and is rarely necessary.

PULMONARY ABSCESS

Lung abscess is the result of either lung parenchymal destruction related to a pulmonary infection or a secondary infection of a structural abnormality in the lung.

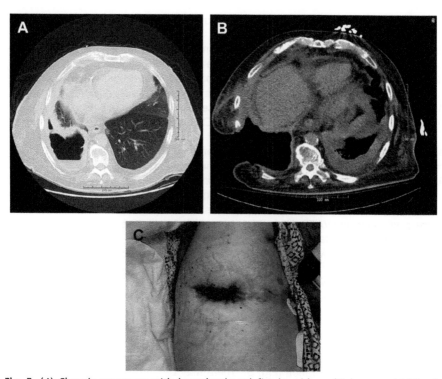

Fig. 5. (*A*) Chronic empyema with bronchopleural fistula with multiple comorbidities in Jehovah's Witness on anticoagulation. He was deemed too high risk for redo thoracotomy and decortication. (*B*) Postoperative CT scan of the same patient revealing the thoracostomy. (*C*) Thoracostomy wound photographed on postoperative day 2 while the patient was lying in the left lateral decubitus position.

Aspiration (**Box 3**) is the most common cause of lung abscess and tends to primarily affect the dependent portions of the lung, including the posterior segment of the right upper lobe and superior segment of the right lower lobe. Community-acquired lung abscesses tend to be polymicrobial[24] and dominated by anaerobic oral flora, including *Peptostreptococcus* species, *Bacteroides* species, *Fusobacterium* species, and *Prevotella* species, in addition to microaerophilic streptococci such as *Streptococcus milleri* and *Streptococcus anginosus*. Hospital-acquired abscesses tend to be more

---

Box 3
Patients at risk for pulmonary abscess

- Altered mental status
- Immunosuppression
- Swallowing disorders
- Prior surgery or upper aerodigestive tract
- Vocal cord dysfunction
- Airway abnormality

commonly associated with aerobic organisms such as *Pseudomonas aeruginosa*, *Staphylococcus aureus*, and *Klebsiella pneumoniae*.[3]

Patients tend to present with symptoms similar to those of pneumonia, including fever, chills, productive cough, and weight loss with an indolent course. Patients may complain of chest pain caused by pleurisy and may report the production of foul-smelling sputum. Chest radiographs may reveal an infiltrative process with air-fluid level. CT scan of the chest will often reveal a cavitary lesion with surrounding consolidation.

The mainstay of therapy for pulmonary abscess is antibiotic therapy. Because of the polymicrobial nature of these infections and the difficulty in isolating anaerobic organisms, sputum cultures may be misleading and should be interpreted with caution. For an uncomplicated community-acquired pulmonary abscess, clindamycin monotherapy is the accepted primary agent, based on 2 randomized trials[25,26] revealing superiority over parenteral penicillin attributed to emerging β-lactamases. An additional note should be made that metronidazole, although effective for anaerobic infections, performed poorly as monotherapy for pulmonary abscesses, likely because of the polymicrobial nature of the infection.[27] For hospital-acquired infections, empiric therapy based on the hospital antibiogram would be acceptable for initial therapy, and bronchoscopically obtained cultures should be considered to tailor therapy. As with community-acquired abscess, appropriate anaerobic coverage should be included. Duration of therapy varies by practitioner, but is generally at least 3 to 4 weeks with careful observation of clinical response.

Various factors can lead to failure of antibiotic therapy, which likely depends on the drainage of the abscess into the tracheobronchial tree. These factors include large abscess cavities (>6 cm),[11,28] bronchial obstruction preventing abscess drainage, and drug-resistant pathogens. In these circumstances intervention is required, and options include percutaneous drainage, endoscopic drainage, surgical drainage (cavernostomy), and surgical resection.

Percutaneous drainage of lung abscess was introduced in the preantibiotic era but is now rarely performed, owing to the 80% to 90% success of antibiotic therapy alone. Wali and colleagues[29] recently presented a meta-analysis of 105 cases of percutaneous drainage of lung abscesses, revealing a success rate of 85%, a complication rate of 9.7%, and a mortality rate of 4.8%. Complications included empyema, bronchopleural fistula, pneumothorax, hemothorax, and intrabronchial hemorrhage.

Endobronchial drainage is an alternative procedure that has been reported on a limited basis.[30] This procedure involves the placement of a transnasal catheter with bronchoscopic guidance into an abscess cavity for subsequent lavage and drainage. Herth and colleagues[30] reported a case series of 42 patients, 38 of whom had successful catheter placement and were subsequently successfully treated over a mean of 6.2 days. The only reported complication was transient ventilation requirement in 2 patients.

Surgical intervention for pulmonary abscess occurs in less than 10% of cases. Indications for surgical intervention include failure of medical therapy, massive hemoptysis, and inability to exclude a cavitary neoplasm with secondary infection. The latter can be a challenging clinical scenario, and highlights the need to follow these patients with serial imaging to ensure that there is gradual reduction in the size of the lung lesion.[30]

Options for surgical resection include segmental pulmonary resection or cavernostomy. Segmental pulmonary resection, often with a lobectomy, is the preferred method to obtain complete resection of the abscess cavity. Segmentectomy and wedge resection may be used for more peripheral lesions. Special considerations for pulmonary resection of an infectious process include careful protection of the unaffected lung by achieving lung isolation with a double-lumen tube or bronchial blocker immediately on induction of general anesthesia. Careful observation of tube position and frequent suctioning of the airway during the procedure is recommended. Furthermore, when an anatomic lung resection is performed, the surgeon should consider use of a vascularized soft-tissue flap, such as an intercostal muscle flap, to buttress the bronchial stump and minimize the risk of bronchopleural fistula.

Often the patient's clinical status will not permit a formal lung resection. In this circumstance drainage can be achieved by placement of drainage catheters, as mentioned earlier, or with surgical drainage. Surgical drainage can be performed either by creating a cavernostomy for external drainage of the abscess or by performing a thoracotomy and unroofing the abscess. In this scenario, the abscess space can then be drained with surgical drains or can be debrided and filled with a muscle flap followed by surgical drainage. Lee and colleauges[31] reported their 8-year experience with 61 patients undergoing surgical treatment of pulmonary abscess. This cohort included 28 patients undergoing resection and 32 undergoing surgical drainage for lung abscess averaging 6.7 cm in size. Major postoperative complications were more frequent in the drainage group (36.3% vs 32.1%; $P = .04$), although selection bias likely contributed. Mortality rate was similar between groups (14.3% vs 18.2%; $P = .7$) and, interestingly, rates of bronchopleural fistula and prolonged air leak were similar.

MYCOBACTERIAL PULMONARY DISEASE

Investigation into the history of treatment of mycobacterial disease of the chest permits the reader a glimpse at the origins of thoracic surgery. The first large-scale efforts at treatment of *Mycobacterium tuberculosis* began in the late nineteenth century with the advent of sanatorium care in the preantibiotic era. Rest, nutrition, and fresh air were considered to hasten the healing related to the disease, although the true benefit was never documented. Collapse therapy was popularized during this time as a means to promote healing of the affected lung, likely through the regional impairment of ventilation and, thus, oxygen deprivation to an obligate aerobe.[32] Various techniques were developed, including artificial pneumothorax, pneumoperitoneum, phrenectomy, plombage therapy, and thoracoplasty, by the pioneers of thoracic surgery.[33] Resectional therapy began to eclipse collapse therapy in the 1940s, following advances including new surgical techniques for hilar ligation, positive pressure ventilation, and endotracheal anesthesia.[34] The advent of the antibiotic era, including the introduction of streptomycin in 1942, isoniazid in 1952, and rifampin in 1966, revolutionized the care of tuberculosis, including a significant reduction in the need for surgical intervention.

Given the high success rates of modern multidrug treatment regimens, surgery is generally relegated to the treatment of complications of tuberculosis infections including bronchial stenosis, massive hemoptysis, bronchopleural fistula, and empyema. Surgery may also be indicated for diagnostic purposes to rule out carcinoma in a thick-walled cavitary lesion. Owing to the emergence of multidrug-resistant tuberculosis (MDR-TB) in the late twentieth century,[35] however, surgery has reemerged as a useful treatment modality for achieving source control of these challenging cases.

MDR-TB is defined as a tuberculosis bacillus demonstrating resistance to both isoniazid and rifampin. Extensively drug-resistant tuberculosis (XDR-TB) demonstrates additional resistance to at least 1 fluoroquinolone and an injectable agent (amikacin, kanamycin, or capreomycin), and was first reported in 2006.[36] Indications for surgery in these patients are listed in **Box 4**. In addition to indications based on sequelae of the disease, surgery has been used for assistance with source control when a localized, persistent focus of disease exists that likely has poor antibiotic penetration.

General principles of surgical management have been meticulously described by Pomerantz and colleagues.[37,38] All patients are managed by a multidisciplinary team including thoracic surgeons, pulmonologists, and infectious disease experts. Patients have an established treatment regimen, including a preoperative antibiotic regimen with duration determined by organism susceptibilities with the goal of achieving negative sputum cultures before surgery. Patients undergo an extensive pulmonary function and nutritional evaluation for medical optimization. Surgery is generally performed with thoracotomy, although VATS techniques may also be applied. Muscle flaps are used to buttress the bronchial stump in the following circumstances: (1) positive sputum culture at the time of surgery; (2) preexisting bronchopleural fistula; (3) polymicrobial contamination of the thoracic cavity; (4) anticipated space problems after lobectomy.[38] In 2001 a series of 180 pulmonary resections were reported over a 17-year period,[38] including 98 lobectomies and 82 pneumonectomies. Fifty percent of patients had negative sputum cultures at the time of surgery. Following surgery, sputum remained positive in only 2% of patients. Major morbidity was 12%, including 5 bronchopleural fistulas, and mortality was 3.3%, including 3 deaths from respiratory failure.

In contrast to *M tuberculosis*, nontuberculous mycobacterial species (NTM; **Box 5**) are opportunistic organisms affecting patients with preexisting structural lung disease and impaired immunity. Similarly to MDR-TB, these organisms are often resistant to many antimicrobial agents, and therefore require multimodality therapy including surgery. Source control of infection and treatment of the sequelae of infection are the main indications for surgery, as mentioned earlier for MDR-TB. Patient selection is equally as important and should focus on single foci of resectable disease. Mitchell and colleagues[37] have reported a series of 236 consecutive cases of anatomic lung resection for NTM. Eighty percent of patients had *Mycobacterium avium* complex and 57% were sputum or tissue culture negative at the time of surgery. The overall mortality rate was 2.6%, although the rate had declined to 0.6% in the final 5 years of the study. There was a major morbidity rate of 11.7% including an overall bronchopleural fistula rate of 4.2%. When looking further at the bronchopleural fistulas, 91%

Box 4
Indications for surgery for multidrug-resistant tuberculosis (TB) and extensively drug-resistant TB

Highly resistant TB with localized disease

Persistent cavitary disease

Persistent sputum positivity

Destroyed lung

Massive hemoptysis

Bronchopleural fistula

Airway stenosis

Data from Pomerantz BJ, Cleveland JC Jr, Olson HK, et al. Pulmonary resection for multi-drug resistant tuberculosis. J Thorac Cardiovasc Surg 2001;121(3):448–53.

Box 5
Nontuberculous mycobacterial species

Mycobacterium avium complex

Mycobacterium kansasii

Mycobacterium xenopi

Mycobacterium simiae

Mycobacterium abscessus

Mycobacterium fortuitum

Mycobacterium chelonae

Mycobacterium gordonae

Mycobacterium malmoense

---

had positive cultures at the time of surgery and 82% occurred after right pneumonectomy. The use of a muscle flap to buttress the right pneumonectomy stump decreased the rate of bronchopleural fistulas from 50% without muscle flap to 26%. All patients were rendered sputum negative after surgery.

PULMONARY ASPERGILLOSIS

Aspergillosis is broadly defined as human illness attributed to *Aspergillus*, a ubiquitous, highly aerobic fungus including more than 100 species with only a minority causing human disease (**Box 6**). Inhalation of fungal spores is the typical means of exposure and, thus, diseases of the respiratory tract are most common. Pulmonary aspergillosis can manifest as several different clinical syndromes, listed in **Table 5**.

Aspergilloma

Aspergillomas most commonly develop in patients with preexisting cavitary lung disease such as bullous emphysema, cavitary tuberculosis, sarcoidosis, or fibrotic lung disease. A second group susceptible to *Aspergillus* infection is immunocompromised hosts, who tend to present with more diffuse pulmonary syndromes.

The clinical presentation ranges from asymptomatic patients with an indeterminate incidental nodule to those with life-threatening hemoptysis. Common symptoms include cough, weight loss, hemoptysis, malaise, and chest pain. Hemoptysis occurs in 54% to 88% of patients, with 10% being massive hemoptysis.[39] Mortality from massive hemoptysis approaches 30%.[40]

CT imaging is essential for the evaluation of patients with suspected mycetoma, and permits the differentiation between simple and complex disease. Simple disease is characterized by thin-walled cavities with the characteristic fungus ball and limited

---

Box 6
***Aspergillus* species causing human disease**

Aspergillus fumigatus

Aspergillus flavus

Aspergillus clavatus

Aspergillus niger

Table 5	
***Aspergillus*-related pulmonary syndromes**	
Allergic bronchopulmonary aspergillosis	Hypersensitivity reaction to airway colonization by *Aspergillus*
Hypersensitivity pneumonitis (also known as extrinsic allergic alveolitis, malt worker's lung)	Immunologic reaction to inhaled *Aspergillus* spores
Aspergilloma	Presence of a mycetoma containing *Aspergillus hyphae* usually in a preexisting lung cavity
Invasive aspergillosis	Disseminated multiorgan infection usually affecting immunocompromised hosts
Chronic cavitary pulmonary aspergillosis	Formation and expansion of more than 1 pulmonary cavity, usually in immunocompetent patients
Chronic necrotizing pulmonary aspergillosis	Similar to chronic cavitary pulmonary aspergillosis but with shorter duration and more rapid progression; associated with invasive fungal hyphae

surrounding parenchymal disease (**Fig. 6**). Complex disease includes thick-walled cavities with extensive surrounding parenchymal disease. Diagnosis can be obtained by sputum culture, which is negative in up to 50% of cases,[39] or visualized hyphae in tissue obtained by bronchoscopic or transthoracic needle biopsy. *Aspergillus* serum antibody analysis, bronchial galactomannan enzyme assay, and quantitative polymerase chain reaction can also be used to enhance the diagnostic yield.[41]

Once an aspergilloma is identified, treatment decisions require a multidisciplinary approach including Infectious Disease, Pulmonary Medicine and Thoracic Surgery. Owing to the relative rarity of this disease, there is a paucity of level I or II data to guide

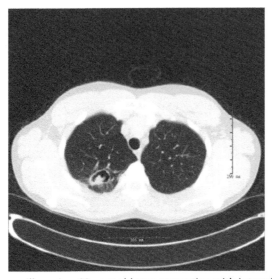

Fig. 6. A simple aspergilloma in a 23-year-old man presenting with intermittent hemoptysis. He underwent an uncomplicated right VATS upper lobectomy with complete resolution of his symptoms.

treatment decisions. For the asymptomatic patient there is debate regarding the value of intervention, although exclusion of malignancy may lead to invasive biopsy including surgical resection. Segmental resection including segmentectomy or lobectomy is curative in this population, and is justifiable in patients with a low surgical risk profile including good functional status and pulmonary function testing. Additional factors favoring surgical resection include failure of prior medical therapy, inability to tolerate medical therapy, and resistant disease.

Symptomatic disease provides a stronger argument for surgical intervention. Additional relative indications are listed in **Box 7**. The most significant of these is hemoptysis, which can be controlled temporarily with bronchial artery embolization,[28] as 90% of cases originate with the bronchial circulation.[39] Unfortunately, up to 50% will recur within 4 years of embolization as a result of recanalization of vessels or recruitment of new blood supply.[42] Jewkes and colleagues[43] noted a significant decline in 5-year survival in patients presenting with mycetoma and massive hemoptysis who underwent medical management as opposed to surgical management (mortality 41% vs 84%; $P<.02$), although underlying disease confounds the results. Surgical evaluation requires an extensive cardiopulmonary evaluation to identify appropriate patients for surgical intervention. Segmental pulmonary resection, by either segmentectomy or lobectomy, is the preferred approach. Wedge resection is reasonable for the rare small, peripheral lesion that can be completely encompassed. Pneumonectomy should be approached with caution because of the significant comorbidities in this patient population and the challenges related to postoperative bronchopleural fistula and empyema. In high-risk patients undergoing pulmonary resection, cavernostomy is a reasonable means to control the infected space. Staged procedures can permit ultimate obliteration of the space with various techniques, including muscle flap transposition and thoracoplasty.

Technical aspects of surgery mirror those previously mentioned for differing infectious conditions. Patients should be prepared carefully for surgery to include careful airway isolation to prevent contamination of healthy lung, adequate intravenous access, and preparation of blood products based on preoperative testing. Thoracotomy is generally necessary owing to long-standing inflammation, although VATS is not contraindicated in appropriate settings. Dense pleural reaction may dictate an extrapleural dissection to avoid violation of the infected cavity. Proximal vascular control,

---

Box 7
Indications for surgical resection for aspergilloma

Hemoptysis

Inability to exclude malignancy

Chronic cough

Immunocompromised host

Pending chemotherapy or hematopoietic stem cell transplantation

Lesions in contiguous with the pericardium or great vessels

Lesions invading the chest wall

Failure of medical management

Growth of cavity on serial imaging

Data from Refs.[28,39,48]

when possible, is advisable before hilar dissection when dense hilar scarring is encountered. Bronchial stump coverage is recommended to decrease the risks of bronchopleural fistula. Finally, control of residual space is important, and various techniques including muscle flap or omental transposition, pleural tenting (when available), phrenic nerve injection, pneumoperitoneum, lower lobe release maneuvers, and thoracoplasty can be entertained.

Cesar and colleagues[44] recently published their 31-year experience including 208 patients treated for pulmonary aspergilloma. Two groups were identified: 111 who underwent segmental resection and 97 who underwent cavernostomy. Not surprisingly, the cavernostomy patients were older and had more significant preexisting lung disease. In both groups, hemoptysis was the most common presenting symptom. Resectional therapy included lobectomy in 55%, pneumonectomy in 29%, and segmentectomy in 5%. Hemorrhagic complications (45% vs 12.4%; P<.01) and recurrence (8.1% vs 0%; P<.01) were more common in the cavernostomy group. Infectious complications predominately related to residual space and fistula were more common in the resection group (24.7% vs 7.2%; P<.01). Similar cure rates were noted in each group (cavernostomy 67.5% vs resection 73.7%; P = .5), and mortality rates (cavernostomy 19.5% vs resection 13.2%; P = .5) were noted. Others have reported mortality rates ranging from 0% to 44%,[39] likely emphasizing the need for careful patient selection to achieve optimal outcomes.

Invasive Aspergillosis

There is evidence that up to 20% of patients with localized aspergilloma will proceed to invasive aspergillosis without appropriate treatment.[39] Invasive aspergillosis is most commonly seen in immunocompromised patients, and is characterized by multifocal involvement in the lungs and multiorgan involvement. Limited data suggest that resection may have a role in multimodal therapy for patients with relatively limited disease.[45]

STERNOCLAVICULAR JOINT INFECTION

Sternoclavicular joint septic arthritis (SCJI) is a rare infection of the chest wall often requiring surgical evaluation. The sternoclavicular joint is a synovial lined joint involving the medial clavicular head, manubrium, and medial aspect of the anterior first rib. Infections generally are the result of hematogenous deposition of bacteria into the joint space, although direct extension from surrounding soft-tissue infection such as a central line infection may occur. Owing to the relatively confined volume of the joint, infections can quickly spread to surrounding structures, resulting in extensive tissue destruction. SCJI has historically been associated with intravenous drug abuse and chronic intravenous access, such as in dialysis patients. In the author's experience these patients are a relative minority, comprising about 20%. The most common associated comorbidities in the author's experience include obesity and diabetes mellitus.

Patients commonly present with swelling and pain overlying the sternoclavicular joint. The patient may also note that the clavicle on the affected side is more prominent, this being related to joint destruction and anterior displacement or a draining sinus tract. Evidence of bacteremia including leukocytosis and fever are common. Prior history of a febrile illness is common but not essential for the diagnosis. Either CT or magnetic resonance imaging is sufficient for further evaluation of the process (**Fig. 7**). Findings include bone destruction with loss of joint integrity and periarticular fluid or phlegmon.

Once the diagnosis has been made, treatment options include joint aspiration, open joint drainage, or sternoclavicular joint resection with or without pectoralis muscle flap

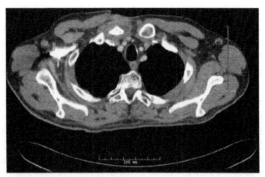

Fig. 7. Right sternoclavicular joint infection. Note the small periarticular collection, surrounding edema, and bone destruction.

transposition. Owing to the rarity of the diagnosis, there are no prospective trials comparing the different treatment strategies. Joint aspiration and drainage are effective means of confirming the diagnosis and obtaining appropriate samples from microbiologic analysis. Unfortunately recurrence has been anecdotally high, and therefore most surgeons prefer complete joint resection. This procedure involves resection of the medial head of the clavicle, hemimanubrium, and the anteromedial portion of the first rib (**Fig. 8**). Careful dissection should be undertaken to avoid injury to the underlying subclavian vein. The wound can then subsequently be managed with dressing changes or closed with or without a pectoralis advancement flap, based on surgeon preference.

Puri and colleagues[46] presented their 7-year experience including 20 patients undergoing 35 operations for SCJI. All patients underwent joint resection; half were managed with wound care including wet-to-dry dressings or negative pressure wound therapy, while the other half had wound closure with a pectoralis muscle advancement flap. S aureus was the most common infecting organism, followed by Streptococcus. The flap group had more unplanned surgical procedures, a higher need for blood transfusion, and a longer hospital stay (10.5 vs 5.5 days). The open wound group had fewer wound complications but did require outpatient wound care for a median of 12 weeks. Burkhart and colleagues[47] reported the Mayo Clinic experience of 26 patients over 13 years. S aureus was again the most common infecting organism.

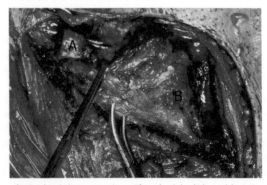

Fig. 8. Right sternoclavicular joint resection. The clavicle (A) and hemimanubrium (B) have been divided (first rib not visualized in photo). Further dissection will separate the specimen from the underlying subclavian vein.

Sternoclavicular joint resection was performed in 77% of patients; 6 had joint debridement and drainage. Eleven (42%) had pectoralis muscle flap transposition, and the wound was treated variably, including primary closure (2), delayed primary closure (12), and secondary intention (6). There were 2 postoperative complications (recurrent infection and unstable angina) and 1 death 3 months after the procedure. Over the long-term follow-up (median 26 months) there were 4 additional deaths from unrelated causes. All living patients denied recurrent infection or significant functional limitations resulting from their surgery.

Clearly clinical judgment is necessary, both preoperatively based on the patient's status and intraoperatively based on the extent of infection, to determine the ideal procedure. The author prefers joint resection in all patients unless they are clinically unstable. If there is extensive soilage including evidence of fasciitis, open wound management is preferred with, ultimately, negative pressure wound therapy once source control is achieved by serial debridement at the bedside or in the operating room. If the infection is more limited, such as in **Fig. 7**, a single-stage procedure including joint resection with pectoralis muscle flap advancement and primary wound closure is acceptable. In this circumstance, drains should be placed above and below the muscle flap and removed once drainage is minimal. When dealing with patients of questionable reliability the author likes to avoid secondary closure techniques, because of the requirement for extensive outpatient care. In this circumstance, either primary closure or repeated operative debridement with ultimate pectoralis muscle flap and secondary closure is recommended.

REFERENCES

1. Davies CW, Gleeson FV, Davies RJ. BTS guidelines for the management of pleural infection. Thorax 2003;58(Suppl 2):ii18–28.
2. Peters RM. Empyema thoracis: historical perspective. Ann Thorac Surg 1989; 48(2):306–8.
3. Mwandumba HC, Beeching NJ. Pyogenic lung infections: factors for predicting clinical outcome of lung abscess and thoracic empyema. Curr Opin Pulm Med 2000;6(3):234–9.
4. de Hoyos A, Sundaresan S. Thoracic empyema. Surg Clin North Am 2002;82(3): 643–71, viii.
5. Patel PA, Ernst FR, Gunnarsson CL. Ultrasonography guidance reduces complications and costs associated with thoracentesis procedures. J Clin Ultrasound 2012;40(3):135–41.
6. Light RW. Parapneumonic effusions and empyema. Proc Am Thorac Soc 2006; 3(1):75–80.
7. Mercaldi CJ, Lanes SF. Ultrasound guidance decreases complications and improves the cost of care among patients undergoing thoracentesis and paracentesis. Chest 2013;143(2):532–8.
8. Joseph J, Badrinath P, Basran GS, et al. Is the pleural fluid transudate or exudate? A revisit of the diagnostic criteria. Thorax 2001;56(11):867–70.
9. Light RW, Macgregor MI, Luchsinger PC, et al. Pleural effusions: the diagnostic separation of transudates and exudates. Ann Intern Med 1972;77(4):507–13.
10. Lee YC, Rogers JT, Rodriguez RM, et al. Adenosine deaminase levels in nontuberculous lymphocytic pleural effusions. Chest 2001;120(2):356–61.
11. Desai H, Agrawal A. Pulmonary emergencies: pneumonia, acute respiratory distress syndrome, lung abscess, and empyema. Med Clin North Am 2012; 96(6):1127–48.

12. Maskell NA, Davies CW, Nunn AJ, et al. U.K. Controlled trial of intrapleural strep-tokinase for pleural infection. N Engl J Med 2005;352(9):865–74.
13. Menzies SM, Rahman NM, Wrightson JM, et al. Blood culture bottle culture of pleural fluid in pleural infection. Thorax 2011;66(8):658–62.
14. Rahman NM, Maskell NA, Davies CW, et al. The relationship between chest tube size and clinical outcome in pleural infection. Chest 2010;137(3):536–43.
15. Cameron R, Davies HR. Intra-pleural fibrinolytic therapy versus conservative management in the treatment of adult parapneumonic effusions and empyema. Cochrane Database Syst Rev 2008;(2):CD002312.
16. Rahman NM, Maskell NA, West A, et al. Intrapleural use of tissue plasminogen activator and DNase in pleural infection. N Engl J Med 2011;365(6):518–26.
17. Coote N, Kay E. Surgical versus non-surgical management of pleural empyema. Cochrane Database Syst Rev 2005;(4):CD001956.
18. Chan DT, Sihoe AD, Chan S, et al. Surgical treatment for empyema thoracis: is video-assisted thoracic surgery "better" than thoracotomy? Ann Thorac Surg 2007;84(1):225–31.
19. Wait MA, Sharma S, Hohn J, et al. A randomized trial of empyema therapy. Chest 1997;111(6):1548–51.
20. Cassina PC, Hauser M, Hillejan L, et al. Video-assisted thoracoscopy in the treatment of pleural empyema: stage-based management and outcome. J Thorac Cardiovasc Surg 1999;117(2):234–8.
21. Pothula V, Krellenstein DJ. Early aggressive surgical management of parapneumonic empyemas. Chest 1994;105(3):832–6.
22. Tong BC, Hanna J, Toloza EM, et al. Outcomes of video-assisted thoracoscopic decortication. Ann Thorac Surg 2010;89(1):220–5.
23. Lardinois D, Gock M, Pezzetta E, et al. Delayed referral and gram-negative organisms increase the conversion thoracotomy rate in patients undergoing video-assisted thoracoscopic surgery for empyema. Am Thora Surg 2005; 79(6):1851–6.
24. Hammond JM, Potgieter PD, Hanslo D, et al. The etiology and antimicrobial susceptibility patterns of microorganisms in acute community-acquired lung abscess. Chest 1995;108(4):937–41.
25. Gudiol F, Manresa F, Pallares R, et al. Clindamycin vs penicillin for anaerobic lung infections. High rate of penicillin failures associated with penicillin-resistant *Bacteroides melaninogenicus*. Arch Intern Med 1990;150(12):2525–9.
26. Levison ME, Mangura CT, Lorber B, et al. Clindamycin compared with penicillin for the treatment of anaerobic lung abscess. Ann Intern Med 1983; 98(4):466–71.
27. Perlino CA. Metronidazole vs clindamycin treatment of anaerobic pulmonary infection. Failure of metronidazole therapy. Arch Intern Med 1981;141(11): 1424–7.
28. Merritt RE, Shrager JB. Indications for surgery in patients with localized pulmonary infection. Thorac Surg Clin 2012;22(3):325–32.
29. Wali SO, Shugaeri A, Samman YS, et al. Percutaneous drainage of pyogenic lung abscess. Scand J Infect Dis 2002;34(9):673–9.
30. Herth F, Ernst A, Becker HD. Endoscopic drainage of lung abscesses: technique and outcome. Chest 2005;127(4):1378–81.
31. Lee CH, Liu YH, Lu MS, et al. Pneumonotomy: an alternative way for managing lung abscess. ANZ J Surg 2007;77(10):852–4.
32. Pezzella AT, Fang W. Surgical aspects of thoracic tuberculosis: a contemporary review—part 1. Curr Probl Surg 2008;45(10):675–758.

33. Naef AP. The 1900 tuberculosis epidemic—starting point of modern thoracic surgery. Ann Thorac Surg 1993;55(6):1375–8.
34. Herbsman H. Early history of pulmonary surgery. J Hist Med Allied Sci 1958; 13(3):329–48.
35. Corbett EL, Watt CJ, Walker N, et al. The growing burden of tuberculosis: global trends and interactions with the HIV epidemic. Arch Intern Med 2003;163(9): 1009–21.
36. Centers for Disease Control and Prevention (CDC). Emergence of *Mycobacterium tuberculosis* with extensive resistance to second-line drugs—worldwide, 2000-2004. MMWR Morb Mortal Wkly Rep 2006;55(11):301–5.
37. Mitchell JD, Bishop A, Cafaro A, et al. Anatomic lung resection for nontuberculous mycobacterial disease. Ann Thorac Surg 2008;85(6):1887–92 [discussion: 1892–3].
38. Pomerantz BJ, Cleveland JC Jr, Olson HK, et al. Pulmonary resection for multidrug resistant tuberculosis. J Thorac Cardiovasc Surg 2001;121(3):448–53.
39. Passera E, Rizzi A, Robustellini M, et al. Pulmonary aspergilloma: clinical aspects and surgical treatment outcome. Thorac Surg Clin 2012;22(3):345–61.
40. Stevens DA, Kan VL, Judson MA, et al. Practice guidelines for diseases caused by Aspergillus. Infectious Diseases Society of America. Clin Infect Dis 2000; 30(4):696–709.
41. Musher B, Fredricks D, Leisenring W, et al. Aspergillus galactomannan enzyme immunoassay and quantitative PCR for diagnosis of invasive aspergillosis with bronchoalveolar lavage fluid. J Clin Microbiol 2004;42(12):5517–22.
42. Joon W, Kim JK, Kim YH, et al. Bronchial and nonbronchial systemic artery embolization for life-threatening hemoptysis: a comprehensive review. Radiographics 2002;22(6):1395–409.
43. Jewkes J, Kay PH, Paneth M, et al. Pulmonary aspergilloma: analysis of prognosis in relation to haemoptysis and survey of treatment. Thorax 1983;38(8): 572–8.
44. Cesar JM, Resende JS, Amaral NF, et al. Cavernostomy x resection for pulmonary aspergilloma: a 32-year history. J Cardiothorac Surg 2011;6:129.
45. Robinson LA, Reed EC, Galbraith TA, et al. Pulmonary resection for invasive Aspergillus infections in immunocompromised patients. J Thorac Cardiovasc Surg 1995;109(6):1182–96 [discussion: 1196–7].
46. Puri V, Meyers BF, Kreisel D, et al. Sternoclavicular joint infection: a comparison of two surgical approaches. Ann Thorac Surg 2011;91(1):257–61.
47. Burkhart HM, Deschamps C, Allen MS, et al. Surgical management of sternoclavicular joint infections. J Thorac Cardiovasc Surg 2003;125(4):945–9.
48. Walsh TJ, Anaissie EJ, Denning DW, et al. Treatment of aspergillosis: clinical practice guidelines of the Infectious Diseases Society of America. Clin Infect Dis 2008;46(3):327–60.

Pneumonia

Challenges in the Definition, Diagnosis, and Management of Disease

Julie Ottosen, MD, Heather Evans, MD, MS*

KEYWORDS

- Hospital-acquired pneumonia (HAP) • Ventilator-associated pneumonia (VAP)
- Pulmonary • Aspiration • Infection

KEY POINTS

- Definitions of the different subtypes of pneumonia are imprecise. Although community-acquired pneumonia is its own entity, ventilator-associated pneumonia (VAP) and hospital-acquired pneumonia (HAP) fall under the umbrella of health care–associated pneumonia. Aspiration pneumonia is a distinct process, which may begin in the communal setting, but is often and sometimes inappropriately labeled a health care–associated event.
- Early HAP may be related to events occurring before hospitalization that are not subject to quality improvement.
- Because VAP is associated with poor outcomes (including longer duration of mechanical ventilation, cost of care, morbidity, and mortality), preventative measures should be used.
- Quantitative lower respiratory tract cultures should be collected from all patients before antibiotic therapy. However, this procedure should not delay initiation of therapy in critically ill patients. Early broad-spectrum antibiotics with appropriate dosing should be used.
- De-escalation of antibiotic therapy should be considered once data from lower respiratory tract cultures are available. Negative lower respiratory tract cultures can be used to stop antibiotic therapy in those who have had cultures obtained in the absence of antibiotic therapy within 72 hours. A shorter duration of antibiotic therapy for uncomplicated HAP (7–8 days) should be used in patients who show an appropriate clinical response.
- Patients with trauma may be at increased risk for VAP because of chest trauma, head injury, depressed levels of consciousness, need for surgery mandating multiple intubations, and aspiration complicating urgent intubation. In patients with lower Injury Severity Scores (ISS), VAP is an independent risk factor for death. More severely injured patients with trauma (ISS >25) seem to succumb to their injuries, and the contributory role of VAP is less clear.

No financial support was received for this publication.
Division of Trauma, Critical Care, and Burns, Harborview Medical Center, 325 Ninth Avenue, Box 359796, Seattle, WA 98104, USA
* Corresponding author.
E-mail address: hlevans@uw.edu

DEFINING PNEUMONIA

Despite thousands of studies devoted to the topic of hospital-acquired pneumonia (HAP), controversies in the definition and management of HAP still remain. Perhaps the most important distinction to be made is what differentiates community-acquired pneumonia (CAP) from HAP, because the treatment paradigms and quality improvement issues vary between the 2.

HAP, or nosocomial pneumonia, arises 48 hours or more after hospital admission in the absence of signs or symptoms of pneumonia at the time of admission. VAP is a subtype of HAP that develops after endotracheal intubation. Because only about 10% of patients with HAP are not mechanically ventilated, the terms HAP and VAP are often used interchangeably. However, the causative organisms of VAP have been isolated from the oropharynx and stomach, and this must be considered when deciding on empirical therapy.[1]

Pneumonia that occurs early in the course of hospital stay is addressed as early onset pneumonia. However, it is difficult to define the cutoff that distinguishes early from late, because it is unknown how long it takes to develop pneumonia after the aspiration of microorganisms. Most studies have used a cutoff of 4 days, or 96 hours. Regardless, when the concept of early versus late is used, it is essential to designate hospital admission, not intubation, as day 1. This designation is based on the premise that the bacterial milieu of the oropharynx is influenced over time by the health care environment and interventions, giving the disease more the bacterial characteristics and antibiotic sensitivities of late onset pneumonia.[2] Late onset pneumonia occurs later in the course of hospital stay (>96 hours) and is associated with poorer outcomes. It is considered a preventable disease and therefore a target for quality improvement. However, it may be difficult to avoid in severely ill patients who are immunocompromised, with poor physiologic reserve and inability to clear secretions. In such situations, it may be considered a terminal event.

In 2005, the American Thoracic Society (ATS) guidelines defined a new category of infections to encompass recent inpatient or on ongoing treatment in a long-term or outpatient health care facility. The health care–associated pneumonia (HCAP) definition includes any patient who was hospitalized in an acute care hospital for 2 or more days within 90 days of the infection; resided in a nursing home or long-term care facility; received recent intravenous antibiotic therapy, chemotherapy, or wound care within the past 30 days of the current infection; or attended a hospital or hemodialysis clinic.[3] Such infections may be caused by community microorganisms, but are designated particularly to alert providers as to the increased risk of multidrug-resistant strains that may be transmitted in health care facilities.

Definitions of HAP, HCAP, and VAP were not designed with quality assessment in mind. They are nonspecific and do not correlate with histopathologic findings of pneumonia, irrespective of the method of microbiological sampling.[4,5] Recently, the Centers for Disease Control and Prevention have implemented an alternative surveillance paradigm for patients who are mechanically ventilated. Recognizing the subjectivity and poor reproducibility of clinical definitions, the working group designed the new surveillance definitions to be more objective, more efficient to collect via electronic medical record data, and more standardized across institutions.[6] However, in practice, these definitions may have little correlation with the clinical practice of the diagnosis of VAP, with poor sensitivity and substantial variation in incidence rates, with subtle changes in electronic implementation (**Table 1**).[7]

To add to the challenge, early onset VAP may be related to aspiration events occurring before intubation and admission to the intensive care unit (ICU) and not

Table 1
Syndromes and definitions

Syndrome	Definition
VAP	New or progressive and persistent infiltrate on chest radiograph plus 2 of the following: abnormal white blood cell count (<4000 or >12,000), presence of fever or hypothermia (<36°C or >38°C), purulent sputum, and deterioration in gas exchange
VAC	An increase in daily minimum positive end-expiratory pressure >3 or an increase of the daily minimum Fio_2 >.20 sustained for $\geq$2 calendar days in a patient who had a baseline period of stability or improvement on the ventilator, defined by $\geq$2 calendar days of stable or decreasing daily minimum Fio_2 or positive end-expiratory pressure
iVAC	An episode of VAC associated with alteration in white blood cell count (>12,000 or <4000) or temperature (>38°C or <36°C) within 2 calendar days of the start of the VAC and >4 d of new antibiotics

Abbreviation: iVAC, infection related ventilator associated condition; VAC, Ventilator associated condition.

necessarily attributable to poor quality of care, and it is unclear as to the impact of early aspiration on the risk of late pneumonia. Lung and general host defenses play a significant role in the development of HAP, and for a given inoculum, the risk of developing pneumonia is highly influenced by these. This finding also confounds the analysis of quality of care.

INCIDENCE

VAP is one of the most common hospital-acquired infections, occurring in 10% to 20% of ICU admissions in large database analyses from the late 1990s.[8,9] In 2010, the US Centers for Disease Control and Prevention reported more than 3500 cases. The reported incidence in patients with trauma is generally higher, up to twice that of the general ICU population.[10] Depressed levels of consciousness secondary to head injury and sedation, need for emergent surgery and anesthesia, and emergent intubation all place this population at particularly high risk for the development of infectious pulmonary disease.[11] Patients with trauma are also at increased risk because of underlying chest trauma and lung injury.[12]

DEFINING SEVERITY OF PNEUMONIA

The severity of pneumonia is, necessarily, contextual. Possible microbial cause, benefit from specific therapies, benefit from experimental therapies, and estimations of morbidity and mortality may be contingent on initial assessment of disease severity. There is considerable interest in the use of novel and potentially disease-specific biomarkers to distinguish pneumonia from other systemic illness, and to classify pneumonia severity. Of these novel biomarkers, most attention has focused on procalcitonin, a prohormone to calcitonin involved in chemoattraction and nitric oxide production. A variety of pulmonary specific biomarkers such as RAGE, HMGB-1, sTREM, and pro-ANP require further study. A variety of nonspecific biomarkers are already used routinely, including serum bilirubin, lactate, and platelet count. For the evaluation of CAP, simple measures of multiple organ dysfunction may be more useful than any of the newer assays, as suggested by the 2007 Infectious Diseases Society of America (IDSA) guidelines, which incorporate platelet count and renal function into the initial patient assessment of illness severity.[13]

DEFINITIONS GUIDING ANTIBIOTIC USE

Delay in treatment with antibiotics is associated with poorer outcomes in sepsis and HAP in particular. Initial treatment with broad-spectrum antibiotics, to be narrowed at a future date, is recommended. Use of antifungals is not routine but should be considered for very high risk populations (ie, immunocompromised patients).

CAUSATIVE ORGANISMS

Bacterial, fungal, or viral agents may be responsible for the onset of CAP. In healthy adults, *Haemophilus influenza* and *Streptococcus pneumoniae* are the most common agents. *Mycoplasma pneumonia*, *Chlamydia pneumoniae*, and *Legionella pneumonia* are rarer but plausible atypical agents. Viruses such as influenza and respiratory syncytial virus should be considered. In immunocompromised patients, fungal infections such as *Pneumocystis jirovecii* (previously *carinii*) must also be suspected.

Likely causative organisms for VAP depend on whether the infection is early or late onset. Early (within the first 96 hours) is more likely to be antibiotic sensitive, whereas VAP developing 96 hours after intubation is associated with more antibiotic-resistant organisms. This finding varies by unit and season, which emphasizes the importance of maintaining current unit-specific antibiograms. Regardless, the later form is associated with a higher morbidity and mortality.

PREDICTIVE MODELS

Critical for early decision making in the treatment of CAP is determination of the level of care required, ranging from outpatient oral antibiotic therapy to intubation and ICU admission. The Pneumonia Severity Index (PSI) is one of many tools devised for the assessment of the severity of CAP at presentation in the emergency department.[14] With the PSI model, patient risk scores are determined by 4 risk categories: demographic factors, comorbid conditions, findings on physical examination, and degree of physiologic derangement as indicated by laboratory results. Points in each category are stratified to 1 of 5 risk classes. For the patient with the lowest risk, outpatient treatment is recommended. For those found to be at high risk (class 4 +), inpatient treatment is recommended. Similar to the PSI, the PIRO (predisposition, insult, response, and organ dysfunction) score incorporates variables classified according to the patient's predisposition, insult, response, and organ dysfunction on presentation with CAP and has been shown to be more predictive of outcome in ICU patients than APACHE II score or ATS/IDSA criteria.[15] Although perhaps not as accurate as the PSI or PIRO, the CURB-65 model (named after confusion, urea, respiratory rate, blood pressure) is a simpler decision support tool for use in determining the level of care required based on the severity of presenting symptoms of CAP.[16,17] A score of 1 or 2 indicates a patient who may be treated in the outpatient setting, whereas a score of 3+ suggests inpatient therapy (**Table 2**).

Table 2	
CURB65 score. One point is assigned for each matched criteria	
C	Confusion
U	Blood urine nitrogen >20
R	Respiratory rate >30 breaths/min
B	Systolic blood pressure <90 or diastolic blood pressure <60
65	Age >65 y

In contrast to the evaluation of CAP, HAP and more specifically VAP, rarely occur without predisposing or contributing factors, and a pneumonia-specific scoring system is not used for outcome prediction. In patients with trauma, some investigators have found a correlation between Injury Severity Score (ISS), severity of brain injury, and chest abbreviated injury score with the development of pneumonia.[18]

Although development of VAP is generally associated with a higher risk of mortality, the attributable mortality of VAP is difficult to ascertain. This situation is because the likelihood of VAP increases with severity of illness, and mortality in critically ill patients may be related to other illnesses. Newer statistical techniques such as multistate models that consider development of VAP as time-dependent show that attributable mortality is highly dependent on case mix and severity of illness at onset.[19] One institution reported that patients with trauma with VAP had significantly better outcomes compared with their surgical ICU patients with VAP treated in the same unit.[20] VAP has also been found to be independently associated with death in less severely injured patients with trauma (ISS <25).[18] More severely injured patients with VAP (ISS>25) show no significant difference in mortality compared with those without VAP. This finding suggests that these patients die because of their injuries, and the contributory role of VAP is nebulous. It is likely that VAP is more a marker of injury severity in this subgroup, and that patient outcomes are less dependent on the development of VAP than on the multiple injuries themselves.

PREVENTION

Because VAP is associated with poor outcomes, including increased ventilator days, cost of care, morbidity, and mortality, much research has focused on identifying interventions aimed at prevention.

General measures for infection control should be used and include alcohol-based hand disinfection, use of microbial surveillance, and early removal of invasive devices. Accumulation of oropharyngeal secretions above the endotracheal tube cuff contributes to the risk for aspiration, and diligent oral care aimed at removing such pooled secretions may reduce the risk for aspiration and early onset VAP.[21] Oropharyngeal colonization, whether present on admission or acquired during ICU stay, has been recognized as an independent risk factor for the development of VAP.[2] Twice-daily care using a chlorhexidine gluconate (CHG) rinse was shown to reduce VAP rates in patients undergoing cardiac surgery.[22] In 2010, the Institute of Health Care Improvement (IHI) added the use of CHG for oral decontamination, but a recent meta-analysis[23] calls into question the usefulness of routine oral care with CHG in all intubated patients, because the prevention of VAP has not been proved outside cardiac surgery cohorts.

Sedation vacations and spontaneous breathing trials should be used to liberate patients from mechanical ventilation as early as possible. The practice of stopping or interrupting sedation on a daily basis has been shown to reduce ventilator days and ICU length of stay.[24] Furthermore, the VAP Guidelines Committee and the Canadian Critical Care Trials group have recommended the following measures for VAP prevention[25]:

- Use orotracheal route for intubation
- Scheduled changes of the ventilator circuits
- Change of heat or moisture exchangers every 5 to 7 days or when clinically indicated

- Subglottic secretion drainage in patients expected to be mechanically ventilated more than 72 hours
- Head of bed elevation to 45° (if possible)

DIAGNOSIS

Diagnostic testing is necessary for 2 purposes:

1. Defining whether a patient's constellation of infectious symptoms are attributable to pneumonia
2. Determining the etiologic pathogen when pneumonia is present to tailor antibiotic therapy

HAP should be suspected in patients with new or progressive radiologic infiltrate along with clinical symptoms suggestive of infection, including fever, leukocytosis, and purulent sputum. Yet, the definitive diagnosis of HAP presents a challenge. Clinical assessment is subjective, and there is substantial variability among clinicians in determining the presence of pneumonia.

The Clinical Pulmonary Infection Score (CPIS), shown in **Table 3**, was developed to aid clinicians in assessing the likelihood of the presence of VAP, based entirely on expert opinion.[26] Its usefulness as a diagnostic aid has been repeatedly called into question, because its specificity is no better than 50%,[27] particularly among patients with trauma.[28]

When possible, bronchoscopy with protected specimen brush or bronchoalveolar lavage (BAL) should be used to obtain quantitative lower respiratory tract cultures. In cases in which bronchoscopy is not immediately available, lower respiratory tract sampling with blind catheterization (mini-BAL) can reliably obtain lower respiratory

Table 3
The Clinical Pulmonary Infection Score

Criterion[a]	Points		
	0	1	2
Temperature (°C)	>36.5 and <38.4 (give 1 point if external cooling)	>38.5 and <38.9	<36 or ≥39
Blood leukocytes, mm3	≥4,000 and ≤11,000	<4,000 or >11,000 (no band forms)	>11,000 and presence of band forms
Tracheal secretions	Absent	Present but nonpurulent	Purulent
Oxygenation (Pao₂/Fio₂)	>240 or acute respiratory distress syndrome		<240 no acute respiratory distress syndrome
Chest radiograph	No infiltrate	Diffuse or patchy infiltrates	Localized infiltrate
Tracheal aspirate culture	Negative		Positive

[a] The modified CPIS score is calculated from the first 5 variables. A score of >6 at baseline is suggestive of pneumonia.

tract secretions for quantitative cultures. In patients with acute respiratory distress syndrome, deterioration of radiographic images because of progression of pulmonary infection may be difficult to detect, and suspicion for pneumonia should be high to avoid delays in treatment. Similarly, patients with chest trauma may have difficult in interpreting radiographs, and a low threshold for microbiological sampling is appropriate.

Blood cultures should be obtained, because VAP with bacteremia is associated with increased mortality compared with VAP alone.[29] However, there are no clear data to support that information from blood cultures either significantly alters treatment or improves outcomes. Ideally, blood and quantitative airway cultures should be obtained before initiating or manipulating antibiotics. This strategy may not be possible in all situations. For instance, a patient may already be on antimicrobial therapy for another source of infection. When this is the case, decreasing the bacterial colony count threshold for defining pneumonia may be of benefit.

Delay in the initiation of appropriate antibiotic therapy may increase disease morbidity and mortality, especially in patients with septic shock requiring ongoing vasoactive agent support. Therefore, under these circumstances, initiation of antimicrobials should not be postponed for the purpose of performing diagnostic workup.

Clinical signs of infection in patients with negative lower respiratory tract cultures should prompt investigation for extrapulmonary sites of infection. By nature, patients managed in an ICU are at risk for several forms of hospital-acquired infection and should be evaluated thoughtfully and broadly.

EMPIRICAL THERAPY

Immediate administration of appropriate antibiotic therapy is essential in the treatment of pneumonia. However, antimicrobial treatment is not without risk. In particular, for a patient receiving prolonged broad-spectrum antibiotics, antibiotic pretreatment shows a considerable microbial selection pressure associated with excess mortality.

The key decision in initial empirical therapy is determining whether the patient has risk factors for multidrug-resistant (MDR) strains. The distinction between early and late onset pneumonia has classically been used to tailor drug therapy. However, patients admitted after recent hospitalization or from long-term care facilities may also be at increased risk for MDR pathogens.

The overall approach to treatment is shown in the algorithm in **Fig. 1**.

INITIAL ANTIBIOTIC SELECTION AND DOSING

Optimal dosing remains a matter of debate. Differences in pharmacokinetics, microbiological characteristics of underlying pathogens, and methodology applied to determine microbial resistance levels all influence the antimicrobial effect of a given dosage. Moreover, penetration into lung tissue is an important factor that should be considered when selecting an antimicrobial regimen. Aminoglycosides are not ideal, because they achieve a lung penetration rate of only 30% to 40%. β-Lactams also have a penetration of less than 50%. Fluoroquinolones, in contrast, show cellular and lung tissue penetration 100% of serum level. Several studies have reported better clinical outcomes using linezolid compared with vancomycin for the treatment of methicillin-resistant *Staphylococcus aureus* (MRSA) pneumonia, supported by the superior lung penetration of the drug.[30]

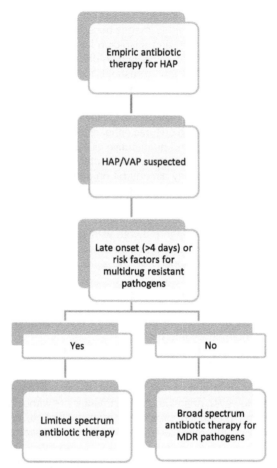

Fig. 1. Approach to empirical therapy for HAP and VAP.

Differences between spontaneously breathing versus ventilated patients are not firmly settled, and drug-resistant organisms may affect both populations. Therefore, recommendations in these 2 settings are frequently similar.

For early onset pneumonia (<4 days from hospital admission) in patients without risk factors for MDR pathogens, likely organism and recommended antibiotics are listed as follows:

Potential Pathogen	Recommended Antibiotic
Streptococcus pneumonia	Ceftriaxone
Haemophilus influenza	or
Methicillin-sensitive *Staphylococcus aureus*	levofloxacin, moxifloxacin, ciprofloxacin
Antibiotic-sensitive enteric gram-negatives	or
• *Escherichia coli*	ampicillin/sulbactam
• *Klebsiella pneumoniae*	or
• *Enterobacter* species	ertapenem
• *Proteus mirabilis*	
• *Serratia marcescens*	

For late onset pneumonia (ie, occurring after hospital day number 4 or in patients at risk for MDR pathogens) likely organisms and suggested therapy are as follows:

Potential Pathogen	Recommended Therapy
Pseudomonas aeruginosa	Antipseudomonal cephalosporin (ie, cefepime,
Klebsiella pneumoniae (extended-spectrum	ceftazidine)
β-lactamase)	or
Acinetobacter species	Antipseudomonal carbapenem (imipenem,
MRSA	meropenem)
	or
	β-lactam/β-lactamase inhibitor (piperacillin/
	tazobactam)
	Linezolid or vancomycin

DOUBLE COVERAGE IS NOT RECOMMENDED

Several studies and meta-analyses have shown that combination therapy for a β-lactam and an aminoglycoside in immunocompetent patients with cancer, neutropenia, or sepsis is not superior to monotherapy for the treatment of sepsis. A recent Cochrane review of 69 trials[31] showed no difference in regard to all-cause clinical fatality and clinical failure; however, rates of nephrotoxicity were higher in the double covered group.

RESPONSE TO THERAPY

Empirical antibiotics should be narrowed as directed by culture results as they become available. If a resistant or unexpected organism is found in a nonresponding patient, coverage may need to be expanded. However, the general trend is to deescalate from broad to the narrowest spectrum of antimicrobials with adequate minimum inhibitory concentration.

DURATION OF TREATMENT

Patients receiving intravenous antibiotics should be switched to an oral regimen as soon as possible. However, this strategy is dependent on how the patient is improving clinically. According to IDSA/ATS guidelines, duration of treatment should factor whether initial antibiotic therapy was effective against the infecting pathogen, or if confounding extrapulmonary infections were present.[3] A minimum of 5 days of treatment is recommended. In addition, the patient should be afebrile for 48 to 72 hours and should meet no more than 1 CAP-associated sign of clinical instability. These signs include the following.

- Temperature greater than 37.8°C
- Heart rate greater than 100 beats per minute
- Respiratory rate greater than 24
- Systolic blood pressure less than 90
- O_2 saturation less than 90% or Pao_2 less than 60 on room air
- Inability to maintain oral intake
- Altered mental status

REASONS FOR TREATMENT FAILURE

There are several potential causes for failure to improve once antibiotic therapy is initiated (**Fig. 2**). One is failure to identify and treat the inciting organism. This is particularly

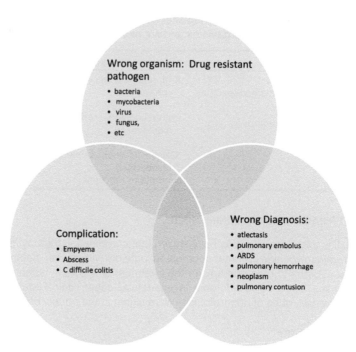

Fig. 2. Reasons for failed treatment of pneumonia.

a problem with MDR pathogens, atypical pneumonias, and more rarely fungal infections.

Treatment failure may also be secondary to a wrong diagnosis. Noninfectious pulmonary disease processes may be mistakenly interpreted as HAP. This situation is particularly true in patients with trauma, who often have coincident conditions related to direct trauma or as a consequence of massive resuscitation, including lung contusion, hemopneumothorax, pulmonary edema, pulmonary embolus with infarction, and aspiration pneumonitis. Missed intra-abdominal injury or postoperative surgical site infection must also be ruled out.

Treatment failure may be related to underlying complications such as empyema or lung abscess, which feature more prominently in patients with blunt injury to the chest, who need multiple chest tube thoracostomies, with resulting retained hemothorax. Targeted imaging with ultrasonography and computed tomographic scans is useful for the evaluation of anatomic reasons for treatment failure and may also be used to guide interventional therapies.

SPECIAL CONSIDERATIONS IN THE POPULATION WITH TRAUMA

Despite recent advances in trauma and critical care, posttraumatic VAP continues to be a significant cause of morbidity and mortality, with death rates reported as high as 25%, although generally in the 10% range. The increased risk of aspiration in the trauma population secondary to depressed levels of consciousness, head injury, need for urgent intubation, and concomitant chest injury create the perfect storm for pulmonary infection to take hold. In addition, it is important to suspect community-acquired aspiration pneumonia early, because delays in diagnosis and treatment lead to worse outcomes.

Incomplete documentation of prehospital aspiration events, including emesis around the time of intubation, makes the diagnosis of community-acquired aspiration pneumonia challenging. Moreover, patients who go on to being diagnosed with pneumonia after aspiration in the prehospital setting (community-acquired aspiration pneumonia) may easily be incorrectly classified as having HAP. This event has particular implications for empirical antibiotic strategies as well as comparison of quality of ICU care across hospitals. Preventative strategies may not be possible in the prehospital setting or in the case of emergent intubation, particularly in the setting of acute aspiration. Intubation in the prehospital setting has not been found to be directly associated with increased risk of pneumonia when compared with intubation in the emergency department.[32]

SUMMARY

Pneumonia in the surgical population continues to be a challenging event. The diagnosis is not always clear, although improvements in this area may be on the horizon, with better techniques for quantification. Early treatment is vital, and antibiotic selection is largely based on the previous duration of hospitalization and local bacterial flora. The duration of therapy is generally 5 to 14 days, with more recent efforts to shorten treatment based on more accurate assessment of physiologic response.

REFERENCES

1. Garrouste-Orgeas M, Chevret S, Arlet G, et al. Oropharyngeal or gastric colonization and nosocomial pneumonia in adult intensive care unit patients. A prospective study based on genomic DNA analysis. Am J Respir Crit Care Med 1997;156(5):1647–55.
2. Ewig S, Torres A, El-Ebiary M, et al. Bacterial colonization patterns in mechanically ventilated patients with traumatic and medical head injury. Incidence, risk factors, and association with ventilator-associated pneumonia. Am J Respir Crit Care Med 1999;159(1):188–98.
3. American Thoracic Society, Infectious Diseases Society of America. Guidelines for the management of adults with hospital-acquired, ventilator-associated, and healthcare-associated pneumonia. Am J Respir Crit Care Med 2005;171: 388–416.
4. Wunderink RG, Woldenberg LS, Zeiss J, et al. The radiologic diagnosis of autopsy-proven ventilator-associated pneumonia. Chest 1992;101(2):458–63.
5. Tejerina E, Esteban A, Fernández-Segoviano P, et al. Accuracy of clinical definitions of ventilator-associated pneumonia: comparison with autopsy findings. J Crit Care 2010;25(1):62–8.
6. Magill SS, Klompas M, Balk R, et al. Developing a new, national approach to surveillance for ventilator-associated events. Crit Care Med 2013;41(11):2467–75.
7. Klein Klouwenberg PM, van Mourik MS, Ong DS, et al. Electronic implementation of a novel surveillance paradigm for ventilator-associated events. Feasibility and validation. Am J Respir Crit Care Med 2014;189(8):947–55.
8. Rello J, Ollendorf DA, Oster G, et al. Epidemiology and outcomes of ventilator-associated pneumonia in a large US database. Chest 2002;122(6):2115–21.
9. Safdar N, Dezfulian C, Collard HR, et al. Clinical and economic consequences of ventilator-associated pneumonia: a systematic review. Crit Care Med 2005; 33(10):2184–93.
10. Rodriguez JL, Gibbons KJ, Bitzer LG, et al. Pneumonia: incidence, risk factors, and outcome in injured patients. J Trauma 1991;31(7):907–12 [discussion: 912–4].

11. Croce MA, Tolley EA, Fabian TC. A formula for prediction of posttraumatic pneumonia based on early anatomic and physiologic parameters. J Trauma 2003; 54(4):724–9 [discussion: 729–30].

12. Michelet P, Couret D, Brégeon F, et al. Early onset pneumonia in severe chest trauma: a risk factor analysis. J Trauma 2010;68(2):395–400.

13. Mandell LA, Wunderink RG, Anzueto A, et al. Infectious Diseases Society of America/American Thoracic Society consensus guidelines on the management of community-acquired pneumonia in adults. Clin Infect Dis 2007;44:S27–72.

14. Fine MJ, Auble TE, Yealy DM, et al. A prediction rule to identify low-risk patients with community-acquired pneumonia. N Engl J Med 1997;336(4):243–50.

15. Rello J, Rodriguez A, Lisboa T, et al. PIRO score for community-acquired pneumonia: a new prediction rule for assessment of severity in intensive care unit patients with community-acquired pneumonia. Crit Care Med 2009;37(2):456–62.

16. Lim WS. Defining community acquired pneumonia severity on presentation to hospital: an international derivation and validation study. Thorax 2003;58(5): 377–82.

17. Aujesky D, Auble TE, Yealy DM, et al. Prospective comparison of three validated prediction rules for prognosis in community-acquired pneumonia. Am J Med 2005;118(4):384–92.

18. Magnotti LJ, Croce MA, Fabian TC. Is ventilator-associated pneumonia in trauma patients an epiphenomenon or a cause of death? Surg Infect (Larchmt) 2005; 5(3):237–42.

19. Nguile-Makao M, Zahar JR, Français A, et al. Attributable mortality of ventilator-associated pneumonia: respective impact of main characteristics at ICU admission and VAP onset using conditional logistic regression and multi-state models. Intensive Care Med 2010;36(5):781–9.

20. Hedrick TL, Smith RL, McElearney ST, et al. Differences in early- and late-onset ventilator-associated pneumonia between surgical and trauma patients in a combined surgical or trauma intensive care unit. J Trauma 2008;64(3):714–20.

21. Munro CL, Grap MJ, Jones DJ, et al. Chlorhexidine, toothbrushing, and preventing ventilator-associated pneumonia in critically ill adults. Am J Crit Care 2009; 18(5):428–37 [quiz: 438].

22. Segers P, Speekenbrink RG, Ubbink DT, et al. Prevention of nosocomial infection in cardiac surgery by decontamination of the nasopharynx and oropharynx with chlorhexidine gluconate: a randomized controlled trial. JAMA 2006;296(20): 2460–6.

23. Klompas M, Speck K, Howell MD, et al. Reappraisal of routine oral care with chlorhexidine gluconate for patients receiving mechanical ventilation: systematic review and meta-analysis. JAMA Intern Med 2014;174(5):751–61.

24. Kress JP, Pohlman AS, O'Connor MF, et al. Daily interruption of sedative infusions in critically ill patients undergoing mechanical ventilation. N Engl J Med 2000; 342(20):1471–7.

25. Muscedere J, Dodek P, Keenan S, et al. Comprehensive evidence-based clinical practice guidelines for ventilator-associated pneumonia: prevention. J Crit Care 2008;23:126–37.

26. Fagon JY, Chastre J, Hance AJ, et al. Detection of nosocomial lung infection in ventilated patients. Use of a protected specimen brush and quantitative culture techniques in 147 patients. Am Rev Respir Dis 1988;138(1):110–6.

27. Luyt CE, Combes A, Reynaud C, et al. Usefulness of procalcitonin for the diagnosis of ventilator-associated pneumonia. Intensive Care Med 2008;34(8): 1434–40.

28. Croce MA, Swanson JM, Magnotti LJ, et al. The futility of the clinical pulmonary infection score in trauma patients. J Trauma 2006;60(3):523–7 [discussion: 527–8].

29. O'Keefe GE, Caldwell E, Cuschieri J, et al. Ventilator-associated pneumonia: bacteremia and death after traumatic injury. J Trauma Acute Care Surg 2012; 72(3):713–9.

30. Wunderink RG, Niederman MS, Kollef MH, et al. Linezolid in methicillin-resistant *Staphylococcus aureus* nosocomial pneumonia: a randomized, controlled study. Clin Infect Dis 2012;54(5):621–9.

31. Paul M, Lador A, Grozinsky-Glasberg S, et al. Beta lactam antibiotic monotherapy versus beta lactam-aminoglycoside antibiotic combination therapy for sepsis. Cochrane Database Syst Rev 2014;(1):CD003344.

32. Evans HL, Zonies DH, Warner KJ, et al. Timing of intubation and ventilator-associated pneumonia following injury. Arch Surg 2010;145(11):1041–6.

Intra-abdominal Infections

Gina R. Shirah, MD[a], Patrick J. O'Neill, PhD, MD[b],*

KEYWORDS

- Antibiotics • Complicated intra-abdominal infections • Damage control surgery
- Resuscitation • Source control • Systemic inflammatory response syndrome
- Uncomplicated intra-abdominal infections

KEY POINTS

- Intra-abdominal infections (IAI) should be suspected in a patient manifesting a systemic inflammatory response syndrome (SIRS) and gastrointestinal dysfunction.
- Uncomplicated IAI are predominantly isolated to an organ and do not involve gastrointestinal disruption, whereas complicated IAI are usually diffuse peritoneal processes that may include disruption of the gastrointestinal tract.
- Adequate treatment of IAI requires early diagnosis combined with resuscitation, appropriate antibiotic therapy, and adequate drainage/debridement of on-going infection or leaking gastrointestinal contents (ie, source control, SC).
- Appropriate and timely empiric antibiotic coverage is imperative because inappropriate or delayed coverage increases morbidity and mortality that cannot be reversed if subsequent appropriate antibiotics are added later.
- In general, β-lactam/β-lactamase antibiotics will provide adequate empiric coverage for low-risk patients; however, high-risk patients are at risk for more resistant microbiologic flora, and empiric coverage should be driven by individual hospital or unit antibiograms.
- Percutaneous drainage is preferred in stable patients with an isolated, anatomically amenable source; surgical debridement (open or laparoscopically) remains the mainstay for failed SC.

INTRODUCTION

Intra-abdominal infections (IAI) represent diverse disease processes and therapies; however, earlier diagnosis with readily available CT imaging, advanced therapeutic techniques of interventional radiology, improvement of antibiotic efficacy, and evolving critical care medicine have all combined to improve patient outcomes.

Disclosure: G.R. Shirah has nothing to disclose. P.J. O'Neill has served as a consultant on the Surgical Review Panel for Cubist Pharmaceuticals.
[a] Division of Trauma & Critical Care Surgery, Department of Surgery, Maricopa Medical Center, 2601 East Roosevelt Street, Phoenix, AZ 85008, USA; [b] Trauma Department, West Valley Hospital, 13677 W McDowell Road, Goodyear, AZ 85395, USA
* Corresponding author. Trauma Department, West Valley Hospital, Goodyear, AZ.
E-mail address: pjoneill@abrazohealth.com

Surg Clin N Am 94 (2014) 1319–1333
http://dx.doi.org/10.1016/j.suc.2014.08.005
surgical.theclinics.com

IAI are divided into uncomplicated and complicated types. Uncomplicated IAI affect a single organ and do not spread to the peritoneum. In these cases, there is no anatomic disruption of the gastrointestinal tract. Complicated IAI describes an extension of the infection into the peritoneal space. It may be localized, as in the case of an intra-abdominal abscess. For the insult that is not contained, diffuse peritonitis may ensue.[1,2] The resultant physiologic response may develop into a systemic inflammatory response syndrome (SIRS) (**Table 1**).[3,4]

In addition to defining type of infection, patient stratification serves as an important guide for treatment and will assist with initial resuscitation, treatment options, and specifically, antimicrobial therapy. Patients are divided into low-risk and high-risk categories that take into account the patient's history, the type of infection, and the resulting physiologic derangements.

Low-risk patients typically have community-acquired infections of mild to moderate severity (perforated appendicitis or diverticulitis). The underlying physiologic status in these patients is not compromised. High-risk patients, on the other hand, are used to define patients who are at risk for multi-drug-resistant organisms,[5–7] failure of source control (SC),[8] and ultimately, increased mortality.[1,5,8–10] Predetermined patient-specific and disease-specific factors act together to determine patient morbidity and mortality (**Box 1**).[6,8,10]

PATHOPHYSIOLOGY

The inner abdomen is lined with a layer of tissue (peritoneum) innervated by the somatic nervous system. Infection begins, followed by inflammation by mast cell degranulation with subsequent increased vascular permeability. This increased vascular permeability causes an influx of complement factors and neutrophils that are responsible for both direct bacterial opsonization and release of cytokines to propagate the host response. This process may be localized to an abscess when the inflammation, chemotaxis, and fibrin formation may form sufficient physical barriers.[10]

Intra-abdominal inflammation may lead to a diffuse paralytic ileus, distention, obstipation, and vomiting.[4] When the host ability to contain the infection is overcome, the infection progresses to diffuse peritonitis. Systemic response to the release of cytokines will lead to a pro-inflammatory state, systemic vasodilation, hypotension, and myocardial depression, manifested clinically as severe sepsis and subsequently as septic shock.[3,10]

DIAGNOSIS

Diagnosis of IAI should be suspected in patients with SIRS and gastrointestinal dysfunction. Essential components of the history include any recent surgeries, and

Table 1 Systemic inflammatory response syndrome criteria[a]	
Finding	**Value**
Temperature	<36°C or >38°C
Heart rate	>90/min
Respiratory rate	>20/min or $Paco_2$ <32 mm Hg
WBC	<4 × 10^9/L, >12 × 10^9/L, or 10% bands

Abbreviations: $Paco_2$, partial pressure of carbon dioxide; WBC, white blood cell count.
[a] Defined as having at least 2 of the above.

Box 1
Characteristics of high-risk intra-abdominal infection patients

Patient-specific factors

- Advanced age (>70 y)
- Immunosuppression
  - Poor nutritional status
  - Corticosteroid therapy
  - Organ transplantation
- Presence of malignancy
- Pre-existing chronic conditions
  - Liver disease
  - Renal disease

Disease-specific factors

- High APACHE II score (>15)
- Health care–associated infection
- Delay in initial intervention (>24 h)
- Inability to obtain source control

---

the presence of vomiting, diarrhea, and obstipation. Although physical examination findings are notoriously nonspecific, particular findings may give insight.[11] Pain out of proportion to examination is classically associated with acute mesenteric ischemia. Inguinal and umbilical hernia examinations are important to rule out the source of obstruction or incarceration. Although minimally invasive surgery is increasingly common, abdominal scars are always important to note.

Laboratory workup begins with the assessment of a complete blood count and serum electrolytes. Liver function tests, amylase, and lipase may be added if clinical concern includes hepatobiliary or pancreatic pathologic abnormality. In patients with SIRS and a concern for sepsis, further assessment of end-organ perfusion or signs of oxygen debt should be assessed (ie, serum lactic acid, superior vena caval/mixed venous oxygenation saturations, arterial blood gas for base deficit).[3,10]

Initial radiographic imaging should include a CT scan with oral and intravenous (IV) contrast to maximize sensitivity and specificity.[4,8,11,12] Oral contrast helps to differentiate bowel loops from adjacent fluid collections and may help guide subsequent drainage procedures.[4] IV contrast helps delineate inflammation, identify hemorrhage, and visualize abscess walls. CT is useful in identifying small areas of free intra-abdominal air (pneumoperitoneum) associated with hollow viscous perforation, air in the biliary tree, and air within the intestinal walls (pneumotosis intestinalis). The exception to this is if biliary pathologic abnormality is suspected (right upper quadrant pain, nausea, and vomiting), then right upper quadrant ultrasound is the higher yield.[11]

Microbiologic diagnosis is not important in community-acquired IAI because empiric antibiotic therapy is initiated based on clinical impression and risk factors.[8,10,12] In the case of high-risk patients, blood and intra-abdominal cultures are necessary to guide antimicrobial therapy due to the higher risk for multi-drug-resistant organisms.

One of the most urgent clinical circumstances is the patient who presents with peritonitis (abdominal rigidity, guarding, and rebound tenderness). These signs are concerning for pending hemodynamic collapse, and urgent evaluation and disposition are necessary. Early hemodynamic assessment is a priority; if adequate (systolic blood pressure >90 mm Hg), there may be time for further workup. On the other hand, unstable patients (systolic blood pressure <90 mm Hg) and the need for vasopressor support indicate the need emergent laparotomy for diagnostic and therapeutic purposes with the understanding that the risk of mortality is higher than in a stable patient.[3]

TREATMENT

The principles of treatment require simultaneous resuscitation, SC, and antimicrobial therapy. If not aggressively managed, IAI may progress to severe sepsis, septic shock, and death.[13]

Resuscitation

Intravascular volume depletion should be expected in patients with IAI. A thorough history and physical examination may aid with guiding resuscitation. Severe nausea and vomiting will cause metabolic alkalosis with relative hypokalemia, whereas a high-volume diarrhea will cause a nonanion gap metabolic acidosis. With peritonitis, the cytokine inflammation causes fluid sequestration both locally and systemically, which may be profound, further contributing to intravascular volume depletion. Fluid accumulation is noted with an ileus by both bowel wall edema and ascites. In addition, patients with fever and tachypnea have more than 700 mL/d of excess fluid loss.[10] These abnormal fluid shifts place patients at risk for intravascular volume depletion, hypotension, and decreased end-organ perfusion. With an increasing severity of illness, more invasive hemodynamic monitoring is indicated (central venous and arterial pressure catheter placement and monitoring).

It has been learned from the Surviving Sepsis Campaign (SSC) that fluid resuscitation should be initiated immediately after the diagnosis of sepsis is suspected.[3] The strategy of early goal-directed therapy has been shown to decrease mortality.[14]

Source Control

SC is a fundamental surgical principle and is defined as the ability to effectively eradicate infection (ie, purulent fluid or tissue) and control leakage (ie, drainage of on-going enteric contamination) by whatever means necessary.[4,6,10] Although resuscitation and treatment with antibiotics are central to the treatment of IAI, SC is paramount. It may be accomplished in a variety of ways, ranging from percutaneous drainage to repeat operations. Timing of SC is generally undertaken as early as safely possible. Although the goal is to remove the driver of the inflammatory response, patients may be in a delicate physiologic state that puts them at high risk for immediate intervention. Nonetheless, SC is directly related to outcome, and inability to provide adequate SC is associated with increased mortality.[8,9] The exception to this rule is acute pancreatitis and pancreatic necrosis, which does not benefit from early SC (see later discussion).

In general, the least invasive procedure that is safely able to eradicate the infection is preferred. Percutaneous image-guided drainage is preferred for isolated IAI that are anatomically amenable to drainage. Surgical debridement, whether laparoscopic or open, remains the mainstay of therapy for failed percutaneous control.

Surgical intervention is required for peritonitis with hemodynamic instability, evidence of uncontrolled, on-going contamination, and/or if bowel necrosis is suspected.[4,5,8,10]

Patients may present with extreme physiologic derangements and multiorgan system failure that requires ICU resuscitation.[10,15] Unfortunately, resuscitation likely will not be successful until SC is achieved. When urgent operative intervention is indicated, intraoperative resuscitation must be continued and this requires close collaboration with anesthesia providers.[8] In these extreme circumstances, one option is to perform damage control surgery (DCS). DSC is a specific type of temporary SC originally described in the trauma setting.[15] Similar concepts are now being applied to the emergency general surgery patient who meets criteria (**Box 2**).

In these DCS patients, the priority is control of on-going contamination that directly decreases mortality.[8] In times of severe contamination and inflammation, definitive surgical treatment may not be safe; the priority is then to perform proximal diversion (if possible) and/or to allow adequate external drainage of any on-going leakage (ie, drains, sub-atmospheric/vacuum pressure dressings).

Options for temporary abdominal closure include a conventional dressing, a subatmospheric pressure dressing, or skin closure alone. The decision to not definitely close someone's abdomen should not be taken lightly. Nonclosure of the fascia is not without complications and puts patients at risk for multiple operations, prolonged intensive care unit stay, infection, fistula formation, and failure of abdominal closure. These complications may potentially negate the beneficial effects of this option if overused.[15]

Relaparotomy should be reserved for patients with specific abnormalities otherwise not recommended.[8] Planned relaparotomy as a management option was thought to be beneficial to allow for complete drainage of intra-abdominal contamination and early detection of anastomotic leaks. A randomized trial found that on-demand re-laparotomy did not have a higher risk of peritonitis-related morbidity, whereas the planned relaparotomy group had an increased use of health care services, costs, and laparotomies.[5,8,16]

Antibiotics

Although secondary to adequate SC, appropriate and timely empiric antibiotic coverage is imperative. Inappropriate coverage increases hospital stay, postoperative abscesses,[10] and mortality that cannot be reversed if subsequent appropriate antibiotics are added later in the clinical course.[2,4] In severe sepsis, appropriate coverage should be started within 1 hour as recommended by the SSC.[3,10] Just as important is the appropriate discontinuation of antibiotics (Antibiotic Stewardship). Unnecessary antibiotic use has contributed to the emergence and spread of drug-resistant microorganisms.

Box 2
Clinical indications for damage control surgery

Hemodynamic instability

On-going contamination or need for further debridement

Tissue/organ ischemia

Loss of abdominal domain

Development of/risk for abdominal compartment syndrome

Initial empiric antibiotic coverage requires both knowledge of normal enteric flora and assessment of potential risk factors. In general, proximal small bowel contains enteric gram-positive streptococcus and gram-negative bacteria, whereas anaerobic bacteria populate the distal ileum and colon (**Table 2**).[8,10,12]

To help guide the clinician, guidelines have been published that standardize the diagnosis and management of IAI.[8,12] The first guideline represents a consensus between the Surgical Infection Society and the Infectious Disease Society of America. Second, worldwide guidelines have been published by the World Society of Emergency Surgery. As previously mentioned, patients with IAI are divided into low-risk and high-risk categories to stratify their risk for developing complicated infections. In general, β-lactam/β-lactamase (penicillin, cephalosporins, carbapenems, monobactams) antibiotics will provide adequate empiric coverage for low-risk patients (**Table 3**).[8,12]

High-risk patients, on the other hand, are at risk for more resistant microbiologic flora. Specifically, this includes gram-negative *Pseudomonas aeruginosa* and *Acinetobacter* species, extended spectrum β-lactamase producing *Klebsiella* species, *Escherichia coli*, *Enterobacter* species, *Proteus* species, methicillin-resistant *Staphylococcus aureus* (MRSA), enterococci, and *Candida* species. Empiric therapies are institution-specific and should be adjusted for individual hospital/unit antibiograms (**Table 4**).

Routine coverage for *Enterococcus faecalis* is only recommended if IAI is health care–associated, if the patient had previously received cephalosporins, if the patient has a history of valvular heart disease/prosthetics, or if the patient is elderly or critically ill. *E faecalis* is seen with frequency in patients with liver disease and infections with a hepatobiliary source.[7] Antibiotics that will provide adequate coverage include ampicillin, piperacillin-tazobactam, and vancomycin. Fungal coverage is necessary in the presence of a nosocomial infection, a critically ill community-acquired infection, a patient on pharmacologic immunosuppression, or isolation of fungi from normally sterile sites. Also, coverage should be considered if there was recent exposure to broad-spectrum antimicrobials. Fluconazole is recommended unless critically ill; then echinocandin is recommended as first-line treatment. MRSA coverage is recommended

Table 2	
Normal enteric flora by gastrointestinal region	
Stomach and duodenum	Streptococcus Lactobacillus
Biliary	E coli Klebsiella sp. Enterococcus sp. (±)
Small intestines	E coli Klebsiella sp. Enterococcus sp. Diptheroid sp. Enterococci sp.
Distal ileum and colon	Bacteroides fragilis Clostridium sp. Enterobacter sp. Enterococcus sp. E coli Klebsiella sp. Peptostreptococcus sp.

Table 3
Empiric antibiotic recommendations for low-risk intra-abdominal infection patients

	Low Risk	High Risk
Single agent	Cefoxitin Ertapenem Moxifloxacin Tigecycline Ticarcillin-clavulanic acid	Imipenem-cilastin Meropenem Doripenem Pipercillin-tazobactam
Combination (with metronidazole)	Cefazolin Cefuroxime Ceftriaxone Cefotaxime Ciprofloxacin Levofloxacin	Cefepime Ceftazidime Ciprofloxacin Levofloxacin

Data from Lopez N, Kobayashi L, Coimbra R. A comprehensive review of abdominal infections. World J Emerg Surg 2011;6:7; and Rivers E, Nguyen B, Havstad S, et al. Early goal-directed therapy in the treatment of severe sepsis and septic shock. N Engl J Med 2001;345:1368–77.

when there is a known history of MRSA, a hospital-acquired infection, or recent, significant antibiotic exposure. Vancomycin is then recommended as treatment.[8]

Duration of antibiotic treatment is an on-going point of discussion in the literature and important to clinically reassess daily.[4,10] General consensus recommendations are a course of 4 to 7 days. Prompt discontinuation of treatment is encouraged if

Table 4
Empiric antibiotic recommendations for high-risk IAI patients

Local Organism	Carbapenems	Piperacillin-Tazobactam	Ceftazidime or Cefepime (+Metronidazole)	Aminoglycoside	Vancomycin
<20% resistant P aeruginosa ESBL-producing Enterobacter sp. Acinetobacter sp. or other MDR GNR	+	+	+		
ESBL-producing Enterobacter sp.	+	+		+	
>20% of P aeruginosa resistant to ceftazidime	+	+		+	
MRSA					+

Abbreviations: ESBL, extended spectrum β-lactamase; MDR GNR, multi-drug-resistant gram-negative rod; MRSA, methacillin-resistant Staphlococcus aureus.

Data from Lopez N, Kobayashi L, Coimbra R. A Comprehensive review of abdominal infections. World J Emerg Surg 2011;6:7; and Rivers E, Nguyen B, Havstad S, et al. Early goal-directed therapy in the treatment of severe sepsis and septic shock. N Engl J Med 2001;345:1368–77.

patients show clinical response because longer treatment has not been associated with improved outcome.[8] Historically, studies have suggested antibiotics should be continued until the patient has resolved their leukocytosis or fever and is tolerating oral diet, but that may not be necessary.[10] Transition to oral antibiotics may be initiated when the patient is taking oral diet without an increased risk of treatment failure.[8,17]

If the patient continues to show signs of fever, leukocytosis, or delayed gastrointestinal function after 7 days, a persistent infection should be suspected and reimaging should be completed to search for on-going infection.[8] In this situation, it is recommended to continue antibiotics and strongly consider a change in covering antibiotic-resistant microorganisms.

SPECIFIC CONSIDERATIONS AND CONTROVERSIES
Appendicitis

Acute appendicitis is the most common source of infection in community-acquired IAI.[4] Antibiotic coverage depends on extent of disease. Prompt discontinuation of antibiotics is recommended after appendectomy if surgery reveals no perforation.[10]

Source Control

In acute appendicitis, nonoperative management has been suggested as an alternative to traditional treatment of appendectomy. Meta-analyses demonstrate antibiotic treatment alone was associated with decreased complications, less pain, and a shorter sick leave. Ultimately, antibiotics were found to have only a treatment success rate of 63% at 1 year and thus remain inferior to surgical management.[10,18,19]

Both the open laparoscopic approach and the laparoscopic approach to appendectomy continue to be accepted treatment modalities and have been extensively compared in the literature. The open approach has been associated with less cost, shorter operative times, and decreased risk of IAI in multiple studies. Alternatively, the laparoscopic approach has been found to have fewer surgical site infections, less pain, shorter hospital stays, and more rapid return to normal activity. For complicated or perforated appendicitis, the laparoscopic approach has been shown to reduce overall mortality.[10,20–22]

Patients who present with a phlegmon or periappendiceal abscess had traditionally required an operation for SC. When patients present during the peak of intra-abdominal inflammation, the safety of surgical intervention comes into question. Treatment with antibiotics and percutaneous drainage, if amenable, have been found to be associated with fewer complications and shorter hospital stay when compared with immediate appendectomy.[10,23] Treatment of periappendiceal abscesses with antibiotics alone has also been suggested but compared with percutaneous drainage has a significant recurrence rate and is therefore not recommended.[24]

For those patients who were treated with percutaneous drainage and antibiotics, generally an interval appendectomy was recommended owing to the variable rates of recurrence (5%–37%).[10,23,25] There is not enough evidence to firmly support interval appendectomy and, in fact, interval appendectomy may be unnecessary in 75% to 90% of cases.[12] Advocates for interval appendectomy argue that there is a significant risk of recurrence and, if no surgical intervention is undertaken, there is a risk of missing a diagnosis of cancer or Crohn disease. A systematic meta-analysis reviewed 61 studies from 1964 to 2005 and found a recurrence rate of only 7.4% and a 1.2% risk of malignancy.[26] Patients who underwent interval appendectomy were found to have a prolonged hospital stay.[26] Interval appendectomy is not strongly supported in the literature.

Acute Cholangitis

Acute cholangitis is defined as a biliary obstruction complicated by infection. The obstruction may be due to calculi, stricture, or a blocked biliary stent. The clinical presentation and subsequent decompensation of a patient may be quite rapid so prompt diagnosis is essential. Rates of mortality have improved over time but remain 11% to 27%.[27] Classic diagnosis is described by Charcot triad: fever, abdominal pain, and jaundice. The complicated form of cholangitis includes septic shock and mental status change (ie, Reynold pentad). The Tokyo Guidelines clarified the diagnostic criteria and in addition graded the severity of cholangitis (**Box 3**).[28]

The severity of disease increases with the presence of organ dysfunction and nonresponse to initial medical treatment. Severe acute cholangitis requires urgent biliary compression with endoscopic retrograde cholangiopancreatography (ERCP).[27]

Source control

No randomized trials have been completed that compare treatment options, but in accordance with the theme of least invasive treatment that may safely provide SC, ERCP-directed internal drainage is the first-line therapy. Recent data suggest that early ERCP (≤24 hours) leads to significantly shorter hospitalization without a significant increase in intervention-related complications.[29] Percutaneous transhepatic drainage is available as a second-line therapy. Operative drainage may be indicated. Recently, endoscopic ultrasound-guided biliary drainage has emerged as an option for biliary decompression.[30]

Antibiotics

Coverage of microorganisms from the proximal bowel is usually sufficient for initial empiric treatment in biliary disease. Anaerobic therapy is added in the case of acute cholangitis and, when there is a biliary-enteric anastomosis, severe physiologic disturbance, or an immunocompromised state. *Enterococcus* species coverage is only necessary if the patient has undergone an extensive hepatic procedure or has other risk factors for enterococcus, such as immunocompromisation.[8]

Box 3
Diagnostic criteria for acute cholangitis

A. Systemic inflammation

  1. Fever and/or chills

  2. Elevated WBC or CRP

B. Cholestasis

  1. Jaundice

  2. Elevated transaminases

C. Imaging

  1. Biliary dilatation

  2. Evidence of cause on imaging (stricture, stone, stent)

Suspected diagnosis: one item in A + one item in either B or C.
Definite diagnosis: one item in A, one item in B, and one item in C.
Abbreviations: CRP, C-reactive protein; WBC, white blood cell count.
  Data from Sartelli M, Viale P, Catena F, et al. 2013 WSES guidelines for management of intra-abdominal infections. World J Emerg Surg 2013;8:3; and Weber DG, Bendinelli C, Balogh ZJ. Damage control surgery for abdominal emergencies. Br J Surg 2014;101:e109–18.

Pancreatitis

Pancreatitis has a variable presentation and if not recognized and treated may result in rapid and severe patient decompensation. Ninety percent of acute pancreatitis is caused by alcohol and gallstones. Simultaneous evaluation of cause should be delineated. Ultrasound and serum alcohol level should be performed in all patients. If these are negative, less common causes should be pursued.[31]

Given the severe inflammatory response seen in these patients, resuscitation is paramount. Worsening hemoconcentration 24 hours after admission is associated with increased morbidity. Lactated Ringer solution should be run at 250 to 500 mL/h within the first 12 to 24 hours of admission, and urine output should be closely monitored.[31,32]

Many scoring systems have been proposed to predict which patients are at risk for complicated pancreatitis. The classic Ranson's criteria on admission and at 48 hours may delay recognizing severe pancreatitis. The Bedside Index for Severe Acute Pancreatitis has been described as easier to use, whereas The Revised Atlanta Classification incorporates both physiologic and radiologic findings. Unfortunately, no system has proven to be all inclusive and therefore the close evaluation of fluid losses, SIRS, and presence of organ dysfunction is absolutely imperative.[31] Radiologic evaluation of pancreatitis is best if performed at least 72 hours after presentation to get a complete evaluation of pancreatic inflammation and necrosis.[32]

Source control

In the setting of gallstone pancreatitis, clearance of CBD with ERCP is strongly recommended within 24 hours. Although the evidence is not as strong as it is in the presence of cholangitis, most recommendations include ERCP.[31,33] If on-going signs of obstruction are present, surgical exploration of the common bile duct may be indicated. Early cholecystectomy (within 48 hours) is recommended in mild gallstone pancreatitis because waiting until complete symptoms and chemical resolution is unnecessary. Aboulian and colleagues[34] found in their randomized study that early cholecystectomy was not associated with increased technical difficulty or complications but resulted in a shorter hospital length of stay. In addition, offering an interval cholecystectomy was associated with a significant increase in biliary readmissions (18%) and is therefore not recommended.[35]

Antibiotics

Unlike other intra-abdominal infectious processes, this disease is not initially secondary to bacterial infection. Unless signs of cholangitis are present, routine use of antibiotics in pancreatitis is not recommended. Prophylactic antibiotics, even in severe necrotizing pancreatitis, do not prevent progression of sterile necrosis to infected necrosis and are therefore not recommended.[8] Ten percent of patients with pancreatitis will ultimately become infected. This number increases to between 30% and 70% if necrosis is present.[1,32]

Infected Pancreatic Necrosis

Infected pancreatic necrosis should be suspected if there is an acute deterioration or failure to improve over a period of 7 to 10 days. Given the underlying SIRS causes fever and tachycardia, ultimately diagnosing infected pancreatic necrosis may be challenging. The diagnostic imaging of choice is a CT scan with IV contrast. Infection is suspected if there is gas in the necrotic cavity.[31]

Source control

With a diagnosis of infected pancreatitis, traditionally this was an indication for operative intervention. Clearly, there is a need for intervention, but image-guided catheter placement with upsizing as necessary has proven to be effective and safe and may be able to successfully avoid surgery in 50% of patients. Multiple approaches have been successfully attempted, including laparoscopic anterior/retroperitoneal or percutaneous radiologic-guided catheter placement followed by endoscopy through the tract.

Ultimately, surgical debridement may be needed to remove infected, necrotic tissue if catheter drainage does not appear to be providing adequate SC. Delayed intervention in pancreatitis, unlike other acute IAI, is associated with improved morbidity. Recommended surgical approach is midline or subcostal and approaches the lesser sac through the gastrocolic ligament. The initial goal of surgery is to obtain aggressive SC and close the abdomen with closed suction drains. Open packing and planned relaparotomies are associated with significant mortality.[32]

Antibiotics

If infection is suspected, broad-spectrum antibiotics should be initiated and CT or US-guided fine-needle aspiration should be obtained for culture material. Carbapenems, fluoroquinolones, metronidazole, and high-dose cephalosporins have best penetrance into pancreatic tissue.[31]

Diverticulitis

The frequency of diverticulosis within the Western population increases with age. Thirty percent of people have diverticulosis by the age of 60. Ten to 25% of these patients will ultimately develop diverticulitis.[36] Diverticulitis is an inflammation and ultimately a microperforation of a diverticula-containing segment of colon. With the great variation in presentation and clinical course, it is imperative to appropriately classify patients. CT scan of the abdomen and pelvis with oral, IV, and rectal contrast is the examination of choice for patients with suspected diverticulitis.[36] The traditional classification was based on clinical and operative findings but, with the widespread use of CT scanning, a modified classification has been proposed (**Table 5**).

Table 5
Hinchey classification with modification

	Hinchey Classification		Modified Hinchey	
Uncomplicated	I	Pericolic abscess or phlegmon	Ia	Confined pericolonic inflammation, phlegmon
			Ib	Confined pericolonic abscess
Complicated	II	Pelvic, intra-abdominal or retroperitoneal abscess	II	Pelvic, distant intra-abdominal or retroperitoneal abscess
	III	Generalized purulent peritonitis	III	Generalized purulent peritonitis
	IV	Generalized fecal peritonitis	IV	Fecal peritonitis

Data from Sartelli M, Viale P, Catena F, et al. 2013 WSES guidelines for management of intra-abdominal infections. World J Emerg Surg 2013;8:3; and Moore LJ, Moore FA, Jones SL, et al. Sepsis in general surgery: a deadly complication. Am J Surg 2009;198:868–74.

Classic presentation is lower abdominal pain, fever, and leukocytosis. Depending on the extent of the disease, peritonitis may be present. Most patients (75%–90%) will experience uncomplicated diverticulitis (Hinchey class I). The goal of therapy has to be tailored around the acute attack as well as the possibility of future episodes. Multiple factors must be taken into account, including underlying patient comorbidities.

Source control

The ideal approach of SC in complicated diverticulitis has been widely debated intensely studied, and ultimately, undergone significant changes in management. Traditional treatment of complicated diverticulitis was managed by surgical intervention up until the 1990s.[37] Current treatment paradigm has shifted to aggressive medical support and, if necessary, nonurgent surgical intervention. Approximately 15% of patients with acute diverticulitis will develop a pericolonic or intramesenteric abscess.[36] Abscesses less than 3 cm have been found to safely resolve with antibiotics alone. Percutaneous drainage is recommended for accessible abscesses greater than 4 cm.[10,38] The ultimate goal for those who are amenable to drainage with percutaneous catheters is to avoid emergency surgery.[36] In fact, nonoperative management has been found successful in 91% of patients with complicated diverticulitis, including patients with large pneumoperitoneum and large abscesses.[37,39] Failure of nonoperative management ultimately requires segmental colectomy. Laparoscopic approach, even for complicated diverticulitis, has been shown as safe even in the setting of longer operative times, demonstrating fewer complications, less pain, and shorter hospital stay.[40,41]

What is not debated is that emergency operative intervention is required for free perforation with peritonitis (Hinchey III or IV) or the presence of hemodynamic instability. Immunocompromised patients are more likely to present with perforation and failed medical management necessitating a lower threshold for urgent surgery. Historically, a Hartmann procedure was standard and necessary. In certain clinical scenarios, primary resection and anastomosis have been proven safe even with diffuse peritonitis.[12] A recent randomized trial compared the Hartmann procedure to resection and primary anastomosis (PA). The PA group was found to have less risk of serious complications, lower in-hospital costs, decreased operating times, and ultimately, decreased hospital length of stay.[42] Another less invasive treatment option that has been proposed is laparoscopic lavage. Laparoscopic lavage has also been proven safe and will be compared with conventional management in the upcoming "LADIES" trial.[43]

Antibiotics

Uncomplicated diverticulitis has a standard treatment with bowel rest and antibiotics for 7 to 10 days, which is successful in 70% to 100% of patients.[10,36,44] Classically, a combination of quinolone and metronidazole are used, but recently Ertapenem, a carbapenem, has been increasingly used and may provide a well-tolerated monotherapy.[44]

The length of treatment has come into question in the literature. A recent study randomized patients with uncomplicated sigmoid diverticulitis to a 4-day versus the traditional 7-day course of antibiotics and found no significant differences in recurrence rate at 1 month and at 1 year. The 4-day group had a significantly shorter hospital length of stay.[44] In the face of increased antibiotic resistance, Chabok and colleagues[45] took the next step and questioned the need for antibiotics at all in uncomplicated acute diverticulitis. In an interesting multicenter randomized trial, patients with acute uncomplicated diverticulitis were given either no antibiotics or the standard 7-day course. Ultimately, they found no differences in complications, operations, recurrences, or hospital stay. Despite lack of adequate evidence to treat with antibiotics, current recommendation for uncomplicated acute diverticulitis is antibiotic coverage for gram-negative and anaerobic organisms for 5 to 10 days.[12]

SUMMARY

IAI arise from many sites and range from a moderate nuisance to life-threatening. Prompt identification, diagnosis, and treatment allow optimal patient outcomes. Resuscitation from shock, early appropriate antibiotic administration, and control of the source of infection are necessary components of a 3-pronged approach. Initial antibiotic administration should be broad spectrum and tailored to the most likely pathogen and then narrowed to the best agent for the appropriate duration. SC may be obtained using radiographically placed percutaneous or traditional operative drains; the choice depends on the anatomic site, site accessibility, and the patient's clinical condition. Patient-specific factors (advanced age and chronic medical conditions) as well as disease-specific factors (health care–associated infections and inability to obtain SC) combine to affect patient morbidity and mortality.

REFERENCES

1. Menichetti F, Sganga G. Definition and classification of intra-abdominal infections. J Chemother 2009;21(Suppl 1):3–4.
2. Sartelli M, Catena F, Coccolini F, et al. Antimicrobial management of intra-abdominal infections: literature's guidelines. World J Gastroenterol 2012;18: 865–71.
3. Dellinger RP, Levy MM, Rhodes A, et al. Surviving sepsis campaign: international guidelines for management of severe sepsis and septic shock: 2012. Crit Care Med 2013;41:580–637.
4. Pieracci FM, Barie PS. Management of severe sepsis of abdominal origin. Scand J Surg 2007;96:184–96.
5. Koperna T, Schulz F. Relaparotomy in peritonitis: prognosis and treatment of patients with persisting intraabdominal infection. World J Surg 2000;24:32–7.
6. Weigelt JA. Empiric treatment options in the management of complicated intra-abdominal infections. Cleve Clin J Med 2007;74(Suppl 4):S29–37.
7. Swenson BR, Metzger R, Hedrick TL, et al. Choosing antibiotics for intra-abdominal infections: what do we mean by "high risk"? Surg Infect (Larchmt) 2009;10:29–39.
8. Solomkin JS, Mazuski JE, Bradley JS, et al. Diagnosis and management of complicated intra-abdominal infection in adults and children: guidelines by the Surgical Infection Society and the Infectious Diseases Society of America. Clin Infect Dis 2010;50:133–64.
9. Wacha H, Hau T, Dittmer R, et al. Risk factors associated with intraabdominal infections: a prospective multicenter study. Peritonitis Study Group. Langenbecks Arch Surg 1999;384:24–32.
10. Lopez N, Kobayashi L, Coimbra RA. Comprehensive review of abdominal infections. World J Emerg Surg 2011;6:7.
11. Crandall M, West MA. Evaluation of the abdomen in the critically ill patient: opening the black box. Curr Opin Crit Care 2006;12:333–9.
12. Sartelli M, Viale P, Catena F, et al. 2013 WSES guidelines for management of intra-abdominal infections. World J Emerg Surg 2013;8:3.

13. Moore LJ, Moore FA, Jones SL, et al. Sepsis in general surgery: a deadly complication. Am J Surg 2009;198:868–74.

14. Rivers E, Nguyen B, Havstad S, et al. Early goal-directed therapy in the treatment of severe sepsis and septic shock. N Engl J Med 2001;345:1368–77.

15. Weber DG, Bendinelli C, Balogh ZJ. Damage control surgery for abdominal emergencies. Br J Surg 2014;101:e109–18.

16. van Ruler O, Mahler CW, Boer KR, et al. Comparison of on-demand vs planned relaparotomy strategy in patients with severe peritonitis: a randomized trial. JAMA 2007;298:865–72.

17. Solomkin JS, Dellinger EP, Bohnen JM, et al. The role of oral antimicrobials for the management of intra-abdominal infections. New Horiz 1998;6:S46–52.

18. Mason RJ, Moazzez A, Sohn H, et al. Meta-analysis of randomized trials comparing antibiotic therapy with appendectomy for acute uncomplicated (no abscess or phlegmon) appendicitis. Surg Infect (Larchmt) 2012;13:74–84.

19. Varadhan KK, Neal KR, Lobo DN. Safety and efficacy of antibiotics compared with appendicectomy for treatment of uncomplicated acute appendicitis: meta-analysis of randomised controlled trials. BMJ 2012;344:e2156.

20. Tuggle KR, Ortega G, Bolorunduro OB, et al. Laparoscopic versus open appendectomy in complicated appendicitis: a review of the NSQIP database. J Surg Res 2010;163:225–8.

21. Tiwari MM, Reynoso JF, Tsang AW, et al. Comparison of outcomes of laparoscopic and open appendectomy in management of uncomplicated and complicated appendicitis. Ann Surg 2011;254:927–32.

22. Page AJ, Pollock JD, Perez S, et al. Laparoscopic versus open appendectomy: an analysis of outcomes in 17,199 patients using ACS/NSQIP. J Gastrointest Surg 2010;14:1955–62.

23. Brown CV, Abrishami M, Muller M, et al. Appendiceal abscess: immediate operation or percutaneous drainage? Am Surg 2003;69:829–32.

24. Zerem E, Salkic N, Imamovic G, et al. Comparison of therapeutic effectiveness of percutaneous drainage with antibiotics versus antibiotics alone in the treatment of periappendiceal abscess: is appendectomy always necessary after perforation of appendix? Surg Endosc 2007;21:461–6.

25. Kaminski A, Liu IL, Applebaum H, et al. Routine interval appendectomy is not justified after initial nonoperative treatment of acute appendicitis. Arch Surg 2005;140:897–901.

26. Andersson RE, Petzold MG. Nonsurgical treatment of appendiceal abscess or phlegmon: a systematic review and meta-analysis. Ann Surg 2007;246:741–8.

27. Wada K, Takada T, Kawarada Y, et al. Diagnostic criteria and severity assessment of acute cholangitis: Tokyo guidelines. J Hepatobiliary Pancreat Surg 2007;14:52–8.

28. Kiriyama S, Takada T, Strasberg SM, et al. TG13 guidelines for diagnosis and severity grading of acute cholangitis (with videos). J Hepatobiliary Pancreat Sci 2013;20:24–34.

29. Jang SE, Park SW, Lee BS, et al. Management for CBD stone-related mild to moderate acute cholangitis: urgent versus elective ERCP. Dig Dis Sci 2013;58:2082–7.

30. Mosler P. Diagnosis and management of acute cholangitis. Curr Gastroenterol Rep 2011;13:166–72.

31. Tenner S, Baillie J, DeWitt J, et al. American College of Gastroenterology guideline: management of acute pancreatitis. Am J Gastroenterol 2013;108:1400–15.

32. Fink D, Alverdy JC. Acute pancreatitis. In: Cameron JL, Cameron AM, editors. Current surgical therapy. 10th edition. Philadelphia: Elsevier Saunders; 2011. p. 383–8.

33. van Geenen EJ, van Santvoort HC, Besselink MG, et al. Lack of consensus on the role of endoscopic retrograde cholangiography in acute biliary pancreatitis in published meta-analyses and guidelines: a systematic review. Pancreas 2013; 42:774–80.
34. Aboulian A, Chan T, Yaghoubian A, et al. Early cholecystectomy safely decreases hospital stay in patients with mild gallstone pancreatitis: a randomized prospective study. Ann Surg 2010;251:615–9.
35. van Baal MC, Besselink MG, Bakker OJ, et al. Timing of cholecystectomy after mild biliary pancreatitis: a systematic review. Ann Surg 2012;255:860–6.
36. Rafferty J, Shellito P, Hyman NH, et al. Practice parameters for sigmoid diverticulitis. Dis Colon Rectum 2006;49:939–44.
37. Dharmarajan S, Hunt SR, Birnbaum EH, et al. The efficacy of nonoperative management of acute complicated diverticulitis. Dis Colon Rectum 2011;54:663–71.
38. Siewert B, Tye G, Kruskal J, et al. Impact of CT-guided drainage in the treatment of diverticular abscesses: size matters. AJR Am J Roentgenol 2006;186:680–6.
39. Costi R, Cauchy F, Le BA, et al. Challenging a classic myth: pneumoperitoneum associated with acute diverticulitis is not an indication for open or laparoscopic emergency surgery in hemodynamically stable patients. A 10-year experience with a nonoperative treatment. Surg Endosc 2012;26:2061–71.
40. Klarenbeek BR, Veenhof AA, Bergamaschi R, et al. Laparoscopic sigmoid resection for diverticulitis decreases major morbidity rates: a randomized control trial: short-term results of the Sigma Trial. Ann Surg 2009;249:39–44.
41. Mbadiwe T, Obirieze AC, Cornwell EE III, et al. Surgical management of complicated diverticulitis: a comparison of the laparoscopic and open approaches. J Am Coll Surg 2013;216:782–8.
42. Oberkofler CE, Rickenbacher A, Raptis DA, et al. A multicenter randomized clinical trial of primary anastomosis or Hartmann's procedure for perforated left colonic diverticulitis with purulent or fecal peritonitis. Ann Surg 2012;256:819–26.
43. Swank HA, Vermeulen J, Lange JF, et al. The ladies trial: laparoscopic peritoneal lavage or resection for purulent peritonitis and Hartmann's procedure or resection with primary anastomosis for purulent or faecal peritonitis in perforated diverticulitis (NTR2037). BMC Surg 2010;10:29.
44. Schug-Pass C, Geers P, Hugel O, et al. Prospective randomized trial comparing short-term antibiotic therapy versus standard therapy for acute uncomplicated sigmoid diverticulitis. Int J Colorectal Dis 2010;25:751–9.
45. Chabok A, Pahlman L, Hjern F, et al. Randomized clinical trial of antibiotics in acute uncomplicated diverticulitis. Br J Surg 2012;99:532–9.

Clostridium Difficile Infection

Prevention, Treatment, and Surgical Management

Jason A. Luciano, MD, MBA[a], Brian S. Zuckerbraun, MD[a,b],*

KEYWORDS

- Vancomycin • Fecal microbiota therapy • Ileostomy • Colectomy

KEY POINTS

- Infection control measures and strategies, including isolation and personal barrier precautions, handwashing, bleach-based environmental cleaning, and antibiotic stewardship, are paramount to prevent *Clostridium difficile* infection.
- Severity scoring and stratification of disease severity is necessary to ensure appropriate therapeutic management.
- Early recognition of patients with complicated disease, with early surgical consultation, improves outcomes.
- Surgical therapies should be considered early in the setting of clinical deterioration.
- Loop ileostomy and colonic lavage should be considered as an alternative to subtotal colectomy in the absence of colonic perforation, necrosis, or abdominal compartment syndrome.

INTRODUCTION

Antibiotic-associated colitis was initially reported in the 1970s after the introduction of clindamycin, and at that time was referred to as clindamycin-associated colitis. Tedesco and colleagues[1] reported endoscopy findings on 200 patients who received clindamycin and showed a 20% incidence of diarrhea and a 10% incidence of pseudomembranous colitis. *Clostridium difficile* as the causative agent of antibiotic-associated pseudomembranous colitis was first reported in 1978 by Bartlett and colleagues,[2,3] and although first reported in patients receiving clindamycin, *C difficile* infection (CDI) has been associated with antibiotic use in general with highest risk

The authors have nothing to disclose.
^a Department of Surgery, University of Pittsburgh, 200 Lothrop St, Pittsburgh, PA 15213, USA;
^b Department of Surgery, VA Pittsburgh Healthcare System, University Drive, Pittsburgh, PA 15240, USA
* Corresponding author. F1271 PUH, 200 Lothrop Street, Pittsburgh, PA 15213.
E-mail address: zuckerbraunbs@upmc.edu

Surg Clin N Am 94 (2014) 1335–1349
http://dx.doi.org/10.1016/j.suc.2014.08.006
0039-6109/14/$ – see front matter © 2014 Elsevier Inc. All rights reserved.

surgical.theclinics.com

following the use of clindamycin, cephalosporins, and fluoroquinolones.[4] Furthermore, the combination of multiple antibiotics and longer duration of antibiotic use is associated with increased risk of developing CDI.[5] The continuation of any nonclostridia antibiotics after initial diagnosis has been shown to be associated with increased rates of recurrent disease.[6,7]

CDI is the most common cause of antibiotic-associated diarrhea and is defined as the acute onset of diarrhea with documented *C difficile* or its toxin, and no other identifiable cause for diarrhea.[8] Reports on incidence of this infection have shown that the incidence of CDI has nearly tripled between 1996 and 2005 from 31 per 100,000 to 84 to 112 per 100,000.[9,10] A more recent survey of US health care facilities from 2008 reported that among hospitalized patients the prevalence rate had continued increasing and was up to 13.1 per 10,000.[11] A 2008 study by Zilberberg and colleagues[10] analyzed CDI trends and stratified the data based on patient age; they noted that whereas adults ages 18 to 44 had an increased incidence from 1.3 to 2.4 per 10,000, the incidence of CDI in adults aged 65 to 84 increased from 22.4 to 49 per 10,000, and the incidence in adults aged greater than 85 also more than doubled from 52 to 112 per 10,000. It is estimated that nosocomial CDI increases the cost of hospitalization four-fold compared with matched cohorts and has been reported to cost between $3.2 and $4.8 billion per year.[12–14] In addition to increasing rates of prevalence, mortality rates associated with CDI have also been increasing significantly, rising from 5.7 per million in 1999 to 23.7 per million in 2004.[15]

Although CDI is frequently thought of in the inpatient setting, studies that have tested the stool of healthy adults found that 5% to 15% of healthy adults are carriers of *C difficile* and 40% of patients who develop community-acquired CDI go on to require subsequent hospitalization.[16–18] When the stool from patients requiring prolonged hospitalization was examined, the rate of colonization jumps significantly to 26% to 50%.[9,19–22] Most of these patients remain asymptomatic with one study, which examined 428 hospitalized patients, reporting a 26% colonization rate among hospitalized patients and that 62% of those patients remained asymptomatic throughout their hospital stay.[23] Overall, patients who develop symptomatic CDI typically have had antibiotic exposure within the past 3 months, have recently been hospitalized, and are older (typically defined as age >65). In addition to increased risk for CDI, advanced age has been shown to be associated with increased rates of recurrence, worse outcomes, and a 68% higher 30-day mortality compared with younger patients.[24,25]

BACTERIAL CHARACTERISTICS

Clostridium difficile is an obligate anaerobic gram-positive spore-forming bacterium that is transmitted via a fecal-oral route. To survive outside of its host and allow for transmission between hosts it produces endospores, which are metabolically inactive and therefore resistant to stomach acid and most classes of antibiotics. The bacterium is noninvasive and produces its pathology through the production of toxin A (a 308-kD enterotoxin) and toxin B (a 269-kD cytotoxin).[26] These toxins inactivate Rho GTPases and work in conjunction to open cellular tight junctions within the intestine leading to increased vascular permeability and inducing the production of tumor necrosis factor and inflammatory cytokines. Additionally, there is a neutrophil chemotactant influence. This results in an extensive inflammatory response and cellular necrosis, which in conjunction with actin depolymerization induced by cytotoxin results in the development of pseudomembranes. Some strains of *C difficile* have also been shown to produce an additional binary toxin, which some studies have reported as being associated with increased severity of CDI, higher mortality rates, and higher rates of recurrence.[27–29] The mechanism of action of binary toxin is not yet fully understood.

Many different *C difficile* strains have been identified. A study by Bauer and colleagues[30] examined CDI across Europe and identified a total of 65 different ribotypes of *C difficile*. Recently newer ribotypes NAP1/RT027 and RT078, which are frequently referred to as hypervirulent strains, have emerged.[31] Both of these strains have been associated with increased toxin production and in the case of NAP1/ribotype 027, toxin upregulation is driven by a deletion of the tcdC gene that is normally responsible for the downregulation of toxin production.[2,32,33] In addition to increased toxin production, the toxin B produced by the NAP1/ribotype 027 strain has been shown to have increased toxicity when compared with control laboratory strains.[34,35] Associated with the increased toxin production and toxin toxicity, the NAP1/ribotype 027 strain has also been associated with increased mortality rates of up to 6.9%.[36]

DIAGNOSIS

Patients with CDI typically present with watery nonbloody diarrhea, leukocytosis, abdominal pain or cramping, and fever. Although many patients with CDI present with diarrhea, patients with fulminant colitis may present with paralytic ileus and sepsis, which increases the risk for development of colonic perforation and peritonitis, which is otherwise typically not commonly seen in CDI.

Testing of stool for *C difficile* should be done in any patient with recent hospitalization and/or antibiotic use who develops diarrhea. Current testing options include enzyme immunoassays (EIA) for toxins A+B, nucleic acid amplification tests (NAAT), toxigenic *C difficile* culture, glutamate dehydrogenase (GDH), and *C difficile* cytotoxin neutralization assay.

In patients without any clinical evidence of diarrhea, stool testing for *C difficile* should not routinely be performed based on low pretest probability, possible identification of an asymptomatic carrier with associated potential for unnecessary treatment for a positive test, and the costs associated with the testing.[5] One exception is patients who have ileus, in which case rectal swabs in conjunction with polymerase chain reaction (PCR) can be used to make the diagnosis.[23]

The gold standard has previously been considered culture confirmation of *C difficile* from stool samples; however, it is typically used as a reference test or in investigational studies and has limited clinical use because of its need for tissue culture and delay of 24 to 48 hours from time of stool collection to diagnosis. EIA for toxins A+B initially gained widespread use, and at one point was the most commonly used diagnostic test. However, since the introduction of newer tests including NAATs, the use of EIA has decreased and it is now used as the primary diagnostic test in approximately 30% of hospital laboratories.[37–39] A large reason for the switch from EIA to NAATs is related to the lower sensitivity rates associated with EIA diagnostic tests for toxin A+B, ranging from 48% to 96%, and current guidelines, which recommend against the use of EIA as a standalone diagnostic test.[5,37,40]

Current guidelines on diagnostic tests advocate for the use of NAAT for the toxin B gene locus as a standalone test or the use of GDH as a screening test followed by subsequent confirmatory tests, such as NAAT or EIA for toxins A+B.[5,41,42] Because strains of *C difficile* that produce toxin B, but not toxin A, have been identified, the TcdB gene locus is the preferred locus for PCR-based diagnostic tests to maximize the sensitivity of the test.

Because of the high sensitivity of GDH- and NAAT-based tests for *C difficile* there is no role for repeat testing in a patient who initially tests negative. Studies have shown that repeat testing after an initial negative result is positive less than 5% of the time.[43–45] Additionally, there is currently no evidence to suggest retesting after the completion of antibiotic treatment because studies have reported positive EIA toxin A+B and toxigenic cultures for up to a month after the clinical resolution of symptoms leading to misleading test results.[46]

Endoscopy and radiologic studies can be used as adjunctive measures. Endoscopy is especially useful in patients with ileus and to rule out other differential diagnoses including inflammatory bowel disease. On sigmoidoscopy or colonoscopy, *C difficile* can be identified by the presence of pseudomembranous colitis. Although pathognomonic for CDI, these lesions are not uniformly present and may not be present throughout the entire colon. Radiologic studies including abdominal radiography and computed tomography scans can identify a thickened edematous colon, with radiographs identifying possible thumbprinting. In general, radiologic studies are primarily used to define the extent of colonic involvement and to rule out alternative sources of infection.

MEDICAL MANAGEMENT OF ACUTE INFECTION

CDI severity is described as being either mild, moderate, severe, or severe-complicated, with management guidelines based on clinical severity as follows[5,47]:

- Mild: CDI with diarrhea as the only symptom.
- Moderate: CDI with diarrhea and additional signs/symptoms, which do not meet the definition for severe or complicated CDI.
- Severe: CDI presenting with two of the following: hypoalbuminemia (<3 g/dL), serum white blood cell (WBC) count greater than 15,000 cells/mm^3, or abdominal tenderness without criteria for complicated disease.
- Severe-complicated: CDI presenting with or developing fever greater than 38.5°C, ileus or significant abdominal distention, mental status changes, WBC greater than 35,000 or less than 2,000, serum lactate level greater than 2.2, any evidence of end organ failure, need for admission to intensive care unit, hypotension with or without need for vasopressors.

There have been several proposed severity scoring systems for CDI in addition to what is referenced previously; however, none have been validated (**Table 1**). The previously mentioned scoring system is based on recent guidelines put forth from the American College of Gastroeneterology.[5] Although somewhat arbitrary, the criteria for severe disease was based on a study by Fujitani and colleagues,[48] which illustrated findings associated with increased severity of disease. The criteria for severe, complicated disease were formulated based on the findings from multiple case series of factors associated with need for surgery and mortality. It is important to stratify the disease severity of CDI to ensure that at-risk patients have an adequate escalation to appropriate care, particularly patients with complicated disease. Additionally, it is important to have criteria to be able to compare patient populations and outcomes from treatment.

Management strategies for management of an initial episode of CDI are based on disease severity and include the following:

- Discontinuation of the inciting antibiotic if the patient is still receiving this. If continued antibiotics for another infectious disease is warranted, preferentially avoid cephalosporins, clindamycin, and fluroquinolones.
- Mild and moderate CDI is treated with 500 mg metronidazole taken orally three times daily for a 10-day course.

Table 1
Severity scoring system and recommended treatment protocols (American College of Gastroenterology Guidelines)

Severity	Criteria	Treatment	Comment
Mild-to-moderate disease	Diarrhea plus any additional signs or symptoms not meeting severe or complicated criteria	Metronidazole 500 mg orally three times a day for 10 d. If unable to take metronidazole, vancomycin 125 mg orally four times a day for 10 d	If no improvement in 5–7 d, consider change to vancomycin at standard dose (vancomycin 125 mg four times a day for 10 d)
Severe disease	Serum albumin <3 g/dL plus ONE of the following: • WBC $\geq$15,000 cells/mm^3 • Abdominal tenderness	Vancomycin 125 mg orally four times a day for 10 d	
Severe, complicated disease	Any of the following attributable to CDI: • Admission to intensive care unit for CDI • Hypotension with or without required use of vasopressors • Fever $\geq$38.5°C • Ileus or significant abdominal distention • Mental status changes • WBC $\geq$35,000 cells/mm^3 or <2000 cells/mm^3 • Serum lactate levels >2.2 mmol/L • End organ failure (mechanical ventilation, renal failure, and so forth)	Vancomycin 500 mg orally four times a day and metronidazole 500 mg IV every 8 h, and vancomycin per rectum (vancomycin 500 mg in 500 mL saline as enema) four times a day	Surgical consultation suggested
Recurrent CDI	Recurrent CDI within 12 wk of completion of therapy	Vanocmycin 14-d course or vancomycin pulse/taper regimen (7 wk)	Consider FMT after three recurrences

Abbreviations: CDI, *Clostridium difficile* infection; FMT, fecal microbiota transplant; IV, intravenous; WBC, white blood cell.[5]

From Surawicz CM, Brandt LJ, Binion DG, et al. Guidelines for diagnosis, treatment, and prevention of *Clostridium difficile* infections. Am J Gastroenterol 2013;108(4):478–98.

- Severe CDI is treated with vancomycin, 125 mg, taken orally four times daily for a 10-day course.
- Severe-complicated CDI should be treated with 500-mg intravenous metronidazole every 8 hours, 125- to 500-mg oral vancomycin four times per day, and 500-mg vancomycin in 500 mL of saline per rectum four times daily with the presence of ileus or significant abdominal distention.
- Severe-complicated CDI should also prompt surgical consultation that would facilitate early surgical management in the case of clinical deterioration.
- Additionally the use of any antiperistaltic agents should be avoided or discontinued if there is any suspicion of CDI because these agents can mask the patient's

symptoms and may also precipitate the development of severe-complicated disease.[8]

The 10-day course of antibiotics used for the management of mild and moderate CDI is largely based on a randomized trial from 1978 by Keighley and colleagues[49] that showed resolution of symptoms, pseudomembranes, and cytotoxin within 10 days of starting oral vancomycin. Since that time additional studies have been conducted examining the optimal treatment duration and have failed to show evidence that extending antibiotic course beyond 10 days results in further clinical improvement.[5] In severe cases of CDI, oral vancomycin is the treatment of choice based on randomized controlled trials, which have shown superiority of vancomycin over metronidazole in the setting of severe CDI.[50,51]

Patients with mild-moderate CDI who are failing to clinically respond to metronidazole by Day 5 to 7 of treatment should be switched to an additional 10-day course of 125 mg vancomycin taken four times daily. Patients who show signs of failure to respond to standard doses of 125-mg vancomycin should be switched to high-dose (500 mg orally four times daily) vancomycin, although the data for this recommendation are relatively weak.[5] In patients with CDI documented in an excluded or diverted portion of a patient's colon, treatment should include vancomycin enemas of 500 mg dissolved in 100 to 500 mL saline administered every 6 hours until the patient shows signs of clinical improvement.[5,52]

Since 2000, failure rates of metronidazole for uncomplicated CDI have increased from 2.5% to more than 18%.[8,9] Because of this increasing antibiotic resistance, numerous studies have attempted to find additional treatment options against CDI. In 2011, fidaxomicin, a macrocyclic-type antibiotic, was approved by the Food and Drug Administration for the treatment of CDI. Like vancomycin, fidaxomicin is not readily absorbed by the gastrointestinal tract and thereby has minimal systemic effects when given orally. Fidaxomicin, which preserves the colonic microbiome to a greater degree than vancomycin, has been shown to have equal efficacy in the treatment of acute infection and is associated with lower rates of recurrence compared with oral vancomycin.[53–55] However, recurrence rates were equal to vancomycin when treating patients infected with the hypervirulent strain. Fidaxomicin has not yet been compared with metronidazole in any side-by-side randomized clinical trials for the treatment of *C difficile*. The current role for fidaxomicin in the algorithm for treating CDI is not yet defined largely because of limitations of the previously cited studies and the significant cost associated with fidaxomicin treatment. Based on reduced rates of recurrence, one possible role may be in patients with recurrent disease and in those patients being treated for an initial infection who are deemed to be at higher risk for recurrence, such as those who must also be continued on nonclostridial antibiotics during their treatment period.

SURGICAL OPTIONS IN THE MANAGEMENT OF ACUTE DISEASE

It is difficult to predict which patients with severe-complicated CDI will ultimately respond to medical management from those whose disease course will progress and require possible surgical intervention. Complicating the decision regarding timing for operative management is that other than colonic perforation or necrosis there are no clear objective indications for surgical intervention and use of surgical subtotal colectomy as a salvage therapy has been associated with mortality rates ranging from 35% to 80%.[56–61] In patients who ultimately undergo colectomy, risk factors associated with increased mortality include the following[57,62,63]:

- Need for vasopressors
- Elevated lactate level >5 mmol/L
- Change in mental status
- End organ failure
- Renal failure
- Need for preoperative intubation

A study by Salihamer and colleagues[56] compared patients with severe-complicated CDI admitted to medical and surgical services and found that patients admitted to a surgical service had decreased mortality compared with similar patients admitted to a nonsurgical service. This is most likely attributable to earlier time from admission to surgical treatment on those patients admitted to the surgical service. Similarly, studies have found that early surgical consultation is also associated with decreased time to operative intervention and improved survival.[58,63–65] Recent guidelines by Surawicz and colleagues[5] recommend that surgical consultation be obtained on every patient that meets the criteria for severe- complicated CDI. Additionally, they recommended that indications for surgery include the following findings associated with complicated CDI:

- Hypotension requiring vasopressor therapy
- Clinical signs of sepsis and organ dysfunction
- Mental status changes
- WBC count ≥50,000 cell/μL
- Lactate ≥5 mmol/L
- Complicated CDI with failure to improve on medical therapy after 5 days

The gold standard surgical intervention has been subtotal colectomy based on higher mortality rates associated with more segmental-based colonic resections.[66,67] More recently, the option of a diverting loop ileostomy with intraoperative colonic lavage and postoperative antegrade vancomycin enemas via the ileostomy for patients with severe-complicated disease was proposed by our group in 2011. This work illustrates that this surgical approach was associated with decreased mortality rates and was able to successfully preserve the colon in 93% of patients. Furthermore, rather than requiring a traditional laparotomy incision, 83% of surgeries were able to be performed laparoscopically.[68] Although in this before-and-after study comparing this approach to colectomy the patient populations had similar severity of critical illness based on Acute Physiology and Chronic Health Evaluation II scores, improvements in outcome were likely in part caused by earlier surgical intervention with the new strategy compared with the colectomy cohort. Absolute and relative contraindications to this approach include the following:

- Colonic necrosis (absolute)
- Colonic perforation (absolute)
- If the patient has an underlying indication that would benefit from colectomy (ie long-standing colonic inflammatory bowel disease)
- Abdominal compartment syndrome that would necessitate a decompressive laparotomy and open abdomen if the colon were not resected

RECURRENT DISEASE

Following an initial infection with *C difficile*, 10% to 25% of patients go on to develop a recurrent CDI within a 12-week period of time. The rate of cure following a recurrent episode falls significantly with 40% to 65% of patients with one episode of recurrence developing a subsequent recurrence and 60% of patients with two or more episodes of recurrence developing further recurrences.[9,69–71]

Recurrent disease is thought to develop largely as a result of an altered colonic microbiome following initial infection.[72,73] Many advocate the treatment regimen of a first recurrence to be the same as an initial episode based on the severity of disease. The guidelines put forth by the American College of Gastroenterology support treating a first recurrence episode with vancomycin, 125 mg orally four times daily. Second recurrences should be treated with a pulsed and tapered regimen of vancomycin (**Table 2**). The recommendation for a third episode after a failed tapered course of vancomycin includes fecal microbiota transplantation (FMT) to repopulate the normal colonic flora.[5]

FMT, which was first reported by Eiseman in 1958, aims to treat recurrent infection by restoring the normal colonic microbiome, which is theorized to provide protection against toxigenic *C difficile*.[72–75] Retrospective studies and systematic reviews have shown an approximately 90% clinical cure rate for recurrent CDI.[76–80] A recent randomized, prospective clinical trial was stopped after interim analysis based on clear superiority in treating patients with recurrent CDI.[81] They compared an initial vancomycin regimen (500 mg orally four times per day for 4 days), followed by bowel lavage and subsequent infusion of a solution of donor feces through a nasoduodenal tube; a standard vancomycin regimen (500 mg orally four times per day for 14 days); or a standard vancomycin regimen with bowel lavage. Based on the clinical cure rates associated with FMT, the FMT workgroup recommends FMT in the settings of recurrent or relapsing CDI defined as at least three episodes of mild to moderate CDI and failure of 6 to 8 weeks of vancomycin.[73] Several resources are being developed to facilitate FMT. These include cultured stool flora that could be delivered in oral, pill form, and banked reservoirs of stool from donors that would be pretested for toxigenic *C difficile* and other infectious diseases. It must be noted that FMT has not yet been approved by the Food and Drug Administration. Despite the idea that probiotics might work similarly to FMT in restoring a normal colonic microbiome, there is currently no strong evidence to suggest that the use of probiotics in either the acute infection or recurrent setting leads to increased cure rates and decreased episodes of recurrence.[5]

Table 2
Strategy for treatment of recurrent CDI

Criteria	Treatment	Notes
First recurrence	Vancomycin 125 mg PO QID for 14 d	
Second recurrence	Pulsed vanco regimen: 125 mg PO QID × 2 wk, then 125 mg PO BID × 1 wk, then 125 mg PO QD × 1 wk, then 125 mg PO QOD × 1 wk, then 125 mg PO every third day × 2 wk	
Three or more recurrences	Consider fecal microbiota therapy	Treat with vancomycin 500 mg orally QID for 4 d), followed by bowel lavage and subsequent infusion of a solution of donor feces through a nasoduodenal tube[81]

Recently the use of monoclonal antibodies against *C difficile* toxins A and B has been suggested as an adjunctive treatment modality to reduce recurrence rates. A randomized controlled trial by Lowy and colleagues[82] reported a reduction in recurrence rate from 25% to 7% when anti-*C difficile* toxin was added to the patient's antibiotic regimen. The decreased recurrence rate was further shown to occur in patients infected with the NAP1 strain (32%–8%) and patients who already had recurrent disease (38%–7%).

PREVENTION

As made famous by Benjamin Franklin, "an ounce of prevention is worth a pound of cure." Toward this goal, current hospital-based infection-control programs most commonly use bleach-based environmental disinfection, antibiotic stewardship programs, and maintenance of strict contact and barrier precautions, all of which have been shown to successfully reduce rates of *C difficile* infections.[8,83] Through antibiotic stewardship, the United Kingdom's National Health Service was able to reduce the use of fluoroquinolones and broad-spectrum cephalosporins, which in conjunction with other infection-control measures was able to reduce the rate of CDI by 60%.[19,84] Measures aimed at maintaining a normal colonic microbiome, such as pre-probiotics, have shown limited success in reducing the rate of CDI. There is currently insufficient evidence to definitively show a clear benefit as a preventative therapy.[85,86]

Because asymptomatic carriers of *C difficile* could ultimately become symptomatic and despite being asymptomatic could still spread the bacterium, it was questioned whether treating asymptomatic carriers would be of benefit. Unfortunately, treatment with metronidazole has been shown to be ineffective in eliminating carriage and treatment of asymptomatic patients with vancomycin resulted in high rates of recolonization, often with new strains of the bacteria.[87]

Currently, there are no approved immunologic therapies for the prevention of CDI. However, the pharmaceutical company Sanofi Pasteur is currently attempting to develop and study a vaccine against *C difficile* that they currently call Cdiffense. The vaccine, which has already completed phase I and II clinical trials, is currently undergoing a phase III clinical trial. This phase III study was started in July 2013 and is currently enrolling adults ages 50 or older who either are anticipating hospitalization for surgical procedures within 60 days of trial enrollment or had multiple hospitalizations and recent antibiotic exposure within the past year. The clinical trial's primary outcome is the development of PCR-confirmed *C difficile* infection within a 3-year period of time and is currently enrolling patients at 200 sites across 17 countries with a target enrollment of 15,000 adults by December 2017.[88]

In addition to the vaccine being studied by Sanofi Pasteur, a European consortium led by Royal Holloway University is attempting to develop an oral vaccine using nonpathogenic bacterial spores to induce an immune response against bacterial antigens. Clinical trials from this consortium are not currently underway; however, they have indicated hopes to start trails by early 2015.

SUMMARY

Clostridium difficile is increasing in incidence and severity with infection rates tripling between 1996 and 2005 and mortality rising more than four-fold over a similar period of time.[9,10,15] Newer strains of *C difficile*, including Nap1, are associated with increased toxin production, increased cytotoxin toxicity, and increased mortality rates.[34–36] Although metronidazole and vancomycin remain the gold standard for medical management, and surgical colectomy the gold standard for surgical management, new treatment alternatives are being investigated that may lead to changes in the current treatment algorithms. Newer antibiotics, such as fidaxomicin, have shown early promise as an alternative to vancomycin, with lower rates of recurrence; however, the studies to date have largely been comprised of patients with mild or moderate disease who are typically treated with metronidazole rather than vancomycin and only a small number of patients had more severe cases of CDI. Therefore, further studies need to be completed including side-to-side comparisons of fidaxomicin and metronidazole and the efficacy of fidaxomicin in the treatment of patients with severe or severe-complicated cases of CDI before any clear determination can be made regarding the ultimate role that fidaxomicin should play in the antibiotic treatment algorithm.

Because of the difficulty in predicting the course progression of CDI, surgical intervention has many times been relegated to a salvage option with mortality rates reported as high as 35% to 80%.[56–61] Although subtotal colectomy remains the gold standard surgical procedure, a study from our institution indicated that the creation of a diverting loop ileostomy with colonic lavage and antegrade vancomycin enemas may serve as a surgical alternative in some patients.[68] This study showed that mortality rates were decreased compared with historical controls and that the procedure was able to be successfully performed laparoscopically more than 80% of the time and was able to preserve the colon in 93% of patients. Although the Acute Physiology and Chronic Health Evaluation II scores of patients undergoing diverting loop ileostomy were comparable with historical controls undergoing subtotal colectomy, it is unclear whether the benefits reported in this study were a result of benefits of the surgical procedure itself or a willingness to intervene at an earlier point in time, partially as a result of the decreased morbidity associated with a laparoscopic loop ileostomy as compared with a laparotomy and subtotal colectomy. Whether it is the procedure itself or physicians' willingness to decrease the threshold for surgical intervention, the possibility of a less invasive surgical alternative is an intriguing possibility and deserves further investigation.

The most exciting development in the treatment options for CDI, however, is likely the development of novel immunologic agents. Lowy and colleagues[82] showed that passive immunization with antitoxin successfully reduced the rates of recurrence in acute and recurrent disease. Numerous animal-based studies have provided preliminary evidence that passive immunization may lead to protection from *C difficile*-induced diarrhea and death; however, to date no human trials have shown improved clinical outcomes other than recurrence rate.[89,90] Although there is not yet an approved vaccine against *C difficile*, it is hoped there will be multiple trials within the next couple of years investigating novel vaccines so that one may become available for generalized use within the foreseeable future. More than advances in treatment options, this holds the potential to reduce the incidence, mortality, and costs associated with *C difficile*.

REFERENCES

1. Tedesco FJ, Barton RW, Alpers DH. Clindamycin-associated colitis. A prospective study. Ann Intern Med 1974;81(4):429–33.
2. Bartlett JG, Chang TW, Gurwith M, et al. Antibiotic-associated pseudomembranous colitis due to toxin-producing clostridia. N Engl J Med 1978; 298(10):531–4.
3. Bartlett JG, Moon N, Chang TW, et al. Role of *Clostridium difficile* in antibiotic-associated pseudomembranous colitis. Gastroenterology 1978;75(5):778–82.

4. Walker KJ, Gilliland SS, Vance-Bryan K, et al. *Clostridium difficile* colonization in residents of long-term care facilities: prevalence and risk factors. J Am Geriatr Soc 1993;41(9):940–6.

5. Surawicz CM, Brandt LJ, Binion DG, et al. Guidelines for diagnosis, treatment, and prevention of *Clostridium difficile* infections. Am J Gastroenterol 2013; 108(4):478–98.

6. Choi HK, Kim KH, Lee SH, et al. Risk factors for recurrence of *Clostridium difficile* infection: effect of vancomycin-resistant enterococci colonization. J Korean Med Sci 2011;26(7):859–64.

7. Garey KW, Sethi S, Yadav Y, et al. Meta-analysis to assess risk factors for recurrent *Clostridium difficile* infection. J Hosp Infect 2008;70(4):298–304.

8. Cohen SH, Gerding DN, Johnson S, et al. Clinical practice guidelines for *Clostridium difficile* infection in adults: 2010 update by the Society for Healthcare Epidemiology of America (SHEA) and the Infectious Diseases Society of America (IDSA). Infect Control Hosp Epidemiol 2010;31(5):431–55.

9. Kelly CP, LaMont JT. *Clostridium difficile*–more difficult than ever. N Engl J Med 2008;359(18):1932–40.

10. Zilberberg MD, Shorr AF, Kollef MH. Increase in adult *Clostridium difficile*-related hospitalizations and case-fatality rate, United States, 2000-2005. Emerg Infect Dis 2008;14(6):929–31.

11. Jarvis WR, Schlosser J, Jarvis AA, et al. National point prevalence of *Clostridium difficile* in US health care facility inpatients, 2008. Am J Infect Control 2009; 37(4):263–70.

12. Vonberg RP, Reichardt C, Behnke M, et al. Cost of nosocomial *Clostridium difficile*-associated diarrhoea. J Hosp Infect 2008;70:15–20.

13. Dubberke ER, Olsen MA. Burden of *Clostridium difficile* on the healthcare system. Clin Infect Dis 2012;55(Suppl 2):S88–92.

14. O'Brien JA, Lahue BJ, Caro JJ, et al. The emerging infectious challenge of *Clostridium difficile*-associated disease in Massachusetts hospitals: clinical and economic consequences. Infect Control Hosp Epidemiol 2007;28(11):1219–27.

15. Redelings MD, Sorvillo F, Mascola L. Increase in *Clostridium difficile*-related mortality rates, United States, 1999-2004. Emerg Infect Dis 2007;13(9): 1417–9.

16. Khanna S, Pardi DS, Aronson SL, et al. Outcomes in community-acquired *Clostridium difficile* infection. Aliment Pharmacol Ther 2012;35(5):613–8.

17. Ozaki E, Kato H, Kita H, et al. *Clostridium difficile* colonization in healthy adults: transient colonization and correlation with enterococcal colonization. J Med Microbiol 2004;53(Pt 2):167–72.

18. Matsuki S, Ozaki E, Shozu M, et al. Colonization by *Clostridium difficile* of neonates in a hospital, and infants and children in three day-care facilities of Kanazawa, Japan. Int Microbiol 2005;8(1):43–8.

19. Walker AS, Eyre DW, Wyllie DH, et al. Characterisation of *Clostridium difficile* hospital ward-based transmission using extensive epidemiological data and molecular typing. PLoS Med 2012;9(2):e1001172.

20. Fekety R, Shah AB. Diagnosis and treatment of *Clostridium difficile* colitis. JAMA 1993;269(1):71–5.

21. Clabots CR, Johnson S, Olson MM, et al. Acquisition of *Clostridium difficile* by hospitalized patients: evidence for colonized new admissions as a source of infection. J Infect Dis 1992;166(3):561–7.

22. Samore MH, DeGirolami PC, Tlucko A, et al. *Clostridium difficile* colonization and diarrhea at a tertiary care hospital. Clin Infect Dis 1994;18(2):181–7.

23. Kundrapu S, Sunkesula VC, Jury LA, et al. Utility of perirectal swab specimens for diagnosis of *Clostridium difficile* infection. Clin Infect Dis 2012;55(11):1527–30.

24. Zilberberg MD, Shorr AF, Micek ST, et al. *Clostridium difficile*-associated disease and mortality among the elderly critically ill. Crit Care Med 2009;37(9): 2583–9.

25. Welfare MR, Lalayiannis LC, Martin KE, et al. Co-morbidities as predictors of mortality in *Clostridium difficile* infection and derivation of the ARC predictive score. J Hosp Infect 2011;79(4):359–63.

26. Hall IC, O'Toole E. Intestinal flora in newborn infants with a description of a new pathogenic anaerobe, *Bacillus difficilis*. Am J Dis Child 1935;49(2):390–402.

27. Bacci S, Molbak K, Kjeldsen MK, et al. Binary toxin and death after *Clostridium difficile* infection. Emerg Infect Dis 2011;17(6):976–82.

28. Barbut F, Decre D, Lalande V, et al. Clinical features of *Clostridium difficile*-associated diarrhoea due to binary toxin (actin-specific ADP-ribosyltransferase)-producing strains. J Med Microbiol 2005;54(Pt 2):181–5.

29. Stewart DB, Berg A, Hegarty J. Predicting recurrence of *C. difficile* colitis using bacterial virulence factors: binary toxin is the key. J Gastrointest Surg 2013; 17(1):118–24.

30. Bauer MP, Notermans DW, van Benthem BH, et al. *Clostridium difficile* infection in Europe: a hospital-based survey. Lancet 2011;377(9759):63–73.

31. Smits TH, Rezzonico F, Lopez MM, et al. Phylogenetic position and virulence apparatus of the pear flower necrosis pathogen *Erwinia piriflorinigrans* CFBP 5888(T) as assessed by comparative genomics. Syst Appl Microbiol 2013; 36(7):449–56.

32. Warny M, Pepin J, Fang A, et al. Toxin production by an emerging strain of *Clostridium difficile* associated with outbreaks of severe disease in North America and Europe. Lancet 2005;366(9491):1079–84.

33. Vedantam G, Clark A, Chu M, et al. *Clostridium difficile* infection: toxins and non-toxin virulence factors, and their contributions to disease establishment and host response. Gut Microbes 2012;3(2):121–34.

34. Lanis JM, Barua S, Ballard JD. Variations in TcdB activity and the hypervirulence of emerging strains of *Clostridium difficile*. PLoS Pathog 2010;6(8):e1001061.

35. Lanis JM, Hightower LD, Shen A, et al. TcdB from hypervirulent *Clostridium difficile* exhibits increased efficiency of autoprocessing. Mol Microbiol 2012;84(1):66–76.

36. Loo VG, Poirier L, Miller MA, et al. A predominantly clonal multi-institutional outbreak of *Clostridium difficile*-associated diarrhea with high morbidity and mortality. N Engl J Med 2005;353(23):2442–9.

37. Planche T, Aghaizu A, Holliman R, et al. Diagnosis of *Clostridium difficile* infection by toxin detection kits: a systematic review. Lancet Infect Dis 2008;8(12): 777–84.

38. Fleshner M. Stress-evoked sterile inflammation, danger associated molecular patterns (DAMPs), microbial associated molecular patterns (MAMPs) and the inflammasome. Brain Behav Immun 2013;27(1):1–7.

39. Barbut F, Delmee M, Brazier JS, et al. A European survey of diagnostic methods and testing protocols for *Clostridium difficile*. Clin Microbiol Infect 2003;9(10): 989–96.

40. Stanley JD, Burns RP. *Clostridium difficile* and the surgeon. Am Surg 2010;76(3): 235–44.

41. Cheng AC, Ferguson JK, Richards MJ, et al. Australasian Society for Infectious Diseases guidelines for the diagnosis and treatment of *Clostridium difficile* infection. Med J Aust 2011;194(7):353–8.

42. Crobach MJ, Dekkers OM, Wilcox MH, et al. European Society of Clinical Microbiology and Infectious Diseases (ESCMID): data review and recommendations for diagnosing *Clostridium difficile*-infection (CDI). Clin Microbiol Infect 2009; 15(12):1053–66.
43. Luo RF, Banaei N. Is repeat PCR needed for diagnosis of *Clostridium difficile* infection? J Clin Microbiol 2010;48(10):3738–41.
44. Debast SB, van Kregten E, Oskam KM, et al. Effect on diagnostic yield of repeated stool testing during outbreaks of *Clostridium difficile*-associated disease. Clin Microbiol Infect 2008;14(6):622–4.
45. Deshpande A, Pasupuleti V, Pant C, et al. Potential value of repeat stool testing for *Clostridium difficile* stool toxin using enzyme immunoassay? Curr Med Res Opin 2010;26(11):2635–41.
46. Surawicz CM, McFarland LV, Greenberg RN, et al. The search for a better treatment for recurrent *Clostridium difficile* disease: use of high-dose vancomycin combined with *Saccharomyces boulardii*. Clin Infect Dis 2000;31(4):1012–7.
47. Gujja D, Friedenberg FK. Predictors of serious complications due to *Clostridium difficile* infection. Aliment Pharmacol Ther 2009;29(6):635–42.
48. Fujitani S, George WL, Murthy AR. Comparison of clinical severity score indices for *Clostridium difficile* infection. Infect Control Hosp Epidemiol 2011;32(3): 220–8.
49. Keighley MR, Burdon DW, Arabi Y, et al. Randomised controlled trial of vancomycin for pseudomembranous colitis and postoperative diarrhoea. Br Med J 1978;2(6153):1667–9.
50. Zar FA, Bakkanagari SR, Moorthi KM, et al. A comparison of vancomycin and metronidazole for the treatment of *Clostridium difficile*-associated diarrhea, stratified by disease severity. Clin Infect Dis 2007;45(3):302–7.
51. Al-Nassir WN, Sethi AK, Nerandzic MM, et al. Comparison of clinical and microbiological response to treatment of *Clostridium difficile*-associated disease with metronidazole and vancomycin. Clin Infect Dis 2008;47(1):56–62.
52. Apisarnthanarak A, Razavi B, Mundy LM. Adjunctive intracolonic vancomycin for severe *Clostridium difficile* colitis: case series and review of the literature. Clin Infect Dis 2002;35(6):690–6.
53. Crook DW, Walker AS, Kean Y, et al. Fidaxomicin versus vancomycin for *Clostridium difficile* infection: meta-analysis of pivotal randomized controlled trials. Clin Infect Dis 2012;55(Suppl 2):S93–103.
54. Louie TJ, Cannon K, Byrne B, et al. Fidaxomicin preserves the intestinal microbiome during and after treatment of *Clostridium difficile* infection (CDI) and reduces both toxin reexpression and recurrence of CDI. Clin Infect Dis 2012; 55(Suppl 2):S132–42.
55. Cornely OA, Miller MA, Louie TJ, et al. Treatment of first recurrence of *Clostridium difficile* infection: fidaxomicin versus vancomycin. Clin Infect Dis 2012; 55(Suppl 2):S154–61.
56. Sailhamer EA, Carson K, Chang Y, et al. Fulminant *Clostridium difficile* colitis: patterns of care and predictors of mortality. Arch Surg 2009;144(5):433–9.
57. Dallal RM, Harbrecht BG, Boujoukas AJ, et al. Fulminant *Clostridium difficile*: an underappreciated and increasing cause of death and complications. Ann Surg 2002;235(3):363–72.
58. Byrn JC, Maun DC, Gingold DS, et al. Predictors of mortality after colectomy for fulminant *Clostridium difficile* colitis. Arch Surg 2008;143(2):150–4.
59. Hall JF, Berger D. Outcome of colectomy for *Clostridium difficile* colitis: a plea for early surgical management. Am J Surg 2008;196(3):384–8.

60. Dudukgian H, Sie E, Gonzalez-Ruiz C, et al. *C. difficile* colitis–predictors of fatal outcome. J Gastrointest Surg 2010;14(2):315–22.
61. Synnott K, Mealy K, Merry C, et al. Timing of surgery for fulminating pseudomembranous colitis. Br J Surg 1998;85(2):229–31.
62. Pepin J, Vo TT, Boutros M, et al. Risk factors for mortality following emergency colectomy for fulminant *Clostridium difficile* infection. Dis Colon Rectum 2009; 52(3):400–5.
63. Ali SO, Welch JP, Dring RJ. Early surgical intervention for fulminant pseudomembranous colitis. Am Surg 2008;74(1):20–6.
64. Butala P, Divino CM. Surgical aspects of fulminant *Clostridium difficile* colitis. Am J Surg 2010;200(1):131–5.
65. Markelov A, Livert D, Kohli H. Predictors of fatal outcome after colectomy for fulminant *Clostridium difficile* colitis: a 10-year experience. Am Surg 2011; 77(8):977–80.
66. Perera AD, Akbari RP, Cowher MS, et al. Colectomy for fulminant *Clostridium difficile* colitis: predictors of mortality. Am Surg 2010;76(4):418–21.
67. Medich DS, Lee KK, Simmons RL, et al. Laparotomy for fulminant pseudomembranous colitis. Arch Surg 1992;127(7):847–52.
68. Neal MD, Alverdy JC, Hall DE, et al. Diverting loop ileostomy and colonic lavage: an alternative to total abdominal colectomy for the treatment of severe, complicated *Clostridium difficile* associated disease. Ann Surg 2011;254(3): 423–7.
69. Petrella LA, Sambol SP, Cheknis A, et al. Decreased cure and increased recurrence rates for *Clostridium difficile* infection caused by the epidemic *C. difficile* BI strain. Clin Infect Dis 2012;55(3):351–7.
70. Pepin J, Saheb N, Coulombe MA, et al. Emergence of fluoroquinolones as the predominant risk factor for *Clostridium difficile*-associated diarrhea: a cohort study during an epidemic in Quebec. Clin Infect Dis 2005;41(9):1254–60.
71. McFarland LV, Elmer GW, Surawicz CM. Breaking the cycle: treatment strategies for 163 cases of recurrent *Clostridium difficile* disease. Am J Gastroenterol 2002;97(7):1769–75.
72. Chang JY, Antonopoulos DA, Kalra A, et al. Decreased diversity of the fecal microbiome in recurrent *Clostridium difficile*-associated diarrhea. J Infect Dis 2008;197(3):435–8.
73. Bakken JS, Borody T, Brandt LJ, et al. Treating *Clostridium difficile* infection with fecal microbiota transplantation. Clin Gastroenterol Hepatol 2011;9(12):1044–9.
74. Eiseman B, Silen W, Bascom GS, et al. Fecal enema as an adjunct in the treatment of pseudomembranous enterocolitis. Surgery 1958;44(5):854–9.
75. Khoruts A, Dicksved J, Jansson JK, et al. Changes in the composition of the human fecal microbiome after bacteriotherapy for recurrent *Clostridium difficile*-associated diarrhea. J Clin Gastroenterol 2010;44(5):354–60.
76. Kassam Z, Lee CH, Yuan Y, et al. Fecal microbiota transplantation for *Clostridium difficile* infection: systematic review and meta-analysis. Am J Gastroenterol 2013;108(4):500–8.
77. Borody TJ, Khoruts A. Fecal microbiota transplantation and emerging applications. Nat Rev Gastroenterol Hepatol 2011;9(2):88–96.
78. Bakken JS. Fecal bacteriotherapy for recurrent *Clostridium difficile* infection. Anaerobe 2009;15(6):285–9.
79. Gough E, Shaikh H, Manges AR. Systematic review of intestinal microbiota transplantation (fecal bacteriotherapy) for recurrent *Clostridium difficile* infection. Clin Infect Dis 2011;53(10):994–1002.

80. Guo B, Harstall C, Louie T, et al. Systematic review: faecal transplantation for the treatment of *Clostridium difficile*-associated disease. Aliment Pharmacol Ther 2012;35(8):865–75.

81. van Nood E, Vrieze A, Nieuwdorp M, et al. Duodenal infusion of donor feces for recurrent *Clostridium difficile*. N Engl J Med 2013;368(5):407–15.

82. Lowy I, Molrine DC, Leav BA, et al. Treatment with monoclonal antibodies against *Clostridium difficile* toxins. N Engl J Med 2010;362(3):197–205.

83. Gouliouris T, Brown NM, Aliyu SH. Prevention and treatment of *Clostridium difficile* infection. Clin Med 2011;11(1):75–9.

84. Jones AM, Kuijper EJ, Wilcox MH. *Clostridium difficile*: a European perspective. J Infect 2013;66(2):115–28.

85. Gao XW, Mubasher M, Fang CY, et al. Dose-response efficacy of a proprietary probiotic formula of *Lactobacillus acidophilus* CL1285 and *Lactobacillus casei* LBC80R for antibiotic-associated diarrhea and *Clostridium difficile*-associated diarrhea prophylaxis in adult patients. Am J Gastroenterol 2010;105(7):1636–41.

86. Hickson M, D'Souza AL, Muthu N, et al. Use of probiotic *Lactobacillus* preparation to prevent diarrhoea associated with antibiotics: randomised double blind placebo controlled trial. BMJ 2007;335(7610):80.

87. Johnson S, Homann SR, Bettin KM, et al. Treatment of asymptomatic *Clostridium difficile* carriers (fecal excretors) with vancomycin or metronidazole. A randomized, placebo-controlled trial. Ann Intern Med 1992;117(4):297–302.

88. Foglia G, Shah S, Luxemburger C, et al. *Clostridium difficile*: development of a novel candidate vaccine. Vaccine 2012;30(29):4307–9.

89. Kink JA, Williams JA. Antibodies to recombinant *Clostridium difficile* toxins A and B are an effective treatment and prevent relapse of *C. difficile*-associated disease in a hamster model of infection. Infect Immun 1998;66(5):2018–25.

90. Babcock GJ, Broering TJ, Hernandez HJ, et al. Human monoclonal antibodies directed against toxins A and B prevent *Clostridium difficile*-induced mortality in hamsters. Infect Immun 2006;74(11):6339–47.

Urinary Tract Infections in Surgical Patients

Rajesh Ramanathan, MD[a], Therese M. Duane, MD, FCCM[b],*

KEYWORDS

- Urinary tract infections • Catheter-associated urinary tract infection • CAUTI
- Urosepsis • Patient safety • Hospital acquired conditions

KEY POINTS

- Short-term catheter-associated urinary tract infections (CAUTI) are associated with increased patient hospital stay, morbidity, and mortality.
- CAUTI negatively impact public reporting of hospital safety and reimbursement.
- CAUTI are increased by unnecessary use of catheters and duration of catheterization.
- Understanding and educating care providers about appropriate indications for catheters and alternatives to indwelling urinary catheters can decrease the incidence of CAUTI.
- Developing institutional guidelines for appropriate use, duration, removal, and alternatives decreases the incidence of CAUTI.

INTRODUCTION

Scope of the problem

- Urinary tract infections (UTI) account for up to 40% of all health care–acquired infections.
- Nearly 80% of all UTI occur in patients with short-term urinary catheters and are tracked as catheter-associated UTI (CAUTI) by regulatory agencies.
- CAUTI increases patient morbidity and mortality, and increases health care costs.
- Hospital incidence of CAUTI is tracked by regulatory agencies and CMS, and affects public reporting on patient safety and hospital reimbursement.

The 2001 Institute of Medicine report, *To Err is Human*, highlighted the opportunity that exists for health care providers to decrease preventable nosocomial events and allow

The authors have nothing to disclose.
[a] Virginia Commonwealth University Medical Center, 1200 East Broad Street, PO Box 980454, Richmond, VA 23298, USA; [b] JPS Health Network, Department of Surgery, 1500 S. Main Street, 3rd Floor OPC Suite 300, Ft. Worth, TX 76104, USA
* Corresponding author. JPS Health Network, Department of Surgery, 1500 S. Main Street, 3rd Floor OPC Suite 300, Ft. Worth, TX 76104.
E-mail address: tduane@jpshealth.org

Surg Clin N Am 94 (2014) 1351–1368
http://dx.doi.org/10.1016/j.suc.2014.08.007
0039-6109/14/$ – see front matter © 2014 Elsevier Inc. All rights reserved.

surgical.theclinics.com

patient outcomes to fully reflect the positive care delivered.[1] This and subsequent reports focused public and regulatory attention on health care practices that are potentially preventable. The federal Agency for Healthcare Research and Quality and the Centers for Medicare and Medicaid Services (CMS) have identified a core set of potentially preventable patient safety events that are increasingly being used as publically reported indicators of hospital safety and quality.[2–4] In 2007, the CMS instituted a change in reimbursement policy whereby hospitals would be held financially responsible, with no increase in reimbursement, for the development of any of 8 preventable, hospitalization-related complications.[4] A subsequent rule change by CMS financially penalizes hospitals for the development of such predefined hospital-related complications.

Catheter-associated urinary tract infection (CAUTI) is a hospital-acquired condition that is recognized by Agency for Healthcare Research and Quality and CMS as a preventable patient safety event. Urinary catheters are widely used with 12% to 16% of all surgical and medical inpatients being exposed during a hospitalization.[5–7] Inpatient urinary tract infections (UTI) account for up to 40% of all health care–acquired infections in the United States.[8,9] Up to 80% of these UTI are urinary catheter associated.[6,10] Specifically, among surgical patients, rates of UTI range from 1.8% to 4.1% based on surgery type, and development of UTI has been associated with increased duration of hospital stay, increased incidence of surgical site infections, increased incidence of prosthetic infections, and increased mortality.[11–15] Financially, nosocomial UTI account for more than $400 million in increased annual health care costs.[16] The development of urinary complications are directly related to urinary catheter use and duration, and thus efforts to more accurately identify, manage, and prevent CAUTI are relevant in the quest to improve patient care and safety.

In addition to those with short-term urinary catheter needs, up to 5% of long-term care facility patients have indwelling urinary catheters, and long-term urinary drainage is a prescient concern for patients with spinal cord injury and other congenital and acquired urologic conditions.[10] Given the magnitude and preventable potential of CAUTI in patients with short-term urinary catheter needs, this review focuses primarily on the pathogenesis, evaluation, definition, management, and prevention of CAUTI in the patient with short-term urinary drainage needs.

PATHOGENESIS

Pathogenesis summary

- The presence and duration of catheterization are the strongest risk factors for bacteriuria development. Approximately 10% to 25% patients with bacteriuria progress to symptomatic UTI and 1% to 4% develop urosepsis.

- Microbial seeding of the urinary bladder occurs during catheter placement and subsequently owing to ascension of microbe-laden biofilms along urinary catheters.

- Biofilms form rapidly, within 1 to 3 days, on the intraluminal and extraluminal catheter surface. Biofilms are dynamic, with changes in the microbial populations and virulence over time.

- Biofilms on catheters encourage microbial growth and ascension into the urinary system, and hinder antimicrobial action.

- Extraluminal microbial colonization likely results from surrounding fecal contamination, whereas intraluminal colonization results from contamination of the closed collection apparatus.

The pathogenesis of UTI and urosepsis begins with bacteriuria—the acquisition of bacteria or fungi in the urinary bladder. In patients with indwelling urinary catheters or in patients with a recent history of indwelling urinary catheterization, the catheter serves as the most common route of access for microorganisms into the bladder. The presence and duration of indwelling urinary catheters is the strongest risk factor for developing bacteriuria, with a 3% to 10% risk of bacteriuria development per urinary catheter day.[17–20] Among patients with bacteriuria, approximately 10% to 25% develop UTI symptoms and 1% to 4% develop urosepsis.[12,17,21]

The initial infection after short-term catheter placement (<1 month) is commonly a monocolonization with *Escherichia coli*; however, in select circumstances, monocolonization with yeast species, *Enterococcus* species and *Pseudomonas aeruginosa* may also occur.[21] In patients with catheters for longer than 1 month, polymicrobial colonization with a variety of enterobacteriaceae and other gram-negative organisms, gram-positive organisms, and yeast is common with an average of 3 to 5 organisms isolated at any time point.[5] The most common yeast species is *Candida albicans*, with a growing incidence of *C glabrata* and *C tropicalis*. Moreover, in patients with longer term catheters, there is a greater incidence of resistant bacteria, particularly vancomycin-resistant enterococci and extended-spectrum β-lactamase–producing enterobacteriaceae.[6,22,23] The incidence of resistant microorganisms is presumably increasing owing to increased health care and antimicrobial exposure. Microbiologic studies have further revealed that the urinary catheter and bladder biofilm is a constantly evolving and dynamic environment with new organisms being continually incorporated in the biofilm, posing further challenges in the management of CAUTI.[21]

Urinary catheters facilitate bacteriuria either through direct inoculation of the bladder during catheter insertion or through biofilm ascension along the catheter. Direct inoculation can occur through breaks in aseptic technique and contamination with skin flora, or through tracking of bacteria along the urogenital tract. Biofilm formation and ascension along the urinary catheter into the urinary bladder is believed to be the primary mechanism for the development of bacteriuria.[6,17] Biofilms are a collection of microbial organisms that organize in a polysaccharide matrix on the extraluminal or intraluminal surface of the catheter.[6,17] Up to 66% of extraluminal biofilms originate from the bacteria on the surrounding tissues, with a majority of these bacteria being of gastrointestinal origin.[21] Formation of biofilms on the intraluminal surface of the catheter occurs mainly through contamination of the closed-system urine collection bag. The microbes identified on the intraluminal surface have been found to match microbes identified on the hands of health care personnel.[21]

Standard latex urinary catheters display a high propensity for biofilm formation owing to a favorable mix of hydrophobic and hydrophilic surface regions that allow for attachment and colonization by a wide variety of microorganisms. Additionally, the flagella and motility of common uropathogens, *E coli* and *P aeruginosa*, facilitate catheter surface attachment and secretion of the glycocalyces matrix needed for biofilm formation.[17,24,25] The ascension of the biofilm from the drainage apparatus to the bladder has been reported to take between 1 and 3 days, but may progress quicker in the setting of swarming urease-producing microorganism like *Proteus mirabilis* and *Providenci stuartii*.[26,27]

The presence of biofilms significantly impacts therapy, because the biofilm matrix reduces the effectiveness of antimicrobials. Microorganisms in biofilms display slower replication rates, thus blunting the effects of antimicrobials. This is particularly detrimental for bacteriostatic antimicrobials. Additionally, chemical signaling within biofilms has been shown to affect gene regulation within bacteria, making them more resistant to antimicrobials.[28,29] Notably, factors affecting the conversion from colonization and bacteriuria to symptomatic bacteriuria and bacteremia remain unclear and do not seem to be associated with bacterial virulence.[17]

EVALUATION

Evaluation summary

- Fevers are often the only symptom of CAUTI.
- Urine culture, with or without urinalysis, is the standard for diagnosis of UTI.
- For catheters indwelling for fewer than 10 days, urine specimens can be collected from the sampling port or tubing puncture.
- For catheters indwelling for longer than 2 weeks, catheters should be replaced and specimens collected through the new catheter.

Evaluation of UTI in a hospitalized patient or a patient in intensive care can be challenging owing to concurrent medical conditions, chemical sedation, and the poor specificity of symptoms. In the unresponsive, chemically sedated, or altered patient, clinical evaluation is limited and a febrile reaction or unexplained leukocytosis should prompt collection of urine for analysis and culture. In the awake, responsive patient, the continued presence of an indwelling urinary catheter may mask the common symptoms of UTI, namely suprapubic tenderness, urinary frequency, dysuria, and stranguria.[5] As a result, other than fever, CAUTI are rarely associated with patient complaints in the awake, responsive patient. Patients with chronic indwelling catheters may experience advanced local symptoms of urethritis, periurethral abscesses, epididymitis or orchitis, and prostatitis.[30]

In patients with unexplained fever, leukocytosis, altered mental status, or clinical deterioration, urine culture with or without urinalysis remains the standard for diagnosis. Urine samples should ideally be obtained before antimicrobial initiation in patients with indwelling catheters and suspected symptomatic UTI. If the urinary catheter has been in place for fewer than 10 days, urine specimens can be collected through the sampling port or tubing puncture. In catheters indwelling for longer than 2 weeks, there is a risk for falsely elevated bacterial counts owing to biofilm contamination.[5,10,31] As a result, urinary catheters should be replaced upon suspicion of symptomatic UTI and a urine specimen collected through the newly inserted catheter.[5]

Accurate interpretation of results from urine culture and urinalysis affects the identification of CAUTI and subsequent therapy. Studies evaluating the correct detection of CAUTI based on US Centers for Disease Control and Prevention (CDC) definitions by general clinicians and infectious disease consultants found poor sensitivity and specificity, advocating for the need to further educate providers on definitions for CAUTI.[32]

DEFINITIONS

The National Healthcare Safety Network and CMS use the US Centers for Disease Control and Prevention definitions for identification and monitoring of CAUTI. Per the Centers for Disease Control and Prevention definitions, a CAUTI is an UTI that develops in a patient who had an indwelling catheter in place at the time of, or within 48 hours before, infection onset. An indwelling catheter is specifically defined as a drainage tube inserted into the urinary bladder through the urethra, left in place, and connected to a closed collection system. As such, it excludes straight catheters, suprapubic catheters, nephrostomy tubes, and condom catheters (**Box 1**).[33]

Diagnosis of symptomatic UTI requires both the presence of symptoms and positive urine culture that is obtained either while the indwelling catheter is in place or within 48 hours of catheter removal. UTI are classified as symptomatic UTI or asymptomatic bacteremic UTI. The diagnosis of symptomatic UTI must include one of the following clinical signs that are not attributable to another source: Fever, suprapubic tenderness, or costovertebral angle tenderness. In patients with catheter removal in the preceding 48 hours, the presence of dysuria, urgency, and urinary frequency qualify as clinical signs of UTI. In addition to clinical signs, patients must have either a urine culture with greater than 10^5 colony-forming units, or a urine culture between 10^3 and 10^5 colony-forming units with a positive urinalysis. Positive urinalysis includes the presence of nitrates, leukoesterases, pyuria, or microorganisms on gram stain (see **Fig. 1**).[33]

Asymptomatic bacteremic UTI are diagnosed in patients without UTI symptoms. These patients must have a urine culture with greater than 10^5 colony-forming units and a positive blood culture with at least 1 matching uropathogen (gram negative bacilli, *Staphylococcus* spp., yeasts, β-hemolytic *Streptococcus* spp., *Enterococcus* spp., *Giardia vaginalis*, *Aerococcus urinae*, or *Corynebacterium* spp.) to the urine culture (see **Fig. 2**).[33] Patients with long-term catheters routinely have asymptomatic microbial colonization, and hence, a consensus conference defined symptomatic UTI as fever, new costovertebral angle tenderness, rigors, or new delirium without an alternative source.[30,34]

The complexities of the definition contribute to the challenge in correctly identifying and treating CAUTI. A strong grasp of the definitions for CAUTI is important, because accurate identification of CAUTI has ramifications on infection tracking, responsible antimicrobial use, performance improvement, and accurate public reporting and reimbursement.

MANAGEMENT

Management summary

- In the absence of clinical symptoms or signs, bacteriuria or funguria should not be treated with antimicrobial therapy.

- For symptomatic bacteriuria, empiric antimicrobial therapy is appropriate in the presence of high suspicion and high severity. Without high suspicion or severity, therapy can be deferred pending urine culture results.

- A 7-day course of antimicrobials is recommended for CAUTI, although shorter durations may be appropriate in select populations. Antimicrobials should be narrowed based on bacterial sensitivities.

- Catheters should be removed as soon as possible. If continued need exists, catheters in place for longer than 2 weeks should be replaced before initiating therapy.

- In patients with continuing epidural analgesia, catheter removal on the first postoperative day could be considered.

> **Box 1**
> **Minimum criteria for CAUTI**
>
> Necessary requirements for CAUTI consideration
>
> - Occurs in a hospital setting
> - Not present or incubating at time of admission
> - Indwelling catheter (does not include straight catheterizations, suprapubic catheters, nephrostomy catheters)
> - CDC CAUTI diagnostic criteria (**Figs. 1** and **2**)
>
> *Abbreviations:* CAUTI, catheter-associated urinary tract infection; CDC, US Centers for Disease Control and Prevention.

Asymptomatic Catheter-Associated Urinary Tract Infection

In patients with afebrile, asymptomatic bacteriuria or funguria, antimicrobial treatment does not alter the natural progression to symptomatic infection or improve outcomes.[5] A randomized trial investigating the effect of antimicrobial therapy and catheter

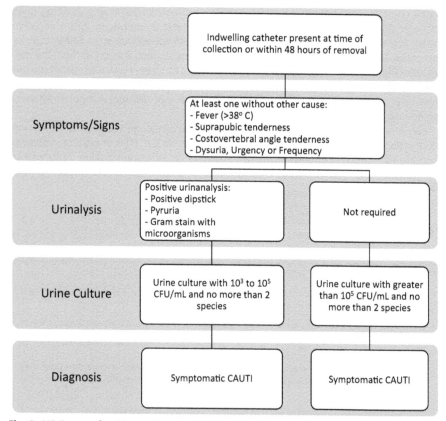

Fig. 1. US Centers for Disease Control and Prevention (CDC) criteria for diagnosis of symptomatic catheter-associated urinary tract infection (CAUTI). (*From* US Centers for Disease Control and Prevention. National Healthcare Safety Network (NHSN) Manual. Atlanta (GA): US Centers for Disease Control and Prevention; 2013.)

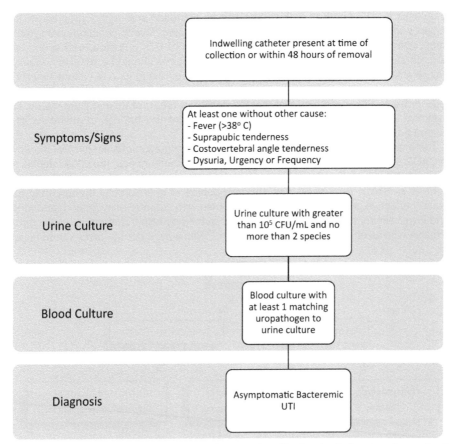

Fig. 2. US Centers for Disease Control and Prevention (CDC) criteria for the diagnosis of asymptomatic bacteremic urinary tract infection (UTI). (*From* US Centers for Disease Control and Prevention. National Healthcare Safety Network (NHSN) Manual. Atlanta (GA): US Centers for Disease Control and Prevention; 2013.)

change on the rates of urosepsis in patients in intensive care with asymptomatic bacteriuria after 48 hours of catheterization found no differences in rates of urosepsis and found no decrease in recurrence of asymptomatic bacteriuria at 7 and 15 days after catheterization.[35] Similarly, the use of azoles to treat asymptomatic funguria revealed initial high eradication rates, but equivalent recurrence of funguria at 2 weeks between treated and untreated patients.[36] Therefore, treatment for asymptomatic CAUTI is not recommended.

In patients with long-term catheters, antimicrobial therapy for asymptomatic bacteriuria similarly does not change the prevalence of bacteriuria or decrease progression to symptomatic UTI.[5] In those undergoing intermittent catheterization, treatment of asymptomatic bacteriuria may contribute to increased frequency of resistant organisms in subsequent symptomatic UTI episodes.[5]

Symptomatic Catheter-Associated Urinary Tract Infection

Specific antimicrobial choice for the treatment of CAUTI should be tailored to institutional susceptibility and resistance patterns. Important biochemical characteristics of antibiotics for UTI ought to include high urinary secretion and urinary drug levels. In patients with high severity of associated symptoms (eg. fevers, constitutional symptoms, hemodynamic instability) and high suspicion of UTI, empiric broad-spectrum parenteral antimicrobial therapy is appropriate. Cultures should be obtained, ideally before antibiotic initiation, and antibiotics narrowed or changed to fit culture sensitivities. In patients with mild symptoms, or patients with other suspected etiologies, it is reasonable to delay antimicrobial therapy until after return of urine culture results to minimize inappropriate antimicrobial use and to minimize the risk of antimicrobial-related adverse effects (**Fig. 3**).

There are varying recommendations regarding the duration of antimicrobial therapy in CAUTI.[10,37] For patients with continued urinary catheter needs, the 2009 Infectious Disease Society of America recommendations suggest a 7-day course.[10] However, there is evidence to suggest that shorter courses of antimicrobial therapy may be equally effective. In a randomized trial of women with catheter-associated bacteriuria and lower urinary tract symptoms, single-dose therapy with trimethoprim–sulfamethoxazole was as effective as a 10-day course.[38] Similarly, a double-blind, randomized

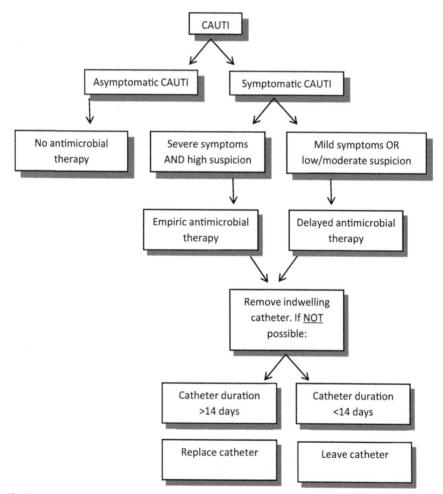

Fig. 3. Management of catheter-associated urinary tract infection (CAUTI).

trial found that a 5-day course of levofloxacin had equivalent therapeutic effect to a 10-day course in treating complicated UTI.[37] The 2009 Infectious Disease Society of America recommendations acknowledge the broad scope of evidence, noting that shorter courses may be appropriate in select patients with only mild lower urinary tract symptoms.[10] For patients with chronic indwelling catheters, longer durations of therapy up to 14 days may be required to prevent recurrence.[39]

If feasible, catheters should be removed before initiation of antimicrobial therapy for source control owing to the presence of biofilms. In patients with an ongoing need for urinary catheters, alternatives to indwelling catheters, as discussed subsequently, should be explored. In patients whom require continued indwelling catheterization, there exists only indirect evidence as to whether catheter replacement is warranted. In a prospective, randomized trial among elderly patients with chronic catheter needs, routine replacement of indwelling catheters before initiation of antimicrobial therapy was associated with a shorter time to fever defervescence, improved clinical status at 72 hours, and lower rate of recurrence in a 28-day follow-up.[31] Although this study was performed in a chronic catheter population, the dynamic of biofilms likely makes the bacterial burden of a long-term catheter similar to a short-term catheter within 3 to 10 days of catheterization.[26,27] Current Infectious Disease Society of America recommendations include replacing the urinary catheter if catheters have been in place for longer than 2 weeks (see **Fig. 3**).[10]

Epidural Analgesia and Urinary Catheters

In patients with postoperative thoracic or lumbar epidural analgesia, urinary catheters are commonly kept in place for the duration of epidural analgesia owing to concerns of urinary retention. However, emerging evidence challenges the need for continuous bladder drainage accompanying epidural analgesia.[40–42] In a prospective study among patients undergoing colorectal surgery with an epidural catheter, urinary catheter removal at 24 hours postoperatively was associated with increased urinary retention in only 12% of patients.[40] In a similar study among surgical patients with thoracic epidurals, patients who had urinary catheter removal on the morning after surgery had a longer return to post void residuals of less than 200 mL (345 vs 169 minutes); however, there were no adverse events or need for recatheterizations.[41] These data suggest that even in the subset of patients with urinary retention, retention is a transient phenomenon that resolves spontaneously without adverse events.

CATHER-ASSOCIATED URINARY TRACT INFECTION PREVENTION

Prevention summary

- Institutional guidelines for the use and maintenance of urinary catheters can reduce unnecessary catheterization, prolonged duration and incidence of CAUTI.

- Use of coated, impregnated, and/or silicone indwelling catheters have not demonstrated reproducible clinical benefits over standard noncoated latex catheters.

- Non-indwelling alternatives to urinary catheters should be considered daily and implemented as soon as feasible.

- Indications for catheter placement should be clearly reviewed before placement. Incontinence and caregiver convenience are not appropriate indications for urinary catheterization.

- Duration of catheterization is the strongest risk factor for catheterization.
- Catheter care should employ aseptic materials and techniques with vigilant maintenance of asepsis of the closed drainage system. Perineal washings may have a role in decreasing fecal contamination of the extraluminal catheter surface.
- Post removal, ultrasonographic bladder scanning can be a useful adjunct in the evaluation of retention. If retention is present, straight catheterization can be employed for up to 48 hours awaiting return of urinary bladder function.
- Systemic reminders and prompts for health care professionals regarding ongoing catheterization is an important element in increasing compliance with guidelines.

Effective prevention of CAUTI requires strict adherence to appropriate indications for placement of catheters, specified duration of catheterization, and proper catheter hygiene. The development of institutional protocols based on published guidelines for the use, maintenance, and removal of urinary catheters is an integral and proven method to reduce CAUTI.[6,7,10,43–45] In patients undergoing abdominal or orthopedic surgery, the institution of a multifaceted intervention to prevent CAUTI resulted in a 64% reduction in CAUTIs and 23% reduction in CAUTI-related antibiotic use, as reported by Stephan and colleagues.[46] Their intervention consisted of operating room guidelines restricting urinary catheter use to operations with anticipated duration of longer than 5 hours, or in older or higher risk patients with hip and knee replacements. In the postanesthesia care unit, voiding requirement and bladder measurement were removed as requisites for discharge, all catheters placed for long operations were removed, and all continuing catheterizations required explicit physician orders. Similarly, there were strict guidelines for removal of catheters on postoperative day 1 or 2 once on the surgical ward. Similar results have been reported in emergency room studies.[47] Prospective and retrospective studies have shown that up to one half of all short-term urinary catheters placed in acute care settings do not have appropriate indications, and that more than one third remained in place beyond the duration of the indication.[48–50] **Fig. 4** displays the authors' institutional guidelines for urinary catheter use.

Types of Urinary Catheters

A variety of alternatives to latex catheters have been investigated to target biofilms, reduce inflammation, and aid in the reduction of CAUTI. Alternatives include silicone-based catheters, or catheters that are silicone coated, antimicrobial impregnated, silver coated, or hydrogel coated. Antimicrobial-impregnated and silver-coated catheters were developed to retard biofilm formation and impede bacterial proliferation.[10,51] The use of silicone was thought to decrease urethral inflammation and consequently UTI development, and the hydrogel surface is theorized to prevent biofilm formation by changing surface affinity for biofilms.[10,52] The efficacy of these alternative catheters over latex catheters have been widely investigated but have yet to yield consistent reductions in CAUTI rates.[5,10] In the UK, a multicenter randomized trial was conducted comparing the efficacy and cost effectiveness of silicone catheters impregnated with nitrofurazone and silver alloy-coated latex catheters compared with standard polytetrafluoroethylene-coated latex catheters in mostly surgical patients requiring shorter term catheterizations. The analysis revealed no improvement in symptomatic CAUTI development in patients with the antimicrobial-impregnated catheter or the silver alloy-coated catheter.[51]

Criteria for the Appropriate Use of Indwelling Urinary Catheters:

A. Review for necessity prior to insertion. Provider (Physician, Nurse Practitioner, or Physician Assistant) will choose indication when ordering.

B. Appropriate choices for indwelling urinary catheters are:

1. Need for accurate urine output monitoring in the physiologically or anatomically unstable patient
2. Chemically paralyzed
3. Stage III/IV pressure ulcers being made worse by incontinence
4. Incontinence associated dermatitis being made worse by incontinence
5. Urinary obstruction or retention
6. Catheter required for surgical procedure (Specific surgical order sets will appear as a drop down for the provider to choose – i.e. cardiac surgery, joint replacement)
7. Other Medical condition (provider must specify)
8. Patient comfort for end of life care

NO — **YES**

Nurse removes urinary catheter and begins trial without catheter. | Maintain urinary catheter and assess daily

Monitor for new onset tachycardia, tachypnea, diaphoresis, restlessness. | Document urinary catheter necessity daily

1a. Offer toileting every 2 hours when age appropriate.

YES

Patient voids after 4-6 hours

NO → Perform Bladder Scan to assess volume. **NO** → Bladder or residual volume >300mL **NO** →

YES / **NO**

Void volume at least 30mL/hr or 1-2 mL/kg/hr in pediatric patients

YES (Bladder or residual volume) **YES**

- Notify Provider
- Perform straight catheterization
- If indwelling catheter needed, restart algorithm
- Consider Urology consul after 48 hours of recurrent retention

Continue to Observe

Fig. 4. Virginia Commonwealth University Health System (VCUHS) guidelines for appropriate indwelling urinary catheter use and monitoring. (*Courtesy of* Virginia Commonwealth University Health System, Richmond, VA.)

Alternatives to Indwelling Urinary Catheterization

Alternatives to indwelling urinary catheters include intermittent catheterization and use of external collection devices like diapers, pads, and condom catheters for men. There are limited studies investigating the safety and efficacy of urethral straight catheterization in patients with short-term needs. In a meta-analysis of patients with short-term non–perioperative need for bladder drainage, suprapubic intermittent catheterization was associated with a lesser risk of bacteriuria than indwelling catheters.[53] Extrapolating from such studies, and based on studies investigating the pathophysiology of bacteriuria development, it is reasonable to estimate that although straight catheterization includes similar risks of bacterial inoculation as indwelling catheter placement, the temporary nature of the straight catheter avoids the duration-related complications of biofilm ascension.[6,17]

In men, an alternative for those with incontinence is the condom catheter. Condom catheters are an external urine collection device that is associated with improved outcomes in a randomized trial by Saint and colleagues.[54] Men hospitalized at a Veteran's Affairs medical center aged 40 years and older were randomized to condom catheter or indwelling catheter, and those with condom catheters had decreased incidence of bacteriuria, symptomatic CAUTI, and death, and had improved patient comfort.[54] In women and men, the use of absorbent external collection devices in conjunction with behavioral interventions like hourly or 2 hourly mandatory toileting can reduce rates of CAUTI and associated patient morbidity.

Indwelling Urinary Catheter Indications

Before the insertion of a urinary catheter, thought should be given to its necessity as well as proposed duration. Appropriate indications include the need for urinary output monitoring in a critically ill patient with fluid status concerns, chemically paralyzed patients, incontinence-related wound concerns, genitourinary surgery, and acute urinary obstruction. Inappropriate uses include patient or nursing inconvenience owing to incontinence, need for urine samples, continued use beyond the perioperative period, or with prolonged epidural use (see **Fig. 4**). In patients with incontinence, alternatives to indwelling catheters should be explored.

Indwelling Urinary Catheter Duration

Duration of catheterization is the strongest risk factor for CAUTI, and therefore the continued need for indwelling urinary catheterization should be assessed daily.[17–20,48,55] In 1978, Garibaldi and associates[18] detailed an 8.1% increased risk of bacteriuria acquisition with each catheter day, adding that the risk in the first 24 hours of 7.4% was similar to the overall daily risk. This further emphasizes the notion that even temporary or very short-term catheterization (<24 hours) carries a continued and equal risk of bacteriuria development. In a more recent analysis of large prospective studies, urinary catheterization for longer than 6 days carried a relative risk of 5.1 to 6.8 of CAUTI development (**Table 1**).[56] In critically ill patients and patients with need for urinary output monitoring, the continued need for urinary catheter and exploration of other alternatives should be reexamined daily. Catheters placed for prolonged duration of surgery should be removed in the postanesthesia recovery unit if feasible, or within the first postoperative day. Similarly catheters should be removed upon cessation of chemical paralysis.

Catheter Care

Catheter care influences the development of bacteriuria and CAUTI. Aseptic materials and technique should be employed during insertion, including gloves, drapes, and periurethal cleaning. Closed drainage systems should be used ensuring that the collection system remains below the level of the bladder and there is no kinking of the tubing. Intraluminal contamination accounts 34% of CAUTI, and intraluminal contamination is almost exclusively owing to breaches in aseptic handing of the urinary collection system.[56]

Table 1
Risk factors for CAUTI

Factor	Relative Risk
Prolonged catheterization >6 d	5.1–6.8
Female gender	2.5–3.7
Catheter insertion outside operating room	2.0–5.3
Urology service	2.0–4.0
Other active sites of infection	2.3–2.4
Diabetes	2.2–2.3
Malnutrition	2.4
Azotemia (creatinine >2.0 mg/dL)	2.1–2.6
Ureteral stent	2.5
Monitoring of urine output	2.0
Drainage tube below level of bladder and above collection bag	1.9
Antimicrobial drug therapy	0.1–0.4

Abbreviation: CAUTI, catheter-associated urinary tract infection.
From Maki DG, Tambyah PA. Engineering out the risk for infection with urinary catheters. Emerg Infect Dis 2001;7(2):342–7.

Perineal washing may also have an impact on CAUTI development. A microbiologic analysis of CAUTI identified a high proportion of gastrointestinal origin bacteria, indicating likely fecal contamination across the perineum.[21] Similarly, genetic studies have suggested similarities between rectal *E. coli* flora and *E. coli* isolated from concurrent UTI.[57] One of the few studies to date investigating the role of perineal washing in UTI prevention in 1985 found no improvement in UTI development with hexachlorophene wipes; however, that study was conducted in women with recurrent UTI and without indwelling catheters.[58] The authors' institution has instituted daily perineal washing with chlorhexidine among patients in intensive care to minimize fecal contamination of the extraluminal surface of the indwelling catheter.

Post-Removal Monitoring

Catheters should be evaluated for the possibility of removal daily, with consideration given to alternatives to continued indwelling catheter use. Upon removal, the authors advocate offering toileting every 2 hours to patients and recording urine output. If patients have not urinated within 4 to 6 hours, or if they have urinated less than 30 mL/h after catheter removal, ultrasonographic bladder scanning should be employed to assess post void residuals or retained urine in the bladder (see **Fig. 4**).[59] In cases of bladder urine volumes of greater than 300 mL, straight catheterization should be employed for up to 48 hours before urologic consultation or replacement of indwelling catheter.[10] If patients have not voided within 6 hours and the bladder scan identifies less than 300 mL, the volume status of the patient should be evaluated.

Prevention Strategies

Strategies to decrease inappropriate use and duration of indwelling catheters, and thereby reduce rates of CAUTI, include the development of institutional protocols for catheter use, care, removal, and alternatives. Lack of awareness among health care providers of their patients' urinary catheterization status contributes to inappropriate, prolonged use of urinary catheters. In a study of health care provider awareness, prescribing providers were unaware of urinary catheters in 22% to 38% of their inpatients. Furthermore, use of a urinary catheter was appropriate significantly more often in patients for whom the prescribing providers were aware of urinary catheter use.[60] Systemic reminder mechanisms can have a large impact on reducing inappropriate catheter use and prolonged duration.[61] In a meta-analysis of reminder systems, duration of catheter use decreased by 37% and CAUTI rates decreased by 52% with the use reminder systems.[62] The meta-analysis included studies that used systems with only reminders, and systems with reminders associated with stop order prompts. The systems with associated stop order prompts included a spectrum of those that prompted physicians to place a discontinue order, those that autogenerated a discontinue order, and those with expiring catheter orders that required active renewal by a physician. A significant reduction in catheter duration was only noted in the systems with reminders associated with stop orders.[62] At the authors' institution, all catheter placements require a physician order with an indication, and urinary catheters placed perioperatively expire automatically at 48 hours postoperatively, requiring active physician justification for continuation. Reminder systems encourage physicians and health care providers to critically assess the requirements of ongoing catheter use lest the presence of urinary catheters be lost in the myriad of decisions and factors to be considered.

SUMMARY

UTI, and particularly CAUTI, have a major impact on surgical patient outcomes, quality and safety reporting, and reimbursement. CAUTI are especially ominous owing to the sequelae of biofilms. Education regarding the diagnosis and definition of CAUTI can improve identification and encourage appropriate use of antimicrobial therapy. Institutional guidelines based on consensus statements can guide and standardize UTI therapy. Prevention of inappropriate use and duration of indwelling catheters is integral. Health care provider ordering and documentation of indication for catheter placement may prevent inappropriate use and limit duration. Additionally, systemic reminders associated with stop orders may encourage timely catheter removal, especially for perioperative indications. Daily systems reviewing urinary catheter use and alternatives to indwelling catheters may also serve to limit duration. Finally, prospective data collection on outcomes including urinary catheter use, duration, CAUTI, and bacteremia will enable quality and process improvement.

REFERENCES

1. Kohn L, Corrigan J, Donaldson M. To err is human: building a safer health system. Washington, DC: Institute of Medicine; 2000.
2. Khuri SF. The NSQIP: a new frontier in surgery. Surgery 2005;138(5):837–43.
3. Agency for Healthcare Research and Quality (AHRQ). AHRQ quality indicators: guide to patient safety indicators. Rockville (MD): AHRQ; 2003.
4. Centers for Medicare and Medicaid Services (CMS), Department of Health and Human Services. Medicare program; changes to the hospital inpatient prospective payment systems and fiscal year 2008 rates. Fed Reg 2007;72(162): 47129–8175.
5. Nicolle LE. Urinary catheter-associated infections. Infect Dis Clin North Am 2012;26(1):13–27.
6. Lo E, Nicolle L, Classen D, et al. Strategies to prevent catheter-associated urinary tract infections in acute care hospitals. Infect Control Hosp Epidemiol 2008;29(Suppl 1):S41–50.

7. Gould CV, Umscheid CA, Agarwal RK, et al. Guideline for prevention of catheter-associated urinary tract infections 2009. Infect Control Hosp Epidemiol 2010; 31(4):319–26.
8. Chenoweth C, Saint S. Preventing catheter-associated urinary tract infections in the intensive care unit. Crit Care Clin 2013;29(1):19–32.
9. National Nosocomial Infections Surveillance System. National Nosocomial Infections Surveillance (NNIS) System Report, data summary from January 1992 through June 2004, issued October 2004. Am J Infect Control 2004;32(8): 470–85.
10. Hooton TM, Bradley SF, Cardenas DD, et al. Diagnosis, prevention, and treatment of catheter-associated urinary tract infection in adults: 2009 International Clinical Practice Guidelines from the Infectious Diseases Society of America. Clin Infect Dis 2010;50(5):625–63.
11. Wald HL, Kramer AM. Nonpayment for harms resulting from medical care: catheter-associated urinary tract infections. JAMA 2007;298(23):2782–4.
12. Saint S. Clinical and economic consequences of nosocomial catheter-related bacteriuria. Am J Infect Control 2000;28(1):68–75.
13. Guillamondegui OD, Gunter OL, Hines L, et al. Using the National Surgical Quality Improvement Program and the Tennessee Surgical Quality Collaborative to improve surgical outcomes. J Am Coll Surg 2012;214(4):709–14 [discussion: 714–6].
14. Trickey AW, Crosby ME, Vasaly F, et al. Using NSQIP to investigate SCIP deficiencies in surgical patients with a high risk of developing hospital-associated urinary tract infections. Am J Med Qual 2014;29:381–7.
15. Regenbogen SE, Read TE, Roberts PL, et al. Urinary tract infection after colon and rectal resections: more common than predicted by risk-adjustment models. J Am Coll Surg 2011;213(6):784–92.
16. Jarvis WR. Selected aspects of the socioeconomic impact of nosocomial infections: morbidity, mortality, cost, and prevention. Infect Control Hosp Epidemiol 1996;17(8):552–7.
17. Saint S, Chenoweth CE. Biofilms and catheter-associated urinary tract infections. Infect Dis Clin North Am 2003;17(2):411–32.
18. Garibaldi RA, Burke JP, Dickman ML, et al. Factors predisposing to bacteriuria during indwelling urethral catheterization. N Engl J Med 1974;291(5):215–9.
19. Platt R, Polk BF, Murdock B, et al. Risk factors for nosocomial urinary tract infection. Am J Epidemiol 1986;124(6):977–85.
20. Shapiro M, Simchen E, Izraeli S, et al. A multivariate analysis of risk factors for acquiring bacteriuria in patients with indwelling urinary catheters for longer than 24 hours. Infect Control 1984;5(11):525–32.
21. Tambyah PA, Halvorson KT, Maki DG. A prospective study of pathogenesis of catheter-associated urinary tract infections. Mayo Clin Proc 1999;74(2):131–6.
22. Sievert DM, Ricks P, Edwards JR, et al. Antimicrobial-resistant pathogens associated with healthcare-associated infections: summary of data reported to the National Healthcare Safety Network at the Centers for Disease Control and Prevention, 2009-2010. Infect Control Hosp Epidemiol 2013;34(1):1–14.
23. Dalhoff A. Global fluoroquinolone resistance epidemiology and implications for clinical use. Interdiscip Perspect Infect Dis 2012;2012:976273.
24. Morris NS, Stickler DJ, McLean RJ. The development of bacterial biofilms on indwelling urethral catheters. World J Urol 1999;17(6):345–50.
25. O'Toole GA, Kolter R. Flagellar and twitching motility are necessary for Pseudomonas aeruginosa biofilm development. Mol Microbiol 1998;30(2):295–304.

26. Donlan RM, Costerton JW. Biofilms: survival mechanisms of clinically relevant microorganisms. Clin Microbiol Rev 2002;15(2):167–93.

27. Sabbuba N, Hughes G, Stickler DJ. The migration of *Proteus mirabilis* and other urinary tract pathogens over Foley catheters. BJU Int 2002;89(1):55–60.

28. Hoyle BD, Wong CK, Costerton JW. Disparate efficacy of tobramycin on Ca(2+)-, Mg(2+)-, and HEPES-treated Pseudomonas aeruginosa biofilms. Can J Microbiol 1992;38(11):1214–8.

29. Donlan RM. Role of biofilms in antimicrobial resistance. ASAIO J 2000;46(6): S47–52.

30. Loeb M, Bentley DW, Bradley S, et al. Development of minimum criteria for the initiation of antibiotics in residents of long-term-care facilities: results of a consensus conference. Infect Control Hosp Epidemiol 2001;22(2):120–4.

31. Raz R, Schiller D, Nicolle LE. Chronic indwelling catheter replacement before antimicrobial therapy for symptomatic urinary tract infection. J Urol 2000; 164(4):1254–8.

32. Hannan EL, Waller CH, Farrell LS, et al. A comparison among the abilities of various injury severity measures to predict mortality with and without accompanying physiologic information. J Trauma 2005;58(2):244–51.

33. US Centers for Disease Control and Prevention. National Healthcare Safety Network (NHSN) manual. Atlanta (GA): US Centers for Disease Control and Prevention; 2013.

34. Loeb M, Brazil K, Lohfeld L, et al. Effect of a multifaceted intervention on number of antimicrobial prescriptions for suspected urinary tract infections in residents of nursing homes: cluster randomised controlled trial. BMJ 2005;331(7518):669.

35. Leone M, Perrin AS, Granier I, et al. A randomized trial of catheter change and short course of antibiotics for asymptomatic bacteriuria in catheterized ICU patients. Intensive Care Med 2007;33(4):726–9.

36. Sobel JD, Kauffman CA, McKinsey D, et al. Candiduria: a randomized, double-blind study of treatment with fluconazole and placebo. The National Institute of Allergy and Infectious Diseases (NIAID) Mycoses Study Group. Clin Infect Dis 2000;30(1):19–24.

37. Peterson J, Kaul S, Khashab M, et al. A double-blind, randomized comparison of levofloxacin 750 mg once-daily for five days with ciprofloxacin 400/500 mg twice-daily for 10 days for the treatment of complicated urinary tract infections and acute pyelonephritis. Urology 2008;71(1):17–22.

38. Harding GK, Nicolle LE, Ronald AR, et al. How long should catheter-acquired urinary tract infection in women be treated? A randomized controlled study. Ann Intern Med 1991;114(9):713–9.

39. Dow G, Rao P, Harding G, et al. A prospective, randomized trial of 3 or 14 days of ciprofloxacin treatment for acute urinary tract infection in patients with spinal cord injury. Clin Infect Dis 2004;39(5):658–64.

40. Stubbs BM, Badcock KJ, Hyams C, et al. A prospective study of early removal of the urethral catheter after colorectal surgery in patients having epidural analgesia as part of the enhanced recovery after surgery programme. Colorectal Dis 2013;15(6):733–6.

41. Zaouter C, Wuethrich P, Miccoli M, et al. Early removal of urinary catheter leads to greater post-void residuals in patients with thoracic epidural. Acta Anaesthesiol Scand 2012;56(8):1020–5.

42. Basse L, Werner M, Kehlet H. Is urinary drainage necessary during continuous epidural analgesia after colonic resection? Reg Anesth Pain Med 2000;25(5): 498–501.

43. Pratt RJ, Pellowe CM, Wilson JA, et al. Epic2: national evidence-based guidelines for preventing healthcare-associated infections in NHS hospitals in England. J Hosp Infect 2007;65(Suppl 1):S1–64.
44. Winter M, Helms B, Harrington L, et al. Eliminating catheter-associated urinary tract infections: part I. Avoid catheter use. J Healthc Qual 2009;31(6): 8–12.
45. Rhodes N, McVay T, Harrington L, et al. Eliminating catheter-associated urinary tract infections: part II. Limit duration of catheter use. J Healthc Qual 2009;31(6): 13–7.
46. Stephan F, Sax H, Wachsmuth M, et al. Reduction of urinary tract infection and antibiotic use after surgery: a controlled, prospective, before-after intervention study. Clin Infect Dis 2006;42(11):1544–51.
47. Gokula RM, Smith MA, Hickner J. Emergency room staff education and use of a urinary catheter indication sheet improves appropriate use of Foley catheters. Am J Infect Control 2007;35(9):589–93.
48. Hartstein AI, Garber SB, Ward TT, et al. Nosocomial urinary tract infection: a prospective evaluation of 108 catheterized patients. Infect Control 1981;2(5): 380–6.
49. Munasinghe RL, Yazdani H, Siddique M, et al. Appropriateness of use of indwelling urinary catheters in patients admitted to the medical service. Infect Control Hosp Epidemiol 2001;22(10):647–9.
50. Gardam MA, Amihod B, Orenstein P, et al. Overutilization of indwelling urinary catheters and the development of nosocomial urinary tract infections. Clin Perform Qual Health Care 1998;6(3):99–102.
51. Pickard R, Lam T, Maclennan G, et al. Types of urethral catheter for reducing symptomatic urinary tract infections in hospitalised adults requiring short-term catheterisation: multicentre randomised controlled trial and economic evaluation of antimicrobial- and antiseptic-impregnated urethral catheters (the CATHETER trial). Health Technol Assess 2012;16(47):1–197.
52. Srinivasan A, Karchmer T, Richards A, et al. A prospective trial of a novel, silicone-based, silver-coated Foley catheter for the prevention of nosocomial urinary tract infections. Infect Control Hosp Epidemiol 2006;27(1):38–43.
53. Niel-Weise BS, van den Broek PJ. Urinary catheter policies for short-term bladder drainage in adults. Cochrane Database Syst Rev 2005;(3):CD004203.
54. Saint S, Kaufman SR, Rogers MA, et al. Condom versus indwelling urinary catheters: a randomized trial. J Am Geriatr Soc 2006;54(7):1055–61.
55. Crouzet J, Bertrand X, Venier AG, et al. Control of the duration of urinary catheterization: impact on catheter-associated urinary tract infection. J Hosp Infect 2007;67(3):253–7.
56. Maki DG, Tambyah PA. Engineering out the risk for infection with urinary catheters. Emerg Infect Dis 2001;7(2):342–7.
57. Yamamoto S, Tsukamoto T, Terai A, et al. Genetic evidence supporting the fecal-perineal-urethral hypothesis in cystitis caused by Escherichia coli. J Urol 1997; 157(3):1127–9.
58. Cass AS, Ireland GW. Antibacterial perineal washing for prevention of recurrent urinary tract infections. Urology 1985;25(5):492–4.
59. Slappendel R, Weber EW. Non-invasive measurement of bladder volume as an indication for bladder catheterization after orthopaedic surgery and its effect on urinary tract infections. Eur J Anaesthesiol 1999;16(8):503–6.
60. Saint S, Wiese J, Amory JK, et al. Are physicians aware of which of their patients have indwelling urinary catheters? Am J Med 2000;109(6):476–80.

61. Fakih MG, Dueweke C, Meisner S, et al. Effect of nurse-led multidisciplinary rounds on reducing the unnecessary use of urinary catheterization in hospitalized patients. Infect Control Hosp Epidemiol 2008;29(9):815–9.
62. Meddings J, Rogers MA, Macy M, et al. Systematic review and meta-analysis: reminder systems to reduce catheter-associated urinary tract infections and urinary catheter use in hospitalized patients. Clin Infect Dis 2010;51(5):550–60.

Index

Note: Page numbers of article titles are in **boldface** type.

Surg Clin N Am 94 (2014) 1369–1378
http://dx.doi.org/10.1016/S0039-6109(14)00181-9
0039-6109/14/$ – see front matter © 2014 Elsevier Inc. All rights reserved.

surgical.theclinics.com

Printed and bound by CPI Group (UK) Ltd, Croydon, CR0 4YY

03/10/2024

01040486-0009